The Female Breast and Its Disorders

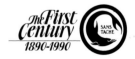

The Female Breast and Its Disorders

Edited by

George W. Mitchell, Jr., M.D.
Professor
Department of Obstetrics and Gynecology
University of Texas Health Science Center
San Antonio, Texas

Lawrence W. Bassett, M.D.
Director
Iris Cantor Center for Breast Imaging
UCLA Medical Center
Professor
Department of Radiological Sciences
UCLA School of Medicine and
Jonsson Comprehensive Cancer Center at UCLA
Los Angeles, California

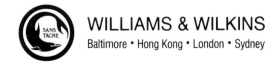

WILLIAMS & WILKINS
Baltimore • Hong Kong • London • Sydney

Editor: Carol-Lynn Brown
Associate Editor: Victoria M. Vaughn
Copy Editors: Elia A. Flanegin, Stephen Siegforth
Designer: Joanne Janowiak
Illustration Planner: Ray Lowman
Production Coordinator: Barbara J. Felton
Cover Designer: Wilma Rosenberger

Accurate indications, adverse reactions, and dosage schedules for drugs are provided in this book, but it is possible that they may change. The reader is urged to review the package information data of the manufacturers of the medications mentioned.

Printed in the United States of America

Library of Congress Cataloging-in-Publication Data

The female breast and its disorders / edited by George W. Mitchell, Jr., Lawrence
   W. Bassett.
     p.   cm.
   Includes bibliographical references.
   ISBN 0-683-06100-3
   1. Breast—Diseases.   I. Mitchell, George W., Jr., 1917–
II. Bassett, Lawrence W. (Lawrence Wayne), 1942–
   [DNLM: 1. Breast Diseases—diagnosis.   2. Breast Diseases—therapy.
3. Mammography.   WP 815 F329]
RG491.F46   1990
618.1'9—dc20
DNLM/DLC
for Library of Congress   89-25051
                                                    CIP

90 91 92 93 94
1 2 3 4 5 6 7 8 9 10

Foreword

Until about 1986 the number of deaths from breast cancer in women exceeded those for any other site. Breast cancer has now been surpassed by lung cancer, a disease which can, for the most part, be prevented. Unfortunately, ways to prevent breast cancer are limited. Although risk factors have been defined and many breast cancers can be detected during their relatively early stages by self-examination, periodic physician examination, breast imaging, and biopsy, there has been relatively little change in death rate from the disease in the last 50 years. Many lesions are still not diagnosed until they have become systemic and can no longer be eradicated. Relatively few women examine their breasts regularly; others do not take advantage of the diagnostic facilities that are available to them; many doctors neither emphasize the importance of early detection nor instruct their patients in self-examination, and some even fail to perform breast examinations regularly.

Although benign breast diseases are common, their diagnosis and management baffle many physicians. These disorders not only produce annoying, or even disabling symptoms, but also may be important precursors of breast malignancy. Like cancer, benign breast diseases cannot be prevented, but symptoms can usually be controlled by appropriate therapy.

Until recently surgeons were primarily responsible for the diagnosis and management of breast diseases. Most family physicians and many obstetrician-gynecologists almost automatically referred patients with breast lesions. This was in part because they knew little about breast diseases; since they have not been emphasized in most residency programs, they did not feel prepared to evaluate women with breast symptoms or masses. Unfortunately, the lack of emphasis led to limited ability to understand and detect disease. The results of studies on the accuracy of breast palpation are alarming; some physicians failed to feel even moderate-sized masses. Obstetrician-gynecologists performed no better than the others. This deficiency in the education of obstetrician-gynecologists, at least, should be corrected in the years ahead. The American Board of Obstetrics and Gynecology now requires experience in the diagnosis and management of breast diseases, and residency program directors have responded by making it available. Residents should now acquire basic competence in managing women with breast disorders. Since family practitioners and internists also see women patients at regular intervals, basic diagnostic procedures should be included as important parts of their residencies.

Doctors Mitchell and Bassett have made an outstanding contribution in "The Female Breast and Its Disorders: Essentials of Diagnosis and Management." They and their collaborators have had extensive experience in managing women with breast diseases and have made their combined expertise available to others. The book is unique in that it deals with breast physiology and the entire array of breast disorders, not with cancer alone. It also comes at an appropriate time, particularly for obstetrician-gynecologists who are becoming more involved with the breast. They, and others who study this publication, can learn to provide more than cursory breast appraisals, to order or perform appropriate examinations, and to treat at least minor breast problems. Information in this book is not limited to basic diagnosis and therapy; there is much that those who perform major operative procedures for benign lesions, for cancer, and for breast reconstruction can learn from studying it. In addition to serving as a practical reference for physicians in practice, it should be required as an important addition to the educational programs for residents in obstetrics-gynecology, surgery, internal medicine, family practice, and diagnostic imaging. It is a welcome and important addition to the literature concerning breast diseases.

J. Robert Willson, M.D.
Professor, Department of Obstetrics &
  Gynecology
The University of New Mexico
School of Medicine
Albuquerque, New Mexico

v

Preface

The many facets of breast function, disease, and treatment are to be found separately in a variety of books, monographs, and articles. The goal of this book is to incorporate all of these facets into a comprehensive whole, containing basic information for physicians and nonmedical personnel who provide health care for women and more specialized insights for those actively involved in the management of breast problems.

Although the chapters have been ordered traditionally, beginning with anatomy, physiology, and pathology and progressing to diagnosis, medical, and surgical treatment, broader headings might include: the breast in pregnancy and during lactation, of particular interest to the obstetrician and midwife; benign breast disease, a problem for primary care physicians as well as the laity; screening and diagnosis of breast cancer, a vital concern of all; and the modalities of breast cancer treatment and their results, important for evaluating progress and counseling patients.

Because of the wide ramifications of these subjects, representatives from gynecology and obstetrics, diagnostic radiology, pathology, surgery, medicine, therapeutic radiology, and psychiatry have contributed chapters pertaining to their particular areas of expertise. Understandably there are some overlaps and even some differences of opinion, but these lend a more academic quality than would a consistent party line by a single author and show that, as in other aspects of medicine, personal opinions thrive on unresolved issues. The editors believe that the essential facts have been covered and appreciate the effort and erudition of the authors. They wish to thank also the staff at Williams & Wilkins for recognizing the need for a breast book, for their helpfulness in the publication, and for their patience.

Contributors

Barrie Anderson, M.D.
Associate Professor and Director of the
  Division of Gynecologic Oncology
Department of Obstetrics and Gynecology
University of Iowa Hospitals and Clinics
Iowa City, Iowa

Lawrence Bassett, M.D.
Director, Iris Cantor Center for Breast Imaging
Professor of Radiological Sciences
Department of Radiological Sciences
UCLA School of Medicine
Los Angeles, California

Fritz Beller, M.D.
William C. Keettel Professor of Obstetrics and
  Gynecology
Department of Obstetrics and Gynecology
University of Iowa College of Medicine
Iowa City, Iowa

Geeta Chhibber, M.D.
Director of Maternal-Fetal Medicine
Albert Einstein Medical Center
Associate Professor
Temple University School of Medicine
Philadelphia, Pennsylvania

Claude Denham, M.D.
Staff
Texas Oncology
Dallas, Texas

Mara J. Dinsmoor, M.D.
Assistant Professor
Department of Obstetrics and Gynecology
Medical College of Virginia
Virginia Commonwealth University
Richmond, Virginia

Martin Farber, M.D.
Senior Vice President and Director of Medical
  Education
Oakwood Hospital
Dearborn, Michigan

Armando E. Giuliano, M.D.
Associate Professor of Surgery
Division of General Surgery
Department of Surgery
UCLA School of Medicine
Los Angeles, California

Richard H. Gold, M.D.
Professor of Radiological Sciences
Department of Radiological Sciences
UCLA School of Medicine
Los Angeles, California

Lori S. Gormley, M.D.
Staff
St. Barnabas Hospital
Livingston, New Jersey

Guy Hewlett, M.D.
Chief Resident
Department of Obstetrics and Gynecology
Albert Einstein Medical Center
Philadelphia, Pennsylvania

David H. Hussey, M.D., F.A.C.R.
Professor and Director
Division of Radiation Oncology
University of Iowa College of Medicine
Iowa City, Iowa

Carolyn R. Kaplan, M.D.
Staff
Women's Medical Group of Santa Monica
St. John's Hospital
Santa Monica Hospital
Santa Monica, California

W. David McInnis, M.D., F.A.C.S.
Private Practice
San Antonio, Texas

Douglas Marchant, M.D.
Professor
Departments of Obstetrics and Gynecology
  and Surgery
Tufts University School of Medicine
Boston, Massachusetts

George W. Mitchell, Jr., M.D.
Professor
Department of Obstetrics and Gynecology
University of Texas Health Science Center
San Antonio, Texas

Barbara Monsees, M.D.
Assistant Professor of Radiology
Washington University School of Medicine
Mallinckrodt Institute of Radiology
St. Louis, Missouri

Edward R. Newton, M.D.
Associate Professor
Department of Obstetrics and Gynecology
University of Texas Health Science Center
San Antonio, Texas

C. Kent Osborne, M.D.
Professor of Medicine
Department of Medicine
University of Texas Health Science Center
San Antonio, Texas

Ibrahim Ramzy, M.D.
Professor of Pathology and Obstetrics and
  Gynecology
Department of Pathology
Baylor College of Medicine
Chief of Anatomic Pathology
The Methodist Hospital
Houston, Texas

Robert S. Schenken, M.D.
Jane and Roland Blumberg Professor
Division Director
Division of Reproductive Endocrinology and
  Infertility
Department of Obstetrics and Gynecology
University of Texas Health Science Center
San Antonio, Texas

Elizabeth Small, M.D.
Professor of Psychiatry
Associate Clinical Professor of Obstetrics and
  Gynecology
Department of Psychiatry
University of Nevada School of Medicine
Chief of Psychiatry
Reno Veteran's Administration Medical
  Center
Reno, Nevada

Elaine Smith, M.D.
Associate Professor of Epidemiology
Department of Preventive Medicine
University of Iowa College of Medicine
Iowa City, Iowa

Antonio P. Vigliotti, M.D.
Assistant Professor
Division of Radiation Oncology
University of Iowa College of Medicine
Iowa City, Iowa

Contents

Development and Anatomy of the Breast

Fritz Beller

EMBRYOLOGY

The origin of the breast is thought to be related to that of the sweat glands and the integument. During the 5th week (6 to 10 mm) of development, the ectodermal primitive milk streak appears as a thickening on each side of the ventral midline, from the axilla to the groin, on the embryonic trunk. The primitive milk streak regresses during the 9- to 15-mm stage, usually remaining only in the region of the thorax, where it forms a mammary ridge (Fig. 1.1). Between months 3 and 4, bud-shaped or globular primordia develop by self-proliferation in the cranial part of the milk ridge, forming small prominent hillocks, which then push down into the underlying mesenchyme (1, 12).

At 16 weeks, desquamation of the epithelium causes the nipple groove to appear, and further epithelial proliferations, in 15 to 25 bands, branch out into the subcutaneous tissue and form the anlage of the ductal system and secretory alveoli (3). At 15 mm, the primordium enlarges and extends to the subcutis (1,2).

The secondary mammary anlage develops with the differentiation of hair follicle and sebaceous and sweat gland elements. Specialized apocrine glands also develop at this time to form Montgomery's glands around the nipple. Even though some data suggest a role for testosterone in the development of the fetal mammary gland (2), hormones are probably not required to achieve this level of development. The canalization stage requires placental sex hormones, which enter the fetal circulation at the 20th to 32nd week (4). At term, 15 to 25 mammary ducts are formed, which unify with sebaceous glands near the epidermis. Lobularalveolar structures containing colostrum also

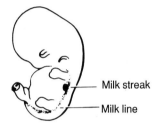

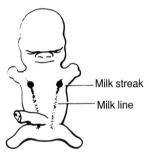

Figure 1.1. Milk streak development in the embryo. (From Wagner H. Topographische Anatomie derweblichen Bust. In: Beller FK. Atlas der Mamma Chirurgie, Stuttgart: Schattauer, 1985.)

develop in the 3rd trimester. Vascular changes are readily apparent by the 20-mm stage, when capillaries develop into a network within the connective tissue and differentiate into three principal zones (1).

The nipple and areola at birth are pigmented, and, in the center, the openings of 15 to 25 mammary ducts lead into the lactiferous sinuses, from which the infundibular branches gradually narrow toward the periphery. Colostral milk, also called witch's milk, is produced in 80 to 90% of newborns, beginning about postpartum day 4 to 7, and can easily be ex-

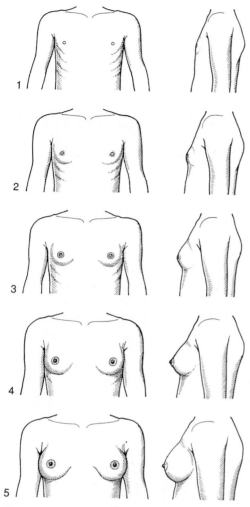

Figure 1.2.   Tanner's stages of breast development.

pressed from the nipple. The secretion lasts for 3 to 4 weeks and is due to stimulation of the end vesicles by luteal and placental hormones. Repeated expression of colostrum can delay its cessation. After the first neonatal month, breast tissue regresses to approximately 4 to 8 mm in size.

The mammary glands consist of four major tissues: fat, connective tissue epithelium, and myoepithelial cells, which constitute the contractile elements for the expulsion of milk. The epithelial ducts and the myoepithelial component are the fastest proliferating tissues within the breast (5).

PUBERTY

There is no further growth until puberty, when the onset of hormone secretion causes the breast tissue to grow. Relatively little is known about the sequential influence of any given hormone, but recent animal data suggest that neither estrogen nor progesterone alone produces uniform development. It is apparent that many hormones are involved, some more important than others, and the four cellular components react differently to each (4). Numerous studies have demonstrated a primary role for the ovary in breast development via secretion of estrogens and progesterone. Based on animal experiments, estrogens seem to influence the growth of the duct system, whereas lobuloalveolar development depends on progesterone (4, 6). Genetic, environmental, and dietary factors are also known to influence the growth of the breast (7).

In 1962, the British pediatrician J.M. Tanner was the first to study and describe sexual characteristics, breast and pubic hair development, and the menarche in a longitudinal fashion in 143 girls (8, 8a). From his study emerged the five Tanner stages, which are widely used: (Fig. 1.2):

Stage 1—The infantile stage, which persists from the immediate postnatal period until the onset of puberty.
Stage 2—The "bud" stage. The breast and papilla are elevated as a small mound, and the diameter of the areola is increased. This appearance is the first indication of pubertal development of the breast.
Stage 3—The breast and areola are further enlarged and present an appearance similar to that of a small adult mammary gland, with a continuous rounded contour.
Stage 4—The areola and papilla continue to expand and form a secondary mound projecting above the corpus of the breast.
Stage 5—The typical adult stage with a smooth rounded contour, the secondary mound present in Stage 4 having disappeared (Fig. 1.3).

In 1987, Beller and coworkers repeated the longitudinal study on 700 girls in Hungary and Germany (9). They confirmed Tanner's data and other reports derived from 180 Swiss and 90 Swedish girls, comprising the only other longitudinal studies in the literature (10, 11). The mean age of thelarche was 11.2 years, and breast development ended at 13.2 years (Fig. 1.4). In a study of Turkish girls, thelarche occurred at the age of 9.8 years and menarche at 10.8 years, earlier than in other studies (12). The median age of menarche in Beller's study was 12.5 years. In Tanner's study, the median age of menarche was 13.5, and the end point of breast development was later. The difference in the age of menarche was not statistically sig-

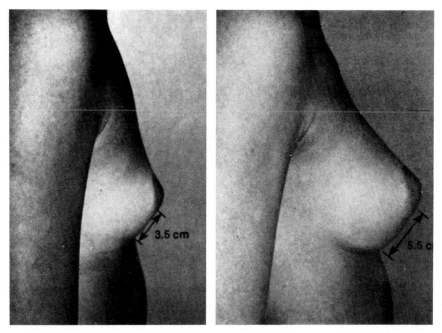

Figure 1.3. Breast development, stage 3 to 5 (Beller). (From Bostwick J. Aesthetic and reconstructive breast surgery. St. Louis: CV Mosby, 1982:23.)

nificant. Thelarche was the first sex characteristic to appear, followed by pubarche, axillarche, and finally menarche (Fig. 1.5) (13).

In Western culture breast development ceases 2 years after menarche. At that time dif-

ferentiation of the mammary gland into ductal, lobular, and alveolar parts has occurred. The breast is essentially a skin appendage contained within layers of superficial fascia (5, 14).

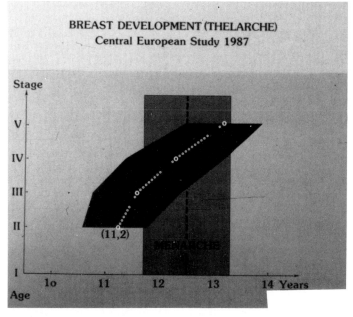

Figure 1.4. Breast development Central European Study. (From Beller FK, Borsos A, Csoknyay T, Schlummer A, Kieback D, Lampe L. Data of the Central European Study: Breast development. Breast Dis 1989; 2:19–25.

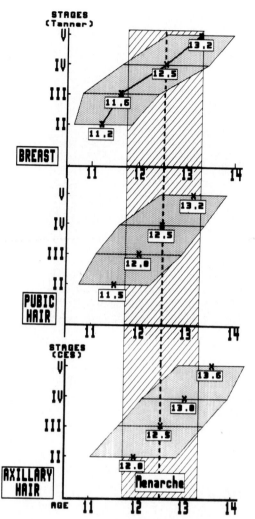

Figure 1.5. Development of puberty, Central European Study. (From Beller FK, Borsos A, Csoknayay T, Schlummer A, Kieback D, Lampe L. Data of the Central European Study: Breast development. Breast Dis 1989; 2:19–25.)

The size, form, and consistency of the breast are determined not only by glands but also by connective and adipose tissue. Each of these elements can be predominant in a given individual. For instance, the well-formed breasts in individuals with testicular feminization contain predominantly adipose tissue.

ANATOMY

The female breast is located between the second or third and the sixth or seventh ribs and between the parasternal and anterior axillary lines. However, glandular tissue spreads beyond the breast outline and nearly always

into the axilla. It may cross the midline or extend down to the epigastrium. It lies on the pectoral fascia and, to a lesser degree, on the serratus anterior muscles. The skin of the breast contains hair follicles, sebaceous glands, and sweat glands. Hair follicles are not present on, but exist around, the areola, which varies from 2 to 12 cm in diameter, with a mean of 5 cm in the reproductive age group. Morgagni's tubercles are located near the periphery of the areola and consist of elevations formed by the openings of the ducts of Montgomery's glands. The latter lubricates the nipple for nursing and are also capable of secreting milk; they represent an intermediate stage between sweat and mammary glands. The areola and nipple are developed in a three-dimensional organization, consisting of an external ring comprising sebaceous glands and connective tissue above middle and inner rings of both longitudinal and circular muscle fibers, responsible for the erection of the nipple in response to stimulation. This is supported by arteriovenous anastomoses. The skin and the sheets of underlying fascia enveloping the glandular parenchyma are connected by thin fascial bands, called Cooper's ligaments, which support the breast. The breast tissue is surrounded by a layer of fat 1 to 3 mm in diameter, the adipose panniculum, which is thicker laterally and thins as it approaches the front. Fifteen to twenty radially arranged lobes, converging at the nipple, are also enclosed in fat, producing a smooth contour (Fig. 1.6).

The lobes are composed of lobules, and the lobules of grape-like clusters of from 10 to 100 alveoli, with interlocking excretory ducts lined by a single layer of columnar epithelium on a basement membrane. Alveolar epithelium resembles that of the ducts. The lobes vary in size and are of pyramidal shape, with the apices toward the nipple. Each lobe has one duct leading to the nipple, and it increases in diameter until it empties into the larger lactiferous sinus and then into the ampulla (Figs. 1.6 and 1.7). The larger ducts may have two layers of epithelium. Peripherally, the ducts become secretory. Just below the areola the cone-shaped ampulla is lined by stratified squamous epithelium. Around the ducts lie connective tissue and myoepithelial cells, which have no innervation but respond to the stimulus of oxytocin (5, 14).

The breast parenchyma spreads along Cooper's ligaments close to the corium and to the surface of the pectoral fascia, where it is likely to penetrate the muscle. It is most heavily concentrated in the upper outer quadrants. This spoke-like arrangement causes skin retraction when cancer occurs in gland or duct, since

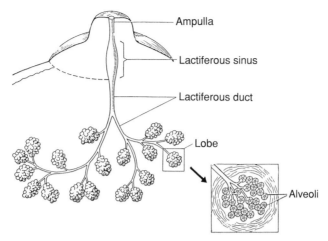

Figure 1.6. Schematic representation of the milk duct system. (From Wagner H. Topographische Anatomie derweiblichen Bust. In: Beller FK. Atlas der Mamma Chirurgie. Stuttgart: Schattauer, 1985.)

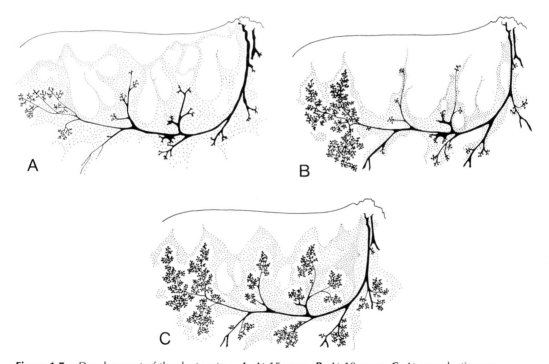

Figure 1.7. Development of the duct system. **A**, At 15 years. **B**, At 19 years. **C**, At reproductive age.

connective tissue does not lengthen as the tumor enlarges. The density of the breast produced by intermingling connective and epithelial tissue compels sharp rather than blunt dissection during surgical procedures.

Arteries

The arterial blood supply of the breast is derived from three main sources (Fig. 1.8). The third, fourth, and fifth intercostal branches of the thoracic aorta supply the skin and parenchyma of the lateral portion of the breast. They perforate the muscles at the side of the chest and divide, with the anterior branches going to the breast and the posterior to the underlying muscles. The internal mammary branches of the subclavian artery send perforators between the six underlying ribs to the medial breast. Branches of the pectoral division of the thoracoacromial trunk of the axillary artery descend along the lower border of the pectoralis

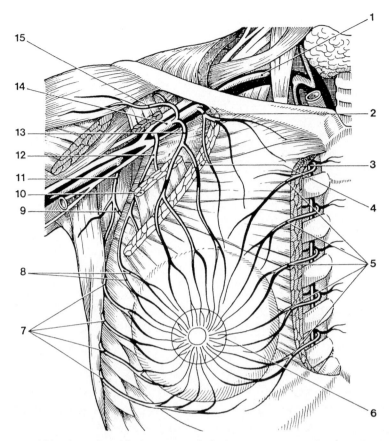

Figure 1.8. Arterial blood supply to the breast. *1*, subclavian artery; *2*, superior thoracic artery; *3*, internal thoracic artery, *4*, major pectoralis muscle; *5*, perforating branches of the internal mammary artery; *6*, arterial plexus around areola; *7*, intercostal arteries; *8*, pectoral branches of the lateral thoracic artery; *9*, circumflex scapular artery; *10*, minor pectoralis muscle; *11*, subscapular artery; *12*, lateral thoracic artery; *13*, pectoral branch of the thoracoacromial artery; *14*, axillary artery; *15*, deltoid branch of the thoracoacromial artery.

minor muscle and enter the breast from below. They supply the upper outer quadrant and tail of the breast. Extensive anastomoses ensure two or three sources to all parts.

Veins

The veins follow a similar pattern. Like the arteries they form an anastomotic circle around the base of the papilla, known as the circulus venosus. A second plexus lies deeper in the gland (15).

Lymphatics

The lymph of the peripheral breast is drained by the subepithelial or papillary channels, which are confluent with the lymphatics over the surface of the rest of the body and eventually lead into a large plexus (Sappey's) below the areola (Fig. 1.9) (2). Channels from the central breast also drain to this plexus, and from there the drainage is first to low axillary nodes, second to central axillary nodes, and third to subclavian nodes at the apex, where the axillary and subclavian vessels join.

The deep or fascial plexus drains partly through the pectoral (Rotter's) nodes to the subclavian nodes (Groszman's pathway) and partly via the internal mammary nodes to the mediastinal nodes. Other paths pass through the abdominal lymphatics to the liver and subdiaphramatic nodes (paramammary route of Gerota), and still others cross to the contralateral breast and beneath the sternum to the anterior mediastinum.

Handly and Thackray noted that Halsted's radical mastectomy left the internal mammary chain intact, even though approximately 40% of the lymph is drained by that route (16). This observation led to an ultraradical approach to surgery with removal of the internal mammary nodes, but this did not improve the prognosis. The axillary lymph nodes drain approximately

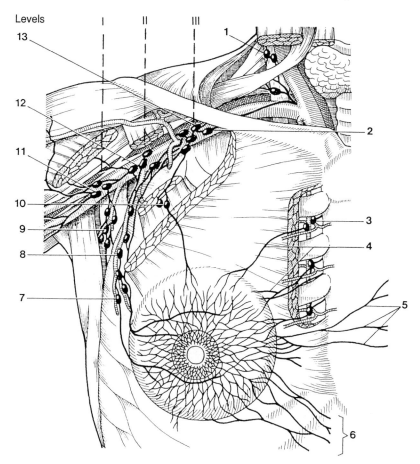

Figure 1.9. Lymph drainage of the breast. *1*, deep cervical nodes; *2*, infraclavicular nodes; *3*, sternal nodes; *4*, pathway to the mediastinal nodes; *5*, pathway to the contralateral breast; *6*, pathway to the sub-diaphragmatic nodes and liver; *7*, anterior pectoral lymph nodes; *8*, central axillary nodes; *9*, subpectoral axillary nodes; *10*, interpectoral nodes (Rotter's); *11*, brachial vein nodes; *12*, axillary vein nodes; *13*, subclavian vein nodes.

60% of the lymph from the mammary gland and the major and minor pectoralis muscles. The lymph nodes are conventionally grouped in three levels (Fig. 1.9). Radical resection of the axillary nodes was an integral part of the classical radical mastectomy, which is now seldom performed since it has not been shown to prolong survival or time of first recurrence. Tumor-containing lymph nodes at level III are rarely present when levels I and II are negative. Most surgeons therefore resect only level I and II lymph nodes for staging purposes.

Nerves

The sensory supply of the breast comes from the third to the sixth lateral intercostal nerves. The second intercostal nerve crosses the axilla to the medial upper arm, and an injury to it during lymphadenectomy causes paresthesia of that area. Supraclavicular branches from the cervical plexus supply the upper portion of the breast and the infraclavicular skin. The medial part of the breast is supplied by branching anterior intercostal nerves.

The nipple-areola complex is supplied by the fourth lateral intercostal nerve and its branches. In general, the skin, especially that of the nipple and areola, is well supplied with sensory nerves. In contrast, the adipose and the glandular parts of the breast have remarkably little nerve supply, which makes local anesthesia appropriate for minor surgical procedures.

NORMAL BREAST DEVELOPMENT

As has been noted, estrogens promote ductal growth, and estrogens and progester-

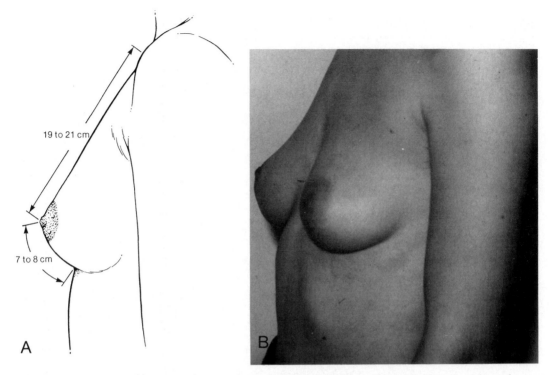

Figure 1.10. **A**, Normal breasts in the reproductive-age female. **B**, Normal breasts. Note the "drop" form.

one together promote lobuloalveolar development. Prolactin and growth hormone are also essential to produce these effects, and adrenal steroids, thyroxin, insulin, and parathyroid hormone may have an adjunctive regulatory effect on mammary growth and function, either directly or synergistically with other hormones (see Chapter 3). Regular variations in the quantity of glandular tissue on a cyclic basis are thus ensured. Vascular engorgement accompanies the premenstrual phase and ductal lumina enlarge, further expanding breast volume.

In the nonpregnant woman the ducts and alveoli of the breast are small and filled with plugs of desquamated granular cells. In pregnancy, the lining cells enlarge, multiply, undergo fatty degeneration, and are eliminated along with the plugs as colostrum in the first milk. The peripheral alveolar cells form oil globules in their cytoplasm and eject them into the ductal lumina as milk. When the alveoli are thus distended, the lining cells become flat. The average breast weighs 400 to 500 g when lactating.

In menopause, involution takes place and glandular tissue reverts toward the infantile state. Fatty tissue disappears more slowly and gradually becomes the chief component. Eventually only redundant skin remains.

APPEARANCE

It is difficult to describe a normal breast, since what constitutes normality is dependent on a variety of ethnic and cultural factors, which include aesthetics as well as function. In Arabian countries large breasts represent fertility, but in the western world favor may vary between small breasts that are actually hypoplastic (Twiggy phenomenon) and large breasts that are hyperplastic (Hollywood phenomenon). Caution must be observed in any description of breast size or shape, especially in the presence of patients, since the observer's evaluation is purely subjective. An average nonlactating breast weighs between 200 and 400 g and measures 10 to 12 cm in diameter and 5 to 7 cm in thickness (Fig. 1.10). Genetic influences cause variations in shape, described as discoidal, hemispherical, pear-shaped, or conical (Fig. 1.11), and cultural practices such as binding or stretching may produce unusual distortion. Ptosis may occur at any age (Fig. 1.12A). The breast tends to become flaccid after pregnancy and with age, unless replaced by fat (Fig. 1.12B).

CONGENITAL ABNORMALITIES

Failure of regression of the milk streak at the embryonic stage leads to the presence of acces-

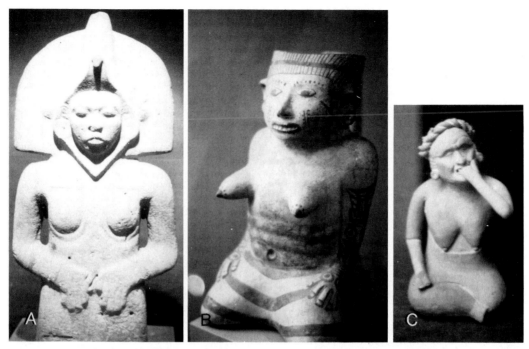

Figure 1.11. **A–C**, Variations in breast form in Aztec sculptures of women of the 15th century. (From the National Anthropological Museum of Mexico.)

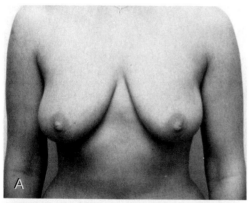

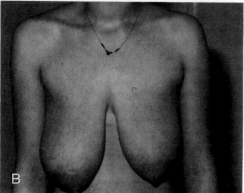

Figure 1.12. **A**, Juvenile ptosis of the breasts. **B**, Normal breasts after two pregnancies.

sory mammary tissue with or without an areola or nipple (polythelia). An accessory nipple found along the milk streak is the most frequent anomaly and can be mistaken for a nevus. Accessory mammary glands (polymastia) are found most often in the axilla but may even extend to the vulva (Fig. 1.13). Postpartum, the small accessory glands may swell to as much as 8 cm in size and, if a nipple is present, may lactate. They regress in the puerperium but occasionally are the site of chronic mastitis. Such accessory glands should be resected when symptomatic or unsightly. They are rarely the site of malignancy.

Hypoplasia

Congenital absence of the breast is termed amastia, and underdevelopment is termed hypoplasia or micromastia. The difference between complete lack of breast tissue and severe hypoplasia can sometimes be determined only during pregnancy, when even hypoplastic breasts increase in size. Athelia, first described by Batchelor in 1888 (17), is the absence of the areola and nipple, a defect rare in the presence of a normal breast and most often observed with hypoplasia. The breast bud may develop earlier on one side and progress more rapidly than the contralateral breast. Major inequities usually disappear by the time development is

3. unilateral hyperplasia, normal contralateral;
4. bilateral hyperplasia with asymmetry;
5. unilateral hypoplasia, contralateral hypoplasia; and
6. unilateral hypoplasia of breast, thorax, and pectoral muscles (Poland's syndrome).

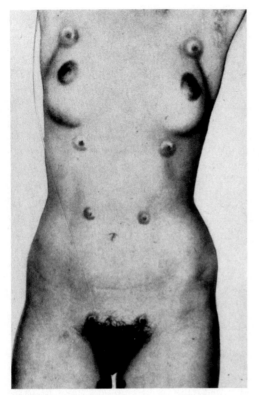

Figure 1.13. Polymastia in a young woman.

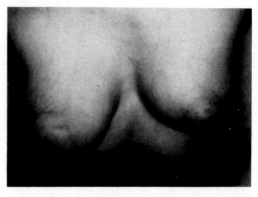

Figure 1.15. Anisomastia of the left breast in an 18-year-old woman. The left breast is smaller with a slightly protruded areola.

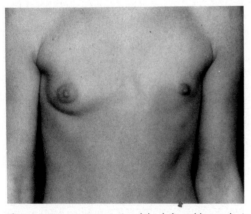

Figure 1.14. Anisomastia of the left and hypoplasia of the right breast in an 18-year-old woman.

complete, but minor differences can be observed in more than 80% of women in the reproductive age (18). If the difference in size between the two breasts is significant, it is termed anisomastia (Figs. 1.14 and 1.15). A wide range of breast abnormalities has been described and classified by Osborne (19):

1. unilateral hypoplasia, normal contralateral;
2. bilateral hypoplasia with asymmetry;

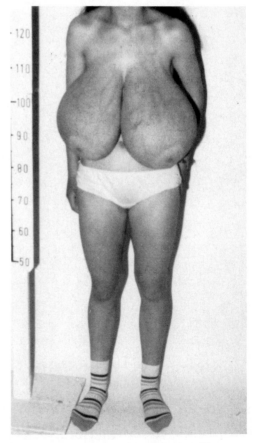

Figure 1.16. Gigantism in a 20-year-old woman, barely 150 cm in height. At reduction mammoplasty 4000 g was resected on each side.

Breast hypoplasias are observed in association with gonadal agenesis and in Turner's syndrome. Iatrogenic reasons for amastia are surgical removal of a breast bud mistaken for a lump or therapeutic irradiation in early childhood.

Breasts with varying degrees of underdevelopment are chiefly psychologic and cosmetic problems. Their treatment is by augmentation mammoplasty (20) (see Chapter 17A).

Hyperplasia

There are usually two groups of women requesting reduction surgery; one comprises young women 16 to 20 years of age with large breasts (pubertal or juvenile macromastia); the other comprises women between 35 and 50 years of age with large, pendulous breasts. The larger breasts in the latter group are usually due to an increase in fatty tissue (21).

Juvenile macromastia is predominantly due to excessive glandular growth and occurs between ages 14 and 16 (Fig. 1.16). Adipose hy-

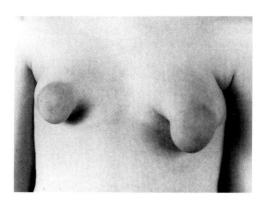

Figure 1.17. A trunk breast in an 18-year-old woman.

perplasia occurs in the older age group, and in most instances the breasts are symmetrically enlarged. Unilateral macromastia is very rare and presents a real challenge to the surgeon. Breasts larger than 600 g provide a medical as well as a cosmetic indication for plastic surgery because of problems related to the heavy weight on shoulders and neck as well as the psychologic impact.

An unusual type of malformation is marked enlargement of the areola relative to the overall size of the breast, with herniation of the anterior parenchyma into it, producing an unsightly protrusion that may stick straight out or hang down from the residual breast (trunk breast) (Fig. 1.17). Attempts at hormonal treatment for this abnormality have not been successful, but there are a variety of surgical techniques available for consideration (22).

PREMATURE THELARCHE

Precocious breast development, or premature thelarche, occasionally occurs in girls less than 8 years of age who do not show any other signs of pubertal development (23, 24). Of the patients observed by Ilicki and coworkers (25), 85% were in the first 2 years of life and 30% were apparent at birth. In 30%, breast development was unilateral. In 44%, the condition eventually disappeared but, when present in the newborn, it lasted an average of 2 years. In the series of patients studied by Mills and coworkers (26), an enlarged breast that persisted after birth continued to progress and, if it did not regress completely by the age of 2, frequently represented the first sign of general precocious puberty (27) (Fig. 1.18). Premature development of glandular breast tissue has been attributed to both endogenous and exogenous causes. Accelerated organ synthesis and the presence of minute concentrations of circu-

Natural History of Premature Thelarche*				
	Outcome			
Type of Onset	Disappeared	Persisted Without Progressing	Continued to Enlarge	Total
Present from birth	3	4	3	10
Onset after neonatal period	10	16	2	28
Regression after birth-later reappearance	1	5	0	6
Total	14 (2 unknown)	25	5	44

*The number of patients was 46.

Figure 1.18. Data regarding premature thelarche. (From Mills J, Stolley P, Davies J, Moshang T. Premature thelarche. Am J Dis Child 1981; 135:743–745.)

lating estrogen have been invoked as etiologic; the latter because an estrogenized vaginal smear was occasionally present in these children (28). It has been suggested that an increased dihydroepiandrosterone (DHEA) level may serve as a precursor for conversion to estrogens in the target tissues. McDonald and coworkers have shown that a low level of conversion of DHEA to estradiol does occur in the peripheral tissue of these patients.

Reports of an epidemic of breast enlargement in Italian children was attributed to the presence of estrogen in ingested meat. This was also the reported cause in 375 girls in Puerto Rico from 1979 to 1981 (29). In Italy, ovarian cysts were also present in 16% of the patients.

Although hyperestrinism has rarely been identified as the cause of premature thelarche, the assumption that it is due to a defect in the maturation of the hypothalamic-pituitary-ovarian axis is supported by treatment results (30, 31). The administration of estrogens produced full breast development in patients with gonadal dysgenesis. In contrast, estrogen treatment of girls with adrenal hypoplasia led only to a bud stage (Tanner's stage 2) after 6 months of treatment, and results were unsatisfactory after 3 years of treatment. Differences in levels of gonadotropins were assumed to be the cause (6).

REFERENCES

1. Knight CH, Peaker M. Development of the mammary gland. J Reprod Fertil 1982; 65:521–536.
2. Patten BM. Human embryology. Philadelphia: Blakiston, 1948: 240.
3. Hughes ESR. Development of the mammary gland. Ann R Coll Surg Engl 1950; 6:99–103.
4. Ceriani RL. Hormones and other factors controlling growth in the mammary gland: a review. J Invest Dermatol 1974; 63:93–108.
5. Mayer G, Klein M. Histology and cytology of the mammary gland. In: Von SK, Cowie AT, eds. The mammary gland and its secretion, vol 1. New York: Academic Press, 1961:47–126.
6. Porter JC. Hormonal regulation of breast development and activity. J Invest Dermatol 1974; 63:85.
7. Taranger J, Engström I, Lichtenstein H, Svennberg-Redegren I. VI. Somatic pubertal development. Acta Paediatr Scand 1976; 258:127–135.
8. Tanner IM. Growth at adolescence. 2nd ed. Oxford: Blackwell and Springfield, Illinois: Charles C Thomas, 1962.
8a. Marshall WA: Puberty in human growth. In: Faulkner F, Tanner JM, eds. New York: Plenum Press, 1978:741.
9. Beller FK, Borsos A, Csoknyay T, Schlummer A, Kieback D, Lampe L. Data of the Central European Study: breast development. Breast Dis 1989; 2:19–25.
10. Largo RH, Prader A. Pubertal development in Swiss girls. Helv Paediatr Acta 1983; 38:229–243.
11. Speroff L, Glass RH, Kase NG. Clinical gynecologic endocrinology and infertility. 3rd ed. Baltimore: Williams & Wilkins, 1983:243.
12. Neyzi O, Alp H, Orhon A. Sexual maturation in Turkish girls. Ann Hum Biol 1975; 2:29–59.
13. Boros A, Beller FK, Kieback D, Csoknyay J, Lampe L, Schlummer A. Pubertal development: the development of sex characteristics—Tanner stages 25 years later. Transact Amer Gyn Obstet Soc 1989; 7:128–134.
14. McKlein MC: Histology and cytology of the mammary gland. In: Von SK, Cowie AT, eds. The mammary gland and its secretion, vol 1. New York: Academic Press, 1961: 47–126.
15. Fara AM, DelCorvo G, Bernuzzi S, et al. Epidemic breast enlargement in an Italian school. Lance 1979; 1:295.
16. Handly RS, Thackray AC. Invasion of internal mammary lymph nodes in carcinoma of the breast. Br Med J 1954; 1:61–63.
17. Batchelor HT. Absence of mammal breast in a woman. Br Med J 1888; 11:876.
18. Nelson KG. Premature menarche in children born prematurely. J Pediatr 1981; 103:756–758.
19. Osborne MP. Breast development and anatomy. In: Harris JR, Henderson IC, Hellman S, Kinney DW, eds. Breast disease. Philadelphia: JB Lippincott, 1987:1–15.
20. Bostwick J. Aesthetic and reconstructive breast surgery. St. Louis: CV Mosby, 1982:23.
21. Beller FK. Atlas der Mamma Chirurgis. New York, Stuttgart: Schattauer, 1985.
22. Seitzer D, Beller FK. The trunk breast (protrusion of the breast) Breast Dis 1988; 1:121–127.
23. Vorherr H. The breast. New York: Academic Press, 1974.
24. Sechel HP. Premature thelarche and premature metrarche followed by normal adolescence. J Pediatr 1980; 57:204–209.
25. Ilicki A, Prager L, Kauli R, Kaufmann H, Schachter A, Laron B. Premature thelarche, natural history and sex hormone. Acta Paediatr Scand 1984; 73:756–762.
26. Mills J, Stolley P, Davies J, Moshang T. Premature thelarche. Am J Dis Child 1981; 135:743–745.
27. Pertzelan A, Yalon L, Kauli R, Laron Z. A comparative study of the effect of estrogen substitution therapy on breast development in girls with hypo- and hyper-gonadotrophic hypogonadism. Clin Endocrinol 1982; 16:359–368.
28. Pasquino AM, Tebaldi L, Cioschi L, et al. Premature thelarche: a follow up study of 40 girls. Arch Dis Child 1980; 60:1180–1192.
29. Saenz De Rodriguez CA, Toro-Sola MA. Anabolic steroids in meat and premature thelarche. Lancet 1982; 1:1300.
30. Pasquino AM, Piccolo F, Scalmandre A, Malvaso M, Oitohani R, Roscheri R. Hypothalamic pituitary—gonadotropic function in girls with premature thelarche. Arch Dis Child 1980; 55:941–944.
31. Reiter EO, Kaplan SL, Conte FA, Grumbach MM. Responsitivity of pituitary gonadotropes to luteinizing hormone-realizing factor in idiopathic precocious puberty, precocious thelarche. Pediatr Res 1975; 9:111–116.

2

History and Physical Examination

George W. Mitchell, Jr.

HISTORY

The family history must include the presence or absence of breast cancer in female relatives of the first degree and, in the event that disease was present, whether it occurred before or after menopause, the former being more significant in terms of genetic predisposition. It is also important to know the level of anxiety imposed on the patient by the presence of the disease in forebears or siblings, since special counseling might be necessary for this condition. Cancer in other organs, such as ovary, colon, and uterine fundus might also have some bearing on probabilities, if it is present in the family to any degree (see Chapter 18).

Asking about breast problems in general terms does not provide sufficient information. Questions regarding the breast must be specific and relate to function, symptoms, previous disease, injury, and nipple discharge. Failure of lactation after pregnancy or inappropriate lactation at other times suggests that there may be an underlying endocrine problem. A history of infection—generalized, unilateral, or localized—may have an etiologic bearing on the presence of skin pigmentation, lumps, or nipple discharge. Ductal and lobular swelling in the second half of the menstrual cycle leads to breast engorgement and pain, especially in the upper-outer quadrants. This commonly occurs in ovulating women and may also be present in those who do not ovulate and who are suffering from prolonged hyperestrinism. Serious discomfort, especially when it is chronic and extends throughout the cycle, suggests the possibility of local pathology, such as fibrocystic change, but psychologic factors must always be considered in the differential diagnosis, as is the case with chronic pelvic pain. Old injuries, including those due to surgery, produce scar tissue and isolated areas of thickening or retraction.

Nipple discharges may be either unilateral or bilateral. Ordinarily, general systemic causes produce bilateral secretion and local causes produce unilateral secretion, but because of variations in end-organ responsiveness this is not invariable. The causes of nipple discharge are listed in Table 2.1. Those related to pregnancy include the "witch's milk" temporarily produced by the newborn in response

Table 2.1. Causes of Nipple Discharge

Hormonal (galactorrhea)
Pregnancy
Neonatal ("witch's milk")
Hypothalamic-pituitary dysfunction
    Adenoma (Forbes-Albright syndrome)
    Other sellar tumors
    Chiari-Frommel syndrome
    Ahumada-del Castillo syndrome
    Chronic renal disease
    Hypothyroidism
    Drugs (phenothiazines, rawolfia alkaloids, tricyclic, antidepressants, methyl dopa, oral contraceptives)
Reflex (galactorrhea)
Sucking
Trauma
Thoracic surgery
Jogging
Garments
Local disease
Cancer
Intraductal papilloma
Cystic change
Ductal ectasia
Galactocele
Infection

to maternal hormones, the thin colostrum of late pregnancy, and the physiologic lactation that follows delivery and persists as long as nursing stimuli continue. Lactation unrelated to pregnancy is termed galactorrhea and may be due to many causes, most of which are associated with high normal or elevated prolactin levels. When a history of galactorrhea unrelated to pregnancy is obtained, blood should be drawn for a serum prolactin level, regardless of other facts in the history or the results of subsequent examination. Possibly the most common cause for this condition is the presence of pituitary micro- or macroadenomas, which oversecrete prolactin. The pressure of extracellular tumors may produce the same effect. In addition to the serum prolactin level, a CT scan of the brain should be obtained to rule out these lesions. Women with galactorrhea may also have other manifestations of a functional endocrinopathy, including postpartum amenorrhea (Chiari-Frommel syndrome) and amenorrhea that is not pregnancy related (Ahumada-del Castillo syndrome) (see Chapter 3).

Since dopamine antagonists increase prolactin secretion, it is to be expected that many drugs used for a variety of medical conditions would produce lactation. Drug administration may also be responsible for defective synthesis of prolactin-inhibiting factor (PIF) and for alterations in receptor binding. Elevated prolactin levels mediated through the PIF system may also be caused by chronic renal disease and hypothyroidism.

Mechanical stimulation of the breast is among the more mundane causes of galactorrhea. Garments that unduly compress or inadequately support the breasts may produce this effect, as can frequent breast manipulation, sucking, or athleticism, such as jogging. Excess prolactin may be released into the blood by reflex stimulation of the thoracic nerves as a result of surgery or trauma.

Nipple secretions other than galactorrhea are often due to local disease and vary widely in appearance and consistency. A brownish discharge suggests the presence of blood and must subsequently be evaluated by microscopic examination. A frankly bloody discharge is pathognomonic of a disease process, most likely an intraductal papilloma, with a 30% probability that malignancy is present. A pale or white discharge, especially when bilateral, may represent excess secretion by lubricating cells or be a manifestation of mild chronic infection. Ductal ectasia, which is common during the perimenopausal and menopausal years and may be classified as a chronic infection (see Chapter 6), may give rise to a green-

ish-yellow, sticky discharge, usually bilateral. Acute infections most commonly occur postpartum and proceed from a diffuse cellulitis to a localized abscess; these and nonpuerperal, generalized infections due to *Staphylococcus aureus* may produce a thick yellow secretion from the nipple.

The most important symptom, and the one that most often brings the patient to the physician, is the suspected or actual presence of a lump in the breast, which she, her spouse, or another physician has detected. It is necessary to know how long the lump has been present, whether it has progressively increased in size or varies with the menstrual cycle, and whether or not it is painful. The patient should be asked exactly where the lump is, whether there are any others, and whether she has felt under her arms for glands. Pain and tenderness in the affected area are important symptoms, although anxiety and constant fingering may have elicited either one. The patient should be asked whether she has noted any changes in the size of the breast or the condition of the skin, areola, or nipple.

Without being asked, patients occasionally allude in a serious or semifacetious way to what they consider to be the small size of their breasts. This may be related to an idealized version and require only reassurance, but it can be a deeper problem needing counseling and perhaps plastic surgery, especially in the young. Marked hypoplasia is rare. Occasionally, pronounced asymmetry is present, causing psychologic distress and necessitating surgical correction (see Chapter 1).

Very large breasts are responsible for downward pull on the neck, shoulders, and back, with resulting strain and chronic discomfort in those areas. Improperly fitting supporting garments may increase the disability, and their straps cause lacerations and scarring across the shoulders. When this history is elicited, the physician must plan to examine the garments both off and on the patient and note points of stress. A list of specialty shops dealing in custom-made supports that might improve the situation should be kept on hand.

An important facet of the history is the frequency and adequacy of self-examinations and the findings on previous examinations by medical personnel. The patient's interpretation of the results of such examinations and of the reports of all previous diagnostic tests should be carefully noted, and the diagnostic aids, especially mammograms, should be requested from available sources for review.

Women who have previously been treated for breast cancer remain at increased risk indefinitely, both for recurrent disease and for new cancer in the contralateral breast. In such a patient, the history must include the time of the last breast examination and the report of the physician who did it, reports of all x-ray examinations and other diagnostic procedures such as liver and bone scans, blood chemistries, and chemical markers. Questions must be asked regarding weight loss, headache, bone pain, hoarseness, cough, weakness, and fatigue, and the necessary steps must be taken to evaluate positive answers.

PHYSICAL EXAMINATION

Self-Examination

Breast self-examination (BSE) has been recommended to women for a generation and, despite caveats by some authorities (1, 2), has gained in popularity among the laity and is endorsed by physicians and other medical personnel, as well as by cancer organizations. A survey by the National Cancer Institute in 1980 showed that 77% of women in the sample had done at least one breast self-examination in the preceding year, and 29% had done the examination on a regular monthly basis (3). Such polls are obviously biased by the type of samples screened, and the extent of education in BSE and the rate of compliance by those who have been educated continue to be speculative. Advocacy of the method by both professionals and consumers is based on the seemingly undeniable assumptions that it is immediately available, noninvasive, and inexpensive and that the benefits are earlier diagnosis and reduction in the mortality of breast cancer (4–8).

Although already firmly embedded in the practices of most medical and paramedical personnel, the scientific debate over these assumptions has been prolonged, with forces aligned on either side producing statistical proof of their beliefs. The basic, and probably insoluble, problem is the fact that all of these studies have been retrospective and subject to criticism because of sample selection and unsatisfactory controls. The possibility of mounting a prospective, randomized controlled study is remote because of what many consider the ethical consideration of denying BSE to controls and the likelihood that such controls would be noncompliant as a result of contamination by widespread advertising of the method. According to one study (8), 69% of women practicing BSE discovered their tumor by that method, and it is generally accepted among physicians that most lumps are discovered by their patients. The question as to whether such discoveries are made by accident or because of self-taught regular examination remains controversial. Figures have been adduced to show that the regular practice of BSE is associated with a reduction in the stage of the disease at the time of diagnosis and in the 5-year survival rate (5–8). Others have seen little or no improvement in early diagnosis or in survival after extensive public and professional education projects devoted to BSE (9, 10).

The most persuasive argument against BSE is that it enhances the risk of further invasive procedures and expense, if the lesion found by the patient is benign. This is particularly true in adolescents and in women in their early 20s, who are most likely to be compliant with the program and are unlikely to have cancer. Even in an age group expanded to include women up to 80 years of age the probability that the self-discovered lesion will be benign is between 80 and 90%, and the predictive value that a positive BSE finding will be cancer is only 6% (9, 11). This implies that the vast majority of women with self-discovered lesions will, in all probability, be subject to repetitive examinations by physicians, diagnostic aids, and invasive procedures, such as aspirations and biopsies. It has also been alleged that a negative BSE might delay a patient visit to a physician for regular physical examination, which is generally regarded as being a superior screening technique. The anxiety-producing aspect of BSE has, perhaps, been overemphasized, since not examining and wondering might be even more stressful.

Age, educational background, and body build have all been shown to be important factors in the success of BSE, and even more important is the educational process itself (3). At what age this process should begin is still conjectural, although the incidence of breast cancer is very low in women under age 25. Benign breast problems do occur in adolescents, and the need to develop healthful habits and become familiar with normal breast anatomy makes learning the technique at an early age seem desirable. The technique should be taught by the best informed professional available and one with whom the patient feels comfortable, probably another female. It is essential that an appropriate amount of time be spent teaching and reinforcing the basic rules; for this purpose, visual aids and artificial models are very helpful, and the former are economical of time, since several patients can view the screen together. Multiple repetitions are necessary for reinforcement, and at each subsequent visit the patient's ability to perform a satisfactory ex-

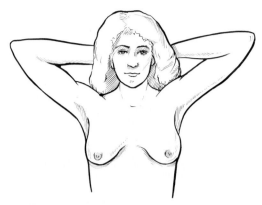

Figure 2.1. Inspection. For either BSE in front of the mirror or professional examination, arms should be up and elbows retracted.

amination should be reassessed. Discrimination between normal and abnormal breast tissue is difficult and requires practice, and this is particularly true premenstrually, when hormonal changes cause swelling, soreness, and lumpiness, especially in the upper outer quadrants. The patient should be well-informed about this and reassured about anatomical variations. She should be told that non-cyclic alterations are of greater concern. Pregnancy produces even greater distortions of the normal anatomy, but practitioners of BSE must be warned that cancer does not respect the pregnant state. Breasts of large size, whether pregnant or nonpregnant, are more difficult to examine and require a greater expenditure of time; even so, accuracy is reduced.

Inspection is done in front of a mirror with the arms upraised and elbows retracted in order to put the skin of the breasts on tension (Fig. 2.1). Pendulous breasts must be uplifted with the hands to expose the undersides. The eye should be trained to detect alterations from the normal in the skin and the nipple-areola complex, particularly elevations and depressions. Palpation of the clavicular areas, the neck, and under the arms can also be done in either the standing or seated position. Palpation must be systematic, compulsive, and repetitive until the entire breast is covered, whether this is done in a clockwise or counterclockwise manner, stripwise across the breast, or by quadrants. Particular attention must be paid to the axillary tail. The examination is best done with the woman supine and her upper back slightly elevated (Fig. 2.2). Some women prefer to do it in the bath, where moisture permits the fingers to slide easily over the breast tissue, and some prefer to use cream or oil for the same pur-

pose. With the fingertips of one hand, the contralateral breast is gently palpated by pressing it against the chest wall. It does not matter whether the three middle fingers or only the index and middle fingers of the hand are used but, since fingernails tend to be long, the pads rather than the tips of fingers are preferable. During the examination the arm is first elevated and then lowered in order to stretch and then relax the breast parenchyma. The process is repeated on the opposite side using the other hand. For women in the reproductive age group, the examination is best done in the days immediately following menstruation, when the breasts are unengorged and relatively flaccid. Even at this time, fairly heavy pressure must be exerted on heavy breasts to palpate tissue close to the chest wall. In postmenopausal women, when the breast tissue is almost entirely replaced by fat, less pressure need be used, and more accuracy can be attained unless the breast is very large.

The patient is instructed to be alert for the presence of a solitary lump, particularly one that is hard, irregular, and nontender. Lumps that are multiple, smooth in outline, and bilateral are likely to be benign but require further investigation. Symmetrical thickened areas in both breasts also suggest benignity, but a hard, dominant projection from one of these areas necessitates professional attention.

In summary, screening for breast cancer by BSE has many shortcomings, but it has become, nevertheless, an established practice. It is inferior to professional examination and far inferior to mammography (8, 12). Sensitivity is high, but specificity is low (13). Current knowledge and usage by the laity being what it is, physicians are advised to recommend it, especially since much of the pressure to do so derives from the American Cancer Society (14). With the recommendation should come emphasis on proper technique, repeat instruction, regular reevaluation, and demonstrations using artificial models and video tapes. A posi-

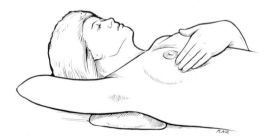

Figure 2.2. BSE. Palpation of the right breast with the left hand while reclining and with the arm raised.

tive attitude on the part of personnel assisting with the process is most helpful. Some teaching aids are listed in the Appendix.

Professional Examination

Careful examination of the breasts is an important part of every physical examination but is sometimes executed in too cursory a manner (15, 16). Lack of proper training in the technique of breast examination is widespread among physicians and, in a recent study, one-third of the 80 physicians drawn from all the major specialties stated that their training in clinical breast examination was not adequate in medical school or residency (17). Eighty-four percent reported that they felt a need to improve their abilities in breast lump detection. How often breast examinations by professionals should be done is speculative, since there are only statistical projections to indicate that a frequency greater than once a year would be beneficial (12). Screening examinations can be done competently by nurses and paramedical personnel, but specific breast problems should be directed to a physician.

The examination should be performed on patients stripped to the waist and without jewelry. Whether for reasons of vanity or modesty, some women dislike being examined while they are seated upright but do not object to the examination while supine. It is important that they be examined in both positions, since they are complementary. With a strong light directed against first one breast and then the other, inspection is carried out with the patient seated and her hands either clasped behind her or raised above her head, while the elbows are retracted (Fig. 2.1). This places tension on the breast skin and reveals imperfections, such as areas of retraction and deviated or inverted nipples. Erythema, edema, nevi, papillomas, warts, furuncles, eczematoid reactions, ulcers, and venous congestion must be noted, both for their own interest and because they might be harbingers of deeper disease. Breast skin is heir to the same dermatologic conditions as the skin of the rest of the body and, although superficial lesions are most often benign, the patient may place a more serious interpretation on them. Significant lesions should be charted for further evaluation. Heavy pendulous breasts must be manually elevated to obtain a view of the underside, and the presence of intertriginous changes due to friction must be noted. For cancer detection the most significant abnormalities are noncongenital nipple retraction or deviation; skin dimpling, which may be isolated or spread over a large area (peau d'orange); and a scaly red eruption around the areola suggestive of Paget's disease.

Inspection must also include attention to abnormalities unrelated to disease. The size and shape of the breasts are compared with the patient's previous observations, and the bra fit is noted. The presence of very large areolae, prominent tubercles, or hair growth are of importance only if the patient has commented on them or requests cosmetic treatment. The breasts of most women are asymmetric, with the left breast more often larger than the right, but the asymmetry may be so marked that the patient appears to be deformed, and a deficiency of this sort is usually associated with psychologic trauma. An even more serious defect is complete aplasia of one or both breasts. At the other end of the spectrum is marked hypertrophy or heavy fatty infiltration, forming pendulous breasts, with nipples pointing downward. These are not only a cause of psychologic problems but are often associated with chronic neck, shoulder, or back pain, symptoms that may not be elicited until the physician asks about their existence, since patients frequently do not make the association on their own. Very large, or protruding, nipples and areolae relative to the overall breast size may be a cause for concern, and supernumerary nipples extending down the milkline on the chest and abdomen, and even to the vulva, are not unusual. Congenital inversion of the nipples, usually but not always bilateral, is very common, and the observer must know the duration of the defect (see Chapter 1).

After inspection, the breasts are palpated, while still on tension, by pressing the breast tissue against the chest wall with the examiner's fingers. As with BSE, it does not seem to be important whether the three middle fingers or only the index and middle fingers are used, nor whether the pressure is applied by the flats or the tips of the fingers (17). The entire breast is covered, either in circles, clockwise, or counterclockwise, stripwise from one side to the other, or by individual quadrants. So long as the examination is done systematically and thoroughly, with particular attention to the axillary tail and the area beneath the areola, the technique can be a matter of personal preference. Variable finger pressure is helpful in detecting deeper lesions. The patient is then asked to place her hands on her hips and relax her shoulders, and the process is repeated, first on one side, then on the other (Fig. 2.3). In older women whose breasts are flaccid as a result of age and fatty infiltration, the breast may be pulled away from the chest wall between the examiner's two hands, and the basal midportion may be gently squeezed to ascer-

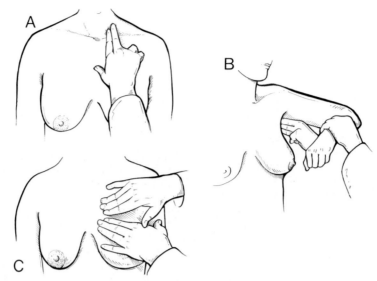

Figure 2.3.   A, Palpation of left supraclavicular area for lymph nodes. **B,** Palpation of left axilla for lymph nodes. **C,** Circumferential palpation with patient seated.

tain whether there are any lesions close to the chest wall.

Palpation of the lymph nodes that drain the breast area can best be done with the patient vertical and bent slightly forward. Some examiners prefer to have the patient place her hands on their shoulders. The anterior and posterior cervical chains are examined first, although there is seldom drainage from the breast to this area (Fig. 2.3). The supra- and infraclavicular lymph nodes may be checked both medial and lateral to the origin of the sternocleidomastoid muscle, using either the first and second fingers together or the thumbs. The axillae are examined by drawing the patient's arm either forward across the chest wall or outward, to relax the pectoralis major muscle, and feeling under its insertion, in the vault of the axilla, and along the inner margin of the latissimus dorsi muscle (Fig. 2.3). Palpable lymph nodes less than 1 cm in diameter are most often unrelated to breast pathology. When they are noted in the absence of any palpable breast disease, careful inspection of areas that drain to the axilla, especially the ipsilateral hand, arm, and thorax, should be done to rule out other etiologies. Lymph nodes that are larger than 1 cm, fixed, hard, multiple, or related to palpable breast disease must be further evaluated either by CT scan, biopsy, or both. The presence of a suspicious mass in the breast and enlarged ipsilateral axillary lymph nodes strongly suggests the presence of cancer.

The patient is next examined in the supine position, with her head comfortably supported, and each shoulder in turn elevated by a

flat pillow (Fig. 2.4). Palpation is repeated on each side, first with the arm up and then down, and the underside of the breast is again inspected. If the patient has felt a lump, that is difficult for the examiner to confirm, the patient must be asked to identify the exact area, and a persistent effort is necessary to ensure the satisfaction of both parties. The examina-

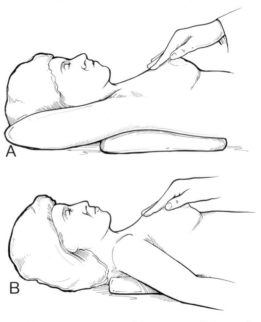

Figure 2.4.   A, Palpation with patient reclining and arm raised. **B,** Palpation with patient reclining and arm at side.

		Date	Age	Parity	Menst. Index	LMP	
		Mo. Day Yr.		G. P. A. LC.	Mo. Day Yr.	Mo. Day Yr.	

Reason for referral: _____

Chief complaint: □ Pain   □ Lump   □ Heaviness   □ Nipple deviation/retraction
Check ✓   □ Swelling   □ Soreness   □ Nipple disch.   □ Other: _____
for positive   □ Redness   □ Lumpiness   □ Skin changes

Past history:

Age, first preg. _____   Breast feed □ Yes □ No   Self-examine □ No □ Yes   Fx _____

Diet:	Y	N	Surgery:	Y	N	Hormones:	Y	N	Med. Hx	Y	N	Fa Hx CA:	Y	N	Age	Relationship
High fat	□	□	Breast	□	□	OC's	□	□	HTN	□	□	Breast	□	□	___	_____
Low fat	□	□	Abdomen	□	□	ERT	□	□	DM	□	□	Uterus	□	□	___	_____
High caffeine	□	□	Pelvis	□	□	HRT	□	□	Ca	□	□	Cervix	□	□	___	_____
Low caffeine	□	□	Chest	□	□	Other	□	□	Other	□	□	Ovary	□	□	___	_____
												Colon	□	□	___	_____

Mammograms: Y   N   Y   N
              □   □   Date: _____   Abnormal: □ □   _____

Physical exam: Breast size: □ Average   □ Small   □ Large   □ Hypertrophic

Nodes:	Y	N	#	Inspection:	Y	N	Inspection:	Y	N
Neck	□	□	___	Symmetric	□	□	Skin normal	□	□
Clavicle	□	□	___	Areola deviation	□	□	Skin retracted	□	□
Axilla	□	□	___	Areola retracted	□	□	Nipple discharge	□	□

RIGHT BREAST   Palpation: **LEFT BREAST**

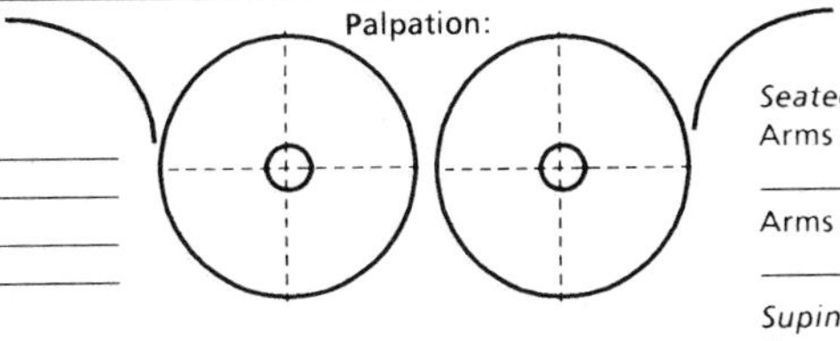

Seated: Norm Abn   Seated: Norm Abn
Arms up □ □ _____   Arms up □ □ _____

Arms dn □ □ _____   Arms dn □ □ _____

Supine: Supine:
Arms up □ □ _____   Arms up □ □ _____

Arms dn □ □ _____   Arms dn □ □ _____

Other: _____

Impression: _____

Recommendations, F/U: _____
_____
_____
_____

Physician Provider _____

Figure 2.5. Form for recording history and physical examination.

tion of the breast with the patient supine is the most critical part of the entire process, and the amount of time spent should be appropriate to the size of the breasts and the feelings of the patient. Examination time has been described as one of the most significant factors in achieving diagnostic accuracy, more important than experience and method (17). From 3 min for breasts of average size to 5 min for very large breasts should suffice.

Some health professionals believe that the patient's breasts should be milked routinely at the time of examination in an attempt to express a discharge from the nipple. This is usually done by quadrants, pressing from the periphery toward the nipple, in order to determine from which geographical area the discharge is produced. Pumps have also been used for the purpose. Exudates are often thin and acellular and should be collected on frosted or albumin-coated slides to prevent run-off. The slide is placed in contact with the nipple and gently rubbed across it. The interpretation is seldom helpful in diagnosing cancer. When the discharge is bloody, further evaluation becomes essential (see Chapter 16).

In general, patients can be relied upon to give a history of nipple discharge, and, when they do, they can usually express it for demonstration more effectively and with less discomfort than the examiner. For this reason, routine squeezing in the absence of a positive history is not recommended.

In summary, professional physical examination of the breasts is a valuable screening tool, although far less sensitive and less specific than mammography. It is essential for the early diagnosis of disease suspected by the patient and must follow screening by other diagnostic aids reported to be positive. Adequate technique requires a learning process that must be supervised and rigorous, preferably using artificial as well as live models, and experience is obviously helpful (17, 18). A sufficient amount of time spent in the process is of the utmost importance. Frowns, exclamations of surprise, or asides to the nurse by the examiner during any part of the process may increase the patient's anxiety and should be avoided.

While the patient is dressing and before the memory fades, a diagram of the breasts should be made and findings charted on it. It should be noted in the record, for legal self-protection, that the patient was examined both seated and supine and with the arms up and down in each position. A description of the findings and the proposed recommendations for reassurance, treatment, or referral should be carefully reported. For staging purposes, the estimated size of any suspicious lesions should be expressed in centimeters; the size and number of palpable lymph nodes should be specified. Fig. 2.5 shows a form that can be used for this purpose.

After the patient is clothed, she should be put at ease for the discussion to follow. Further evaluation of a lesion suspected of being cancerous should be planned for the immediate future. Observation, medical treatment, or surgery should be prescribed for problems associated with benign breast disease. Patients concerned about cosmesis because of underdevelopment should be informed of the risks and benefits of augmentation operations; those suffering from orthopaedic problems or pain associated with heavy breasts need to know the advantages of reduction mammoplasty. Those who are without disease or blemish but have symptoms should be informed of the cyclic nature of many symptoms because of the ebb and flow of hormones, reassured about their condition, and told when to return for the next appointment. Diagnostic aids should be ordered according to current guidelines. Negative mammograms do not preclude biopsy of suspicious areas.

APPENDIX

Code 501	Breast Health Awareness Training Guide and Flip Chart
0208	Teaching Breast Model
528	Physician's Wall Chart on BSE
P4	Early Detection of Breast Cancer—Video or Slide/Tape
P5	BSE: A Special Touch—Video
1097	Finding a Lump in Your Breast—Pamphlet
508	How to Examine Your Breast—Pamphlet
509	Learn to Give Yourself Breast Self-Examinations—Bilingual Pamphlet, Spanish/English

REFERENCES

1. Frank JW, Mai V. Breast self-examination in young women: more harm than good? Lancet 1985;2:654–657.
2. Moore FD. Breast self-examination. N Engl J Med 1978;229(6):304–305.
3. National survey on breast cancer. A measure of progress in understanding. Dept Health and Human Services, Public Health Service, NIH, Bethesda, Md: 1980.
4. Feldman JG, Carter AC, Nicastri AD, Hosat SF. Breast self-examination, relationship to stage of breast cancer at diagnosis. Cancer 1981;47:2740–2745.
5. Foster RS Jr, Costanza MC. Breast self-examination practices and breast cancer survival. Cancer 1984;53:1000–1005.
6. Foster RS Jr, Lang SP, Costanza MC, Worden JK, Haines CR, Yates JW. Breast self-examination processes and breast cancer stage. N Engl J Med 1978;299:265–270.
7. Gastrin G. Program to encourage self examination for breast cancer. Br Med J 1980;ii:193.
8. Greenwald P, Nasea PC, Lawrence CE, et al. Estimated effect of breast self-examination and routine physician examination on breast cancer mortality. N Engl J Med 1978;199:271–273.
9. Saltzstein, SL. Potential limits of physical examination and breast self-examination in detecting small cancers of the breast. An unselected population-based study of 1302 cases. Cancer 1984;54:1443–1446.
10. Health and Policy Committee, American College of Physicians. The use of diagnostic test for screening and evaluating breast lesions. Ann Intern Med 1985;103:147–151.
11. Holliday H, Roebuck EJ, Doyle PJ. Initial results from a program of BSE. Clin Oncol 1983;9:11–16.
12. Kirch RLA, Klein M. Prospective evaluation of periodic breast examination programs. Cancer 1976;38:265–272.
13. Huguley CM Jr, Brown RL. The value of breast self-examination. Cancer 1981;47:989–995.
14. American Cancer Society. Breast Self-Examination Subcommittee BSE. Breast self-examination, a health practice for everyone. New York: American Cancer Society, Form 246.
15. Byrd BF: Close up: standard breast examination. CA 1974;24:290–293.
16. Haagensen CD. Carcinoma of the breast: a monograph for the physician. New York: American Cancer Society, 1958:7.
17. Fletcher SW, O'Malley MS, Bunce LA. Physicians' abilities to detect lumps in silicone breast models. JAMA 1985;253(15):2224–2228.
18. Hall DC, Adams CC, Stein GH, et al. Improved detection of human breast lesions following experimental training. Cancer 1980;46:408–414.

3

Endocrinology of the Breast

Carolyn R. Kaplan
Robert S. Schenken

The mammary gland is a unique endocrine organ that undergoes growth, differentiation, and lactation in response to hormones. The hormonal regulation of mammogenesis occurs throughout fetal, adolescent, and adult life. The endocrine milieu of pregnancy has an important effect on the breast that is critical for normal lactation. After delivery of the newborn, a complex neuroendocrine feedback system controls milk ejection and maintains lactation until weaning. Involution follows, with a gradual return to the resting state, until pregnancy again stimulates a cycle of secretory activity. In this chapter, the hormonal control of mammary development, lactation, and the regulation of milk secretion and ejection will be discussed.

DEVELOPMENT OF THE HUMAN BREAST

Mammogenesis—the growth and differentiation of the mammary gland—begins in early fetal life. In classic experiments using hypophysectomized, adrenalectomized, ovariectomized rats, Lyons' studies demonstrated that many hormones are involved in mammary development. These include prolactin, growth hormone, thyroid-stimulating hormone (TSH), luteinizing hormone (LH), human placental lactogen (hPL), ovarian and adrenal steroids, and insulin (1) (Fig. 3.1). The minimal hormonal requirement for mammary growth and secretory activity in the human is unknown, but estrogen and progesterone exert key roles in the growth and maturation of the gland (1, 2). Administration of estrogen (or alteration of the

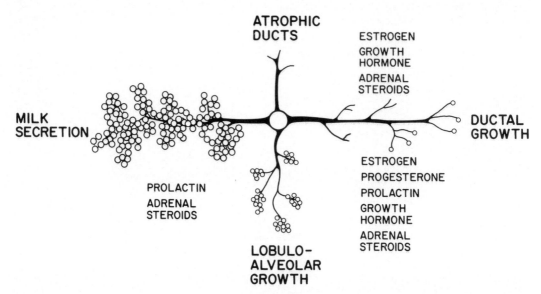

Figure 3.1. Hormones affecting mammary growth and lactation. (Adapted from Lyons WR, Li CH, Johnson RE. The hormonal control of mammary growth and lactation. Recent Prog Horm Res 1958;14:219–250.)

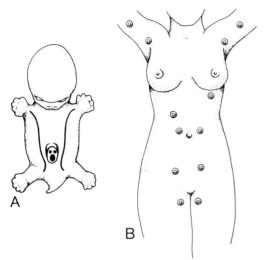

Figure 3.2. **A**, Schematic drawing of "milk line" in human embryos. **B**, The corresponding sites of supernumerary nipples and mammary tissue in women. (Adapted from Patten BM. Human embryology, 3rd ed. New York: McGraw-Hill, 1968:195–205.)

sults from animal studies have, for the most part, been extrapolated to humans.

Embryonic and Prepubertal Development

In humans, the mammary gland is identified 6 weeks after conception as an ectodermal thickening along the ventrolateral aspect of the fetus. With cell growth, a mammary ridge is formed. This ridge soon differentiates into localized areas that represent the paired glands characteristic of the species. Normally, one pair of glands develops in the thoracic region, but supernumerary nipples and breast tissue may develop anywhere along the milk line (6) (Fig. 3.2).

Epithelial cell proliferation and penetration into the underlying mesenchyme form the primitive mammary bud (7) (Fig. 3.3). During the second trimester, projections of ectoderm form the primary sprouts (15 to 25 in the human), which will eventually elongate and arborize to form the lactiferous ducts. This initial growth may be independent of maternal or fetal hormones, as mouse mammary explants grown in vitro will form primary sprouts in the absence of exogenous hormones (2).

Canalization of the lactiferous ducts occurs late in fetal life (Fig. 3.3). Once the ducts canalize, two layers of epithelial cells are identified: the inner layer of cells that forms the secretory component and the outer layer of cells that becomes the myoepithelium (8). Only the main lactiferous ducts are present in the fetus; limited ductal differentiation and secretory activity occur in late gestation under the influence of fetal prolactin and placental steroids (9).

At birth, newborn breast secretions (socalled "witch's milk"), may be seen for several

normal ratio of estrogen to androgen) induces breast development in the human at any phase of life (3, 4). Repetitive suckling stimuli can induce lactation in nulliparous females in the absence of pregnancy or exogenous hormone supplementation (5), and, occasionally, suckling induces lactation in men. The literature detailing hormonal control of mammary growth and development is vast (2), and most information is derived from animal models. There are few studies with human breast tissue, and re-

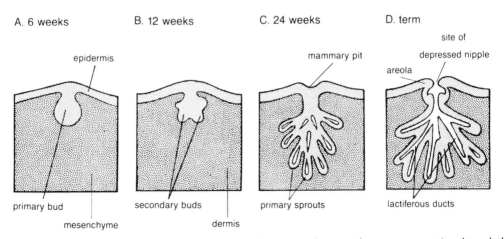

Figure 3.3. Development of the mammary glands. **A**, Schematic drawing of a transverse section through the trunk and mammary ridge at 6 weeks; **B**, **C**, and **D**, Similar sections showing successive development between the 12th week and birth. (Adapted from Moore KL. The developing human. Philadelphia: Saunders, 1977:376–386.)

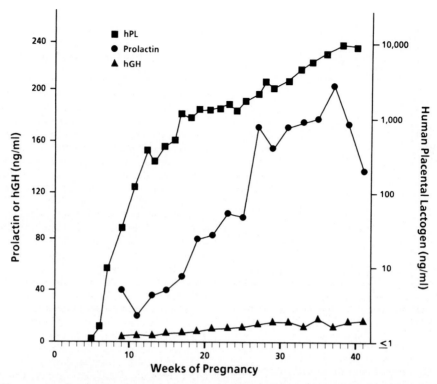

Figure 3.4. Mean values of plasma prolactin, human growth hormone, and human placental lactogen during normal pregnancy. (Adapted from Kletzky OA, Rossman F, Bertolli SI, Platt LD, Mishell DR Jr, Dynamics of human chorionic gonadotropin, prolactin, and growth hormone in serum and amniotic fluid throughout normal human pregnancy. Am J Obstet Gynecol 1985;151:878–884; hPL levels taken from Braunstein GD, Rasor JL, Engvall E, Wade ME. Interrelationships of human chorionic gonadotropin, human placental lactogen, and pregnancy-specific β₁-glycoprotein throughout normal human gestation. Am J Obstet Gynecol 1980;138:1205–1213.)

days with equal frequency in male or female infants (10). Although testosterone induces partial regression of the mammary bud in rodents (2), there are no histologic or functional differences between the human male and female breast until puberty. Shortly after birth, the epithelial cells revert to an undifferentiated state and remain quiescent until puberty. Minimal ductal growth occurs during childhood, and there is no lobuloalveolar development (2).

Puberty

The rise of estrogen levels prior to menarche reinitiates lactiferous duct proliferation. Breast enlargement occurs due to deposition of periglandular adipose tissue (6). Concurrent organization of the stromal connective tissue forms the interlobular septa. Ovarian steroids appear necessary for mammary development in women, as breast enlargement fails to occur at puberty in girls with gonadal dysgenesis (11). Estrogen alone stimulates ductal proliferation but not lobuloalveolar development (12), the latter being dependent on progesterone (2).

Upon establishment of ovulatory menstrual cycles, rising estrogen and progesterone levels during the cycle cause an increase in blood flow and interlobular edema (13). A moderate degree of ductal and lobular proliferation also occurs during each follicular and luteal phase (8). Histologic examination of normal breast tissue shows limited glandular secretion just before menses and milk discharge from the nipple may occur. At menses, a reduction in the number and size of glandular cells occurs, with loss of edema and slight decrease in breast size.

Pregnancy

During pregnancy, the breast undergoes final maturation in preparation for lactation. Early in the first trimester, mammary epithelial cells proliferate, and ductal sprouting and branching are initiated. The ducts proliferate into the fatty pad, and the ductal end buds differentiate into alveoli (8). This growth is accompanied by increased mammary blood flow, interstitial water, and electrolyte concentrations. Growth of the mammary gland occurs

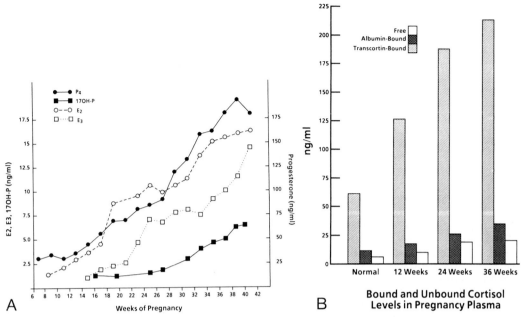

Figure 3.5. **A**, Mean values of plasma estradiol (E_2), estriol (E_3), progesterone (P_4), and 17-hydroxyprogesterone (17-OH-P) during pregnancy. (Adapted from Tulchinsky D, Hobel CJ, Yeager E, Marshall JR. Plasma estrone, estradiol, estriol, progesterone, and 17-hydroxyprogesterone in human pregnancy. 1. Normal pregnancy. Am J Obstet Gynecol 1972;112:1095–1100.) **B**, Bound and unbound cortisol levels in plasma during pregnancy (From Rosenthal HE, Slaunwhite, WR Jr., Sandberg AA. Transcortin: corticosteroid-binding protein of plasma. X. Cortisol and progesterone interplay and unbound levels of these steroids in pregnancy. J Clin Endocrinol Metab 1969;29:352–357.)

primarily in clusters of epithelial cells (lobules) organized into a sphere (alveolus). Proliferation of lobuloalveolar structures occurs throughout pregnancy and, in some species, into early lactation (14).

The alveolar cells become single-layered at midpregnancy, and the alveolar lumina begin to dilate. Lymphocytes, plasma cells, and eosinophils collect in the interstitial spaces (8). The mammary blood supply is enhanced by increasing vascular luminal diameters and by formation of new capillaries around the mammary lobules. During the last trimester, the secretory cells fill with fat droplets, and the alveoli are distended with a proteinaceous, eosinophilic secretion termed colostrum. Mammary epithelial proliferation then declines, and the alveolar epithelium differentiates for secretory function (2).

Hormonal Control of Mammary Development during Pregnancy

Several hormones increase markedly during pregnancy and significantly affect mammary development. In humans, prolactin (15, 16) and hPL (17–19) increase concurrently during pregnancy and reach peak levels prior to parturition (Fig. 3.4). Human prolactin and hPL

have considerable amino acid homology (13%), and the lactogenic activity of the two hormones is very similar (12). Both hormones induce mammary growth in vitro and in vivo (20, 21), and either hormone is sufficient for mammogenesis in humans (22, 23).

The amino acid sequence of hPL also has remarkable homology with human growth hormone. Although more than 80% of amino acid residues are identical (24), hPL has little somatotrophic activity. Growth hormone does appear to be lactogenic in some animals (12), but growth hormone levels remain low during human pregnancy (16) (Fig. 3.4) and lactation (18, 25), and normal mammogenesis and lactation occur in women with growth hormone deficiency (15, 26). Thus, growth hormone does not appear to play an important role in breast development and lactation in women.

Estrogen and progesterone levels increase dramatically during normal pregnancy (27) (Fig. 3.5a). 17β-Estradiol (E_2) is one of the hormones required for mammary growth and epithelial proliferation during pregnancy (2). Evidence for a direct effect of E_2 on mammary cells is lacking, but E_2 does stimulate prolactin release in vitro (28, 29) and in vivo (30), and E_2 increases breast prolactin receptors in some species (2).

During pregnancy, progesterone stimulates lobuloalveolar growth while suppressing secretory activity. High progesterone levels inhibit lactose synthetase and milk protein (casein) mRNA synthesis in vitro (2). Progesterone may also play a positive role in differentiation of the gland. Progesterone sensitizes mammary cells to the effects of insulin and growth factors and may be involved in final preparation of the mammary gland for lactogenesis (14).

Glucocorticoid levels increase during pregnancy (31, 32) (Fig. 3.5b), primarily due to a decreased clearance rate and an increase in corticosteroid binding globulin. However, unbound steroid is also increased (33) (Fig. 3.5b). Although not essential for ductal or alveolar growth, glucocorticoids enhance formation of lobules during pregnancy (2). Insulin is not required for ductal or alveolar growth in vivo, although mammary cells in the mouse gain insulin responsiveness during pregnancy. Insulin acts in synergy with prolactin to stimulate terminal differentiation of insulin-sensitive mammary cells in vitro, and in high concentrations insulin acts as a mitogen (14). Thyroid hormone is not necessary for ductal growth but, in some species, is essential for alveolar growth (2). Thyroid hormones increase the responsiveness of mammary cells to prolactin and may improve lactational performance as discussed below.

INITIATION OF MILK SECRETION (LACTOGENESIS)

Lactogenesis can be divided into two stages, the first occurring prepartum, the second occurring around parturition. In pregnant women, the breast is capable of milk secretion by the second trimester. Enzymatic and cytologic differentiation of the mammary epithelium and limited milk secretion occur during this initial stage of lactogenesis (34). The hormonal stimulus responsible for these changes is unknown, but placental lactogen is a likely candidate, as its maximal secretion coincides with the initial phase of lactogenesis in several species (35).

The concentration of enzymes specific for milk secretion increases within the alveolar cell as parturition approaches. Synthesis of lactose, casein, and α-lactalbumin increases concurrently. α-Lactalbumin, the regulatory subunit of the lactose synthetase enzyme complex (36), is synthetized only by mammary epithelial cells, and its presence indicates that final differentiation has occurred (2). A marked rise in citrate and α-lactalbumin occurs at the onset of the second stage of lactogenesis (37). Histologic evidence of secretion within the alveolar lumen appears, and the breast becomes engorged (8). Secretion of copious quantities of milk occurs immediately preceding (e.g., in cattle) or after (e.g., in women) parturition and signals the second stage of lactogenesis (35).

Hormonal Mechanisms in the Initiation of Lactation

The maternal hormonal milieu changes dramatically at parturition. There are considerable differences between species but, in general, the periparturient period is characterized by falling levels of progesterone and placental lactogen and by increases in estrogen, prolactin, prostaglandin $F_{2\alpha}$, oxytocin, and glucocorticoids (12). Because of concurrent changes in several hormones, it is difficult to identify the specific hormone(s) that controls the onset of lactogenesis.

Rising hormone levels at parturition (especially prolactin and glucocorticoids) are thought to be the trigger for initiating lactation. However, prolactin levels reach their peak shortly before delivery (38), and lactation fails to occur. Also, estrogen treatment inhibits puerperal lactation in the presence of elevated prolactin levels (39). Thus, it appears that placental steroids inhibit secretory activity of the alveolar epithelium during pregnancy, and their removal at parturition is necessary for the mammary gland to respond to lactogenic hormones.

Although progesterone withdrawal is the most likely lactogenic trigger mechanism (40), falling progesterone levels must act in the presence of adequate levels of lactogenic hormones—in particular, prolactin. Binding of prolactin and glucocorticoids to the mammary epithelial cell is essential for full lactogenic activity.

HORMONES AND LACTATION

Lactation normally follows parturition and the removal of placental steroids from maternal serum. During the first few postpartum days, colostrum is secreted in varying amounts. There is a gradual conversion to mature milk secretion, but the onset of copious milk secretion does not occur in humans until the 3rd or 4th postpartum day (41).

Maintenance of established lactation (galactopoiesis) requires milk removal by periodic suckling. Without suckling, breast milk synthesis declines despite an appropriate hormonal milieu. Milk secretion and removal are closely associated processes, but adequate milk removal alone will not maintain lactation indefinitely. The hormonal requirements for the initiation and maintenance of milk secretion will be considered next. Oxytocin, essential for milk removal, is discussed with the milk ejection reflex.

Prolactin

Prolactin is essential for the initiation of lactation in humans and most other species. Hy-

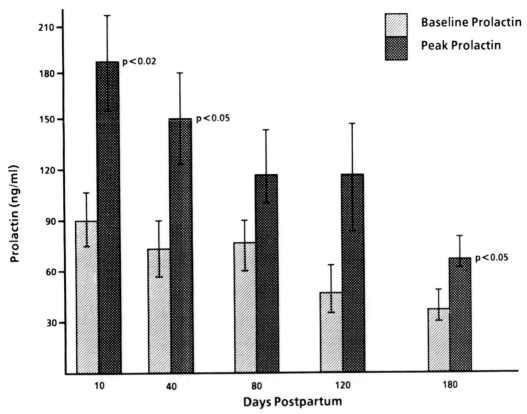

Figure 3.6. Comparison of baseline and peak serum prolactin levels after suckling during the first 180 days postpartum (mean + SEM). (Adapted from Battin DA, Marrs RP, Fleiss PM, Mishell DR Jr. Effect of suckling on serum prolactin, luteinizing hormone, follicle-stimulating hormone, and estradiol during prolonged lactation. Obstet Gynecol 1985;65:785–788.)

pophysectomy in pregnant women and animals markedly suppresses subsequent lactation (35, 42), and isolated prolactin deficiency has been associated with the absence of lactation in women (43, 44). In ovariectomized, adrenalectomized, hypophysectomized rats, the minimal hormonal requirements for milk secretion are prolactin and glucocorticoids (45). In mammary tissue explants primed with insulin and cortisol, prolactin stimulates synthesis of milk fats and proteins, such as casein and α-lactalbumin (21, 46). Prolactin also increases the mammary gland's concentration of IgA-lymphoblasts, possibly through a receptor mechanism that mediates interaction of plasma cells with the mammary gland (47).

Prolactin levels remain low throughout the greater portion of gestation in most animal species. Thus, the early increase in mammary secretory activity in many species is not due to prolactin (35). In women, prolactin levels increase steadily throughout gestation (15, 48, 49), reaching an average of 200 to 300 ng/ml at term (Fig. 3.4). However, lactogenesis does not occur early in human gestation because of the inhibitory ef-

fects of estrogen and progesterone on prolactin receptors in mammary epithelial cells (50, 51).

Prolactin's effects on the mammary cell are mediated through specific hormone-binding receptors (12). The number of prolactin receptors in breast tissue remains relatively constant throughout pregnancy (52). Since prolactin increases the concentration of its own receptor, the prepartum surge of prolactin is probably important for the second stage of lactogenesis and the onset of milk secretion (35).

Prolactin levels fall rapidly in postpartum women who are not breast-feeding and usually decline to prepregnant levels within 4 to 6 weeks (15, 49). In women who breast-feed, basal prolactin levels remain significantly elevated for 1 to 2 weeks and exhibit further modest increases with suckling. Basal prolactin levels remain slightly elevated from 2 weeks to 3 months postpartum, with relatively dramatic increases of prolactin in response to breast-feeding (15, 53, 54) (Fig. 3.6). After the 3rd postpartum month, basal prolactin levels are usually normal, and only small increases occur with suckling (55–57). Basal prolactin levels are

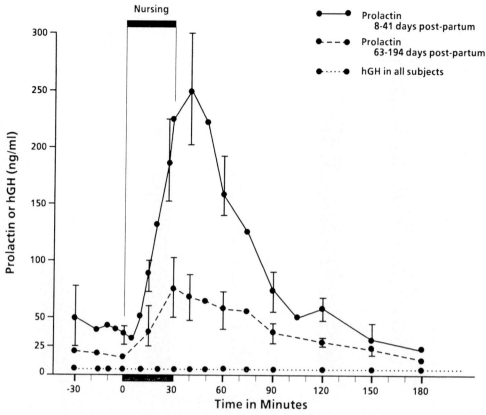

Figure 3.7. Plasma prolactin and growth hormone levels (mean±SEM) in response to suckling in the early (8 to 41 days) and late (63 to 194 days) postpartum periods. (Adapted from Noel GL, Suh HK, Frantz AG. Prolactin release during nursing and breast stimulation in postpartum and nonpostpartum subjects. J Clin Endocrinol Metab 1974;38:413–423.)

proportional to the frequency and duration of suckling, especially in long-term breast-feeding. Elevated baseline prolactin levels are reported up to 2 years postpartum in some cultures where breast milk is the infant's sole source of nutrition (58–60). Continued prolactin release in response to suckling is seen even in the late postpartum period (>60 days) if breast-feeding provides the majority of nutrition for the infant (54, 56, 57) (Fig. 3.7).

Prolactin is necessary for maintenance of lactation in several species, including humans. Extensive evidence attests to the importance of prolactin. Neutralization of prolactin by prolactin antisera (61) or prolactin-receptor antisera (50) results in decreased milk production in rats and mice. Administration of the dopamine agonist bromocriptine immediately postpartum lowers prolactin levels and prevents milk secretion in women and nonruminant animals (39, 50, 62). In ruminants, ergot alkaloids block the prepartum surge of prolactin and partially inhibit milk secretion; however, with continued milking, milk yields gradually return to normal despite very low serum prolactin concentrations

(35). Administration of bromocriptine to women at any time postpartum will decrease circulating prolactin levels and completely inhibit lactation (39, 63). Therefore, it appears that even late in the postpartum period, prolactin is necessary for continued lactation in women.

Growth Hormone

Growth hormone is galactopoietic in ruminants but not in humans (12). Injection of human growth hormone into women with lactational insufficiency increases milk yields, but this is probably due to the intrinsic prolactin activity of human growth hormone (64). Growth hormone does not increase in women in response to suckling (Fig. 3.7) (55), and successful lactation occurs in women with growth hormone deficiency (26, 55). Thus, growth hormone is not essential for lactogenesis in humans.

Placental Lactogen

Human placental lactogen rises continuously throughout pregnancy and appears to parallel the increases in placental mass (65).

Women have significant hourly fluctuations in plasma hPL levels, possibly due to changes in placental blood flow (66). However, the role of hPL and its secretory vagaries in human lactation are incompletely understood.

Placental lactogens appear in sera of many species coincident with early phases of lactogenesis and while prolactin levels are low (35). In humans, placental lactogen levels are 100-fold greater than prolactin throughout pregnancy (67) (Fig. 3.4). Because of its short half-life, hPL is rapidly removed from maternal circulation and is generally undetectable 24 hours after delivery (68). Thus, hPL concentrations are highest when the breast's lactogenic responsiveness is inhibited by high estrogen and progesterone levels.

Placental lactogens may suppress lactation by binding to prolactin receptors and blocking the effects of prolactin (69). However, prolactin receptors in ewes are specific for prolactin and have minimal binding affinity for placental lactogen (70). In humans, it is unclear whether placental lactogen has an inhibitory effect on lactogenesis during pregnancy. Furthermore, it is unclear whether removal of this potential inhibition with expulsion of the placenta is important in the second stage of lactogenesis.

Estrogens

There is no conclusive evidence that estrogens directly stimulate the mammary gland to secrete milk. However, estrogens do mediate the mammary gland response to lactogenic hormones (12). The effect of estrogen on the mammary gland in experimental studies is highly dependent on the dosage and the physiologic state of the animal. Estrogen administration to virgin animals causes a pituitary-dependent increase in mammary cell prolactin binding (12) and stimulates lobuloalveolar development of the mammary glands (2). Estrogen receptors are present in mammary tissue of lactating animals (12, 35) and in human mammary tumors (71), but the regulatory role of estrogen in the lactating mammary gland is obscure.

Estrogens are known to promote synthesis and release of prolactin (30, 72) and to stimulate prolactin receptors in breast tissue (70). Estrogens may also have a lactogenic effect through stimulation of prostaglandin $F_{2\alpha}$ release (73), as this substance is known to initiate lactogenesis in the rat (35-40).

Estrogens increase gradually throughout gestation and, in many species, a rapid increase in estrogen is coincident with the onset of lactogenesis in late gestation. In women, there is no prepartum estrogen surge, and estrogen levels decline rapidly postpartum (27). Estrogen administration postpartum inhibits lactogenesis, probably by interfering with prolactin binding (39, 50). Thus, estrogen is necessary for preparing the breast for milk production but must be removed postpartum for lactation to occur.

Progesterone

In 1905, Halban observed that milk secretion did not occur during pregnancy or in some women with placental retention after delivery. He suggested that the placenta secreted a substance that prevented lactogenesis (74). Observations in several animal species identified progesterone as the specific inhibitory factor (40) and correlated the prepartum fall in progesterone with lactose production and the onset of lactogenesis (35). Similarly, in humans, plasma progesterone falls after delivery of the placenta, and only then does lactogenesis begin (40).

Progesterone blocks the lactogenic effects of glucocorticoids (12, 40) and antagonizes the induction of prolactin receptors by prolactin (51). Progesterone binding to mammary tissue also prevents the prolactin-induced secretion of lactose, α-lactalbumin, and casein (75) and blocks induction of casein mRNA in vitro (46). Progesterone does not inhibit established lactation, probably because of the absence of progesterone receptors in mammary tissue of lactating animals (76).

Adrenal Glucocorticoids

Adrenal steroids, especially glucocorticoids, are essential for normal lactation. Adrenalectomy inhibits milk production in animals (12), and administration of glucocorticoids to pregnant or pseudopregnant rabbits and heifers induces precocious milk secretion (35). These animal studies suggest that glucocorticoids are a hormonal trigger for lactogenesis. However, the doses of glucocorticoids required to initiate lactation are pharmacologic, not physiologic (40). It appears that glucocorticoids act in synergy with prolactin to induce final differentiation of mammary epithelial cells (46, 77). Similarly, the high levels of glucocorticoids associated with parturition act in concert with prolactin to stimulate casein production and milk secretion (78).

Glucocorticoids (31) and mammary glucocorticoid receptors (35) are increased in late pregnancy and lactation. Progesterone binds to glucocorticoid receptors but does not translocate to the nucleus, thus acting as a glucocorticoid antagonist (76, 79). Presumably, progesterone withdrawal at parturition permits glucocorticoids to exert their lactogenic effects (12). Glucocorticoids increase with suckling in the rat and may play a role in the release of prolactin in response to suckling in women (80). The role of adrenal steroids in human lactation has not been extensively studied, and their importance is still unknown.

Prostaglandins

The mammary gland produces prostaglandins in large quantities. In spite of extensive in vivo and in vitro studies, the role of prostaglandins in primate lactogenesis is unclear (35). Increased estrogen levels at parturition stimulate the release of prostaglandins (73). Exogenous prostaglandin $F_{2\alpha}$ stimulates release of prolactin, growth hormone, and glucocorticoids and inhibits progesterone secretion in rodents (35). Lactation frequently follows therapeutic abortion in women treated with prostaglandin $F_{2\alpha}$ but does not occur in women undergoing dilation and extraction (81). These observations suggest that prostaglandins initiate lactation by increasing the secretion of hormones that play a direct role in lactogenesis. In contrast to the lactogenic effects of prostaglandin $F_{2\alpha}$, prostaglandin E_2 reduces prolactin levels and inhibits lactation in postpartum women (82). Clearly, the role of prostaglandins requires further study.

Thyroid Hormone and Parathyroid Hormone

Thyrotropin-releasing hormone (TRH) acts as a galactopoietic agent by stimulating secretion of prolactin, growth hormone, and thyroxine (12). Administration of TRH to fully lactating women has little effect on milk yields but may be beneficial in women experiencing lactational insufficiency (83). The increase in milk yield after TRH administration to cattle or women is not large, and it is unknown whether the effect of TRH is due to increases in prolactin, growth hormone, or thyroxine (35).

Thyroid hormone deficiency suppresses milk yields in ruminants, whereas exogenous thyroxine or triiodothyronine stimulates milk production in normal animals (35). Thyroid supplementation increases catabolic work and loss of body fat and protein and is therefore not a useful galactagogue (12). Although thyroid hormone appears necessary for complete breast development and lactational performance, it probably plays a permissive rather than a regulatory role.

Removal of parathyroids from lactating animals suppresses lactation (35). In cows, despite the large amounts of calcium secreted in milk, parathyroid gland activity is depressed during lactation.

Insulin and Serum Growth Factors

Insulin is requisite for lactogenic hormones to exert their effects in vitro (2) and is probably necessary for maintenance of normal lactation (12). Insulin may exert its effects at the mammary cell level or via the overall metabolism of the lactating animal. Insulin stimulates mammary epithelial cell metabolism and increases synthesis of lactose, fats, and casein (84). Human breast tissue has insulin receptors (2), but their regulatory role in human lactation remains to be defined.

Serum contains a number of factors that stimulate mammary epithelial cell replication. Epidermal growth factor, a potent mitogen originally isolated from the mouse submaxillary gland, is present in the serum of pregnant women (85). This factor causes proliferation of mouse mammary glands and mammary carcinomas in organ culture (86). Its role in lactogenesis is unknown.

THE MILK EJECTION REFLEX

Milk removal from the breast requires suckling by the infant and contraction of the myoepithelial cells surrounding the alveoli. The milk ejection reflex occurs when direct stimulation to sensory neurons in the areola results in release of oxytocin from the posterior pituitary. This causes contraction of myoepithelial cells, which forces milk into the ductal system. Impulses from the cerebral cortex, ears, and eyes may also elicit release of oxytocin through exteroceptive stimuli.

Afferent Neural Pathway

Impulses triggered by suckling travel along mammary afferent nerve fibers and enter the spinal cord via the dorsal roots. The nerves ascend, primarily uncrossed, and terminate in the paraventricular and supraoptic nuclei of the hypothalamus (12). Oxytocin is synthesized within specialized magnocellular neurons of both nuclei, along with its binding protein, neurophysin 1 (87).

Efferent Pathway

The paraventricular and supraoptic nuclei receive excitatory (cholinergic) and inhibitory (noradrenergic) neurons from other parts of the brain, allowing rapid control of oxytocin synthesis and release. Neurosecretory granules containing oxytocin and neurophysin 1 are transported along axons to terminals in the posterior lobe of the pituitary gland and stored until afferent impulses stimulate their release by exocytosis (87) (Fig. 3.8).

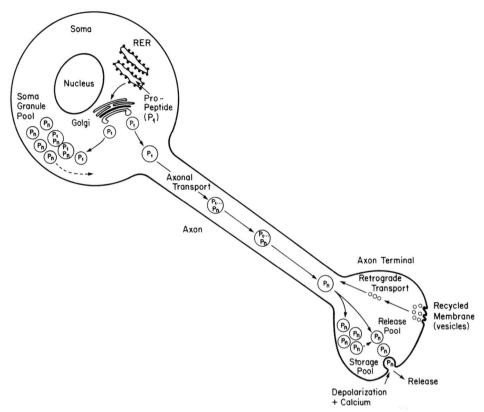

Figure 3.8. Oxytocin synthesis, processing, and release. Diagrammatic representation of a magnocellular neuron with its cell body, axon, and terminal. Translation of messenger RNA occurs on the rough endoplasmic reticulum (*RER*) in the neuronal soma, yielding a propeptide or precursor protein molecule (P_1) in the cisternal space of the endoplasmic reticulum. The packaging of P_1 into secretory granules occurs in the Golgi body. The secretory granule is the site of posttranslational processing to smaller peptide products ($P_1 \ldots P_n$), which can occur either in the cell body or in the axon during axonal transport. The peptide products (P_n) are stored in the granules in nerve endings in the posterior pituitary. (From Browstein MJ, Russell JT, Gainer H. Synthesis, transport and release of posterior pituitary hormones. Science 1980;207:373–378.)

Suckling stimulates the pulsatile release of oxytocin (53, 88, 89), without concurrent release of vasopressin (54). Oxytocin release in response to nursing is maintained throughout the late postpartum period in women (54, 56). Peak blood levels following nursing average 5 to 15 units/ml (90), and approximately 100 mU of oxytocin is released during a 10-minute nursing episode (89). Oxytocin has a half-life of only 1.5 to 2 minutes; therefore, it is important to commence nursing shortly after nipple stimulation.

Myoepithelial cells surrounding the alveoli are the effector cells for oxytocin (91). These cells are not innervated but contain specific, high-affinity binding sites for oxytocin (12). Local oxytocin induces myoepithelial cell contraction and forces milk into the mammary ducts. Myoepithelial cells also contract in response to direct mechanical stimulation (35).

MILK YIELDS AND RESPONSE TO SUCKLING

Prolactin Release

Prolactin levels increase markedly during nursing in women with normal lactation, although prolactin levels in response to suckling gradually diminish in the late postpartum period (54–57) (Fig. 3.6). The secretion of prolactin appears to be proportional to the amount of suckling in both humans and rats (41), and prolactin release may control the amount of milk secreted with suckling. A number of observations support this possibility. Inhibition of prolactin secretion with bromocriptine inhibits milk production (39), and low milk yields in postpartum women are associated with reduced prolactin secretion (92). Administration of metoclopramide (44), sulpiride (93), or TRH

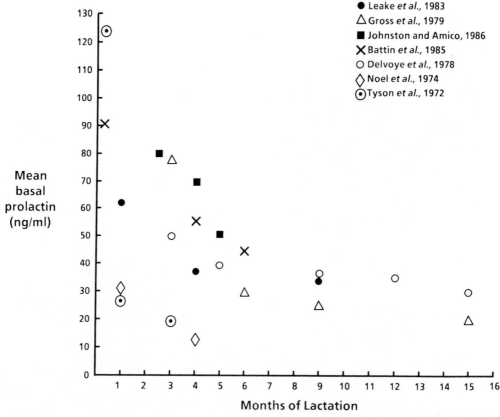

Figure 3.9. Mean prolactin values in breastfeeding women. (Data from refs. 15, 54–60.)

(83) to women with lactational insufficiency results in increased prolactin levels, accompanied by higher milk yields.

Plasma prolactin levels vary widely in lactating women however (Fig. 3.9), and basal levels do not always correlate with milk yield. Furthermore, in a careful study of prolactin release in response to nursing, Howie and colleagues were unable to correlate milk yields with peak prolactin levels (94). Normal lactation has been observed in women with low prolactin levels in the late puerperium (60) and in women subsequent to pituitary surgery (22) or bromocriptine therapy (95) for pituitary adenoma. Therefore, while basal levels of prolactin may be necessary to maintain the functional differentiation of the mammary epithelium, the actual amount of milk produced is probably regulated by other mechanisms, especially in the late puerperium.

Oxytocin Release

Whereas prolactin release in response to nursing is diminished in the late postpartum period (54), suckling induces an increase in oxytocin throughout the lactational period (53, 54). The milk ejection reflex, including release of oxytocin, is essential for transfer of milk from the breastfeeding mother to the infant (53).

Although oxytocin and prolactin are released in response to suckling, the patterns of release are clearly different (54, 55) (Fig. 3.10). Oxytocin is normally released before the start of suckling, as a conditioned response to tactile, auditory, or visual stimuli; prolactin release occurs only in response to direct stimulation of the nipple (53, 55). Although release of the two hormones appears to be independent (54), oxytocin does stimulate prolactin release in vitro (96). Oxytocin is present in hypophysial portal blood in high concentrations (97) and may play a physiologic role in the control of prolactin secretion, independent of a dopaminergic effect (98).

Other neuroendocrine mechanisms may control prolactin release. TRH stimulates release of TSH and prolactin (99), and administration of TRH antiserum attenuates prolactin release in response to suckling (100). TRH may not be a major physiologic prolactin-releasing factor, as release of TRH does not appear critical for the suckling-induced rise of prolactin (101). Hypothalamic opioids and glucocorticoids are involved in the prolactin response to

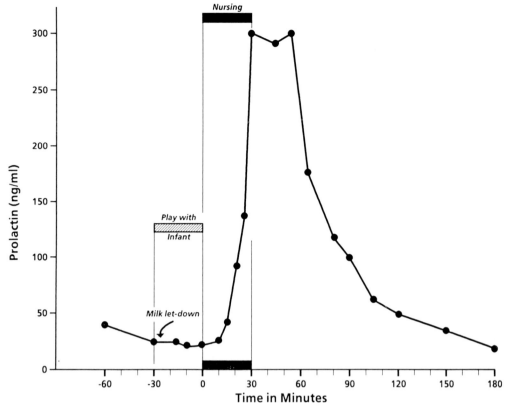

Figure 3.10. Plasma prolactin levels before, during, and after nursing, 22 to 26 days postpartum. Milk let-down occurs during play with infant, but prolactin does not rise until the actual onset of nursing. (Adapted from Noel GL, Suh HK, Frantz AG. Prolactin release during nursing and breast stimulation in postpartum and nonpostpartum subjects. J Clin Endocrinol Metab 1974;38:413–423.)

suckling in the rat (80), but the physiologic role for these pathways in humans is unclear (102).

DISORDERS OF LACTATION

Lactation Failure

Lactation failure most often results from inadequate suckling by the infant and/or feedings that are too infrequent or of too short duration to stimulate milk supply. Without regular emptying of both breasts, especially in the early postpartum period, there may be insufficient stimulation to generate adequate milk production. The introduction of supplemental food further jeopardizes the tenuous supply-demand control of milk yield, and milk production declines further. Proper education and support with appropriate intervention by health care personnel may prevent this decline in milk yields and ensure adequate lactation in the majority of motivated women.

Primary medical barriers to lactation are rare, but prompt identification is important to prevent malnutrition in the breast-fed infant

and guilt and disappointment among women with lactational insufficiency due to physiologic reasons.

Maternal Factors

Augmentation mammoplasty rarely interferes with successful lactation, although inadvertent operative nerve damage to the nipple-areola complex may affect the neurohumeral reflexes involved in normal lactation (103). Reduction mammoplasty often involves auto-transplantation of the nipple, which disrupts the innervation of the nipple and areola and severs the lactiferous ducts as they enter the nipple, thus preventing normal milk drainage.

Primary lactational insufficiency due to inadequate mammary glandular tissue has been reported (104). This diagnosis was made from a constellation of historical and physical features in several patients, albeit without histologic documentation. Prolactin levels were in the expected range during pregnancy and 5 to 10 days postpartum. Oxytocin nasal spray failed to improve milk yields, despite adequate frequency and duration of breast-feeding.

Complete absence of lactation, or agalactia, is rare and is usually associated with prolactin deficiency. Absence of lactation may be the first sign of Sheehan's syndrome, or acute postpartum pituitary necrosis (105). More recently, isolated prolactin deficiency has been identified as a cause for alactogenesis (44).

Infant Factors

The most common infant-related factor that adversely affects breast milk supply is inadequate suckling during the early puerperium. Prematurity, neonatal illness, birth defects, and neurologic disorders may all result in insufficient emptying of the breast with stasis and gland atrophy. Regular use of a breast pump to facilitate complete milk removal ensures an adequate milk supply and can be gradually discontinued as the infant becomes able to suck effectively. Infants with cleft palates may be fitted with a dental prosthesis to permit successful nursing.

Relactation

Relactation is the reinitiation of human lactation after a hiatus in postpartum milk production (106). Due to maternal or infant factors, the breast-feeding relationship may be interrupted or not established early in the puerperium. The result is inadequate milk supply. Attempts to improve lactational performance or, in the case of an adoptive mother, to stimulate lactation in a nonpuerperal setting have involved use of a variety of galactagogues. Pharmacologic agents, including phenothiazines (43, 106) and TRH (83), increase serum prolactin concentrations and are used to stimulate milk production. Metoclopramide (10 or 15 mg given three times daily) improves milk yields in women with inadequate lactation (107), although placebo is equally effective in women with normal lactation (108). Galactagogues must be critically evaluated prior to empiric therapy because most drugs enter breast milk.

Increasing the frequency of nursing is often sufficient to improve milk yields, and use of a regular suckling stimulus may initiate milk secretion, even in nulliparous women who adopt (5). Although supplementation with formula is often necessary for the adoptive mother, breast-feeding may be highly desirous for psychologic reasons and for women in underdeveloped countries where clean water and adequate supplements are unobtainable (106). When galactagogues are used, emphasis should be placed on increasing breast stimulation and on short-term drug therapy.

Suppression of Lactation

The simplest method of lactation suppression is avoidance of breast stimulation, thereby reducing the milk ejection reflex and decreasing the prolactin secretion necessary for continued milk production. Inhibition of the milk ejection reflex results in distension of alveoli, milk stasis, and eventual suppression of lactation. Mechanical compression of the breast may hasten these changes, but engorgement and significant pain commonly occur (109). Increasing or decreasing fluid intake and the use of diuretics have been advocated to suppress postpartum lactation. However, comparison of these treatments shows no differences in the rate of breast engorgement (109).

Pharmacologic attempts to suppress lactation began in the late 1930s with the use of estrogen compounds. A variety of estrogen and estrogen-androgen preparations have been used to suppress physiologic lactation (109). The best results are obtained when treatment is started prior to or shortly after delivery, as estrogen preparations cannot suppress milk secretion once lactation has commenced. Initial high doses of estrogens and gradual tapering are necessary to avoid delayed engorgement. Steroid contraceptives may reduce milk yields somewhat, especially if administered before lactation is fully established. Progestogen-only compounds have little effect on lactation (110).

The high doses of estrogens required for suppression of lactation increase the risk of venous thrombosis (111). Also, rebound engorgement occurs frequently after completing therapy. Estrogens have therefore been supplanted by other medications. Bromocriptine, a specific dopamine receptor agonist, suppresses prolactin secretion by a direct effect on the pituitary. When administered postpartum, bromocriptine lowers prolactin levels to normal within 24 to 48 hours, blocks initiation of lactation, and prevents breast engorgement and mastodynia (112). Administration of bromocriptine at any time in the postpartum period will suppress lactation with less rebound engorgement than estrogens (39). However, a 25% incidence of rebound engorgement is reported in women treated with bromocriptine for only 8 days (113). The most effective dosage schedule for suppression of lactation and prevention of rebound engorgement is 2.5 mg twice daily for the 1st 2 weeks postpartum, followed by 2.5 mg daily for a 3rd week (112). Side effects such as postural hypotension and gastrointestinal upset are infrequent in postpartum women, but the cost of a 2- to 3-week course of bromocriptine may be prohibitive.

Administration of prostaglandin E_2 in the early puerperium reduces plasma prolactin levels

Table 3.1. Pathologic Causes of Inappropriate Prolactin Secretion

- Structural hypothalamic lesions
    - Craniopharyngioma
    - Sarcoidosis
    - Irradiation
    - Head trauma
    - Metastatic or primary neoplasms
    - Surgical stalk section
- Functional hypothalamic-pituitary disorders
- Structural pituitary lesions
    - Prolactinomas
    - Empty-sella syndrome
    - Acromegaly
    - Cushing's disease
- Endocrine-metabolic
    - Hypothyroidism, primary
    - Addison's disease
    - Adrenal carcinoma or hyperplasia
    - Renal disease
    - Nelson's syndrome
    - Sheehan's syndrome
- Chest wall trauma or infection
- Other described causes
    - Hysterectomy/oophorectomy
    - Dilatation/curettage
    - Polycystic ovarian syndrome
    - Pseudotumor cerebri
    - Pseudocyesis
- Ectopic production
    - Bronchogenic carcinoma
    - Hypernephroma

Table 3.2. Pharmacologic Causes of Inappropriate Prolactin Secretion

- Estrogens/progestogens
- Dopamine receptor blockers
    - Phenothiazines
    - Haloperidol
    - Metoclopramide
    - Sulpiride
    - Domperidone
    - Methadone
- Dopamine reuptake inhibitors
    - Amphetamine
    - Tricyclic antidepressants
- Dopamine receptor stimulants
    - Apomorphine
- Dopamine-depleting agents
    - Reserpine
    - α-methyldopa
    - MAO inhibitors
- Histamine H_2-receptor antagonists
    - Cimetidine

(82) and suppresses lactation with less rebound engorgement than does bromocriptine (114). Prostaglandin E_2 is not effective in reducing prolactin levels in the late puerperium.

Galactorrhea

Galactorrhea is the secretion of milk under nonphysiologic circumstances. The amount of milk secreted varies greatly and may be either spontaneous or in response to manual expression. Galactorrhea may occur alone or in association with amenorrhea, ovulatory dysfunction, and infertility. The relationship between galactorrhea and reproductive dysfunction has been noted for centuries. Hippocrates observed that "if a women who is not with child nor has brought forth has milk, her menses are obstructed" (86). Several eponyms for galactorrhea syndromes are recognized (115–117).

Chiarri, in 1855, and Frommel, in 1882, described a syndrome consisting of persistent postpartum amenorrhea and lactation (115). Subsequently, Argonz and del Castillo noted estrogen insufficiency and decreased urinary estrogens in association with galactorrhea (116). Forbes, around 1951, noted low urinary follicle-stimulating hormone (FSH) in patients

with amenorrhea and galactorrhea (117). These were the first observations linking galactorrhea to pituitary dysfunction. The development of a radioimmunoassay (RIA) for prolactin and the identification of prolactin as an entity separate from growth hormone were critical to our understanding of these syndromes (48). Advances in hormone measurements by means of RIA, radiographic techniques, and transsphenoidal microsurgery have made classifications based on eponyms obsolete.

Nonpuerperal galactorrhea is associated with a variety of endocrine and nonendocrine disorders. Galactorrhea may be due to increased prolactin levels or altered responsiveness of the breast to normal hormone levels (118). When prolactin levels are elevated, the primary diagnostic problem is differentiating pituitary prolactin-secreting adenomas from "idiopathic" hyperprolactinemia, i.e., when a pituitary tumor cannot be identified. The problem is compounded by the wide variety of drugs and organic disorders associated with hyperprolactinemia (Tables 3.1 and 3.2).

ETIOLOGY OF GALACTORRHEA

Physiologic

As discussed earlier, the hyperprolactinemia of pregnancy rarely results in lactation until postpartum clearance of placental steroids from maternal serum. Persistent galactorrhea for more than a year after delivery or cessation of breast-feeding may indicate the presence of a slow-growing pituitary adenoma. Eventual resolution of galactorrhea usually occurs and, as with nonpostpartum patients, avoidance of breast stimulation and reassurance are adequate therapy if prolactin levels and menstrual cyclicity are normal. Several physiologic states other than pregnancy and nursing may result in galactorrhea. Prolactin levels increase during sleep, surgical or exercise-induced stress, and sexual intercourse (119). Breast stimulation, either manually or by a breast pump, also increases prolactin in a significant proportion of normally menstruating women who are not postpartum (55).

Pharmacologic

Numerous drugs increase prolactin secretion either by direct stimulation of the lactotroph or by altering endogenous dopamine activity. Oral contraceptives or postmenopausal E_2 replacement therapy increase plasma prolactin levels (30, 120) and result in proliferation of breast glandular elements. Galactorrhea during oral contraceptive therapy may be noted throughout the cycle or only at menses when hormone withdrawal results in secretion in the steroid- and prolactin-primed breast, a situation similar to that of postpartum milk secretion (120).

A variety of drugs inhibit the synthesis, metabolism, reuptake, or receptor binding of dopamine, thereby reducing dopamine availability and increasing prolactin secretion. Galactorrhea is a common side effect of phenothiazines, metoclopramide, reserpine, α-methyldopa, and other drugs (4, 119). The mechanism of action of these drugs appears in Table 3.2.

Pathologic

Hypothalamic

Infiltrative or degenerative lesions of the hypothalamus may result in hyperprolactinemia and galactorrhea due to a decrease in hypothalamic dopamine (118). Hypothalamic dysfunction may cause amenorrhea due to abnormalities in gonadotropin-releasing hormone secretion of FSH and LH pulsatile release. Functional hypothalamic disorders, such as anorexia nervosa, may cause similar symptoms (4).

Pituitary

Prolactin-secreting tumors (prolactinomas) are the most common endocrine tumors of the pituitary gland, accounting for 30% of all pituitary tumors (121). Patients with prolactinomas usually present with galactorrhea and/or menstrual abnormalities such as amenorrhea or anovulation. Subtle alterations of ovulatory function, such as luteal phase defects, may also occur (122, 123). Prolactin levels range from normal to well over 1000 ng/ml (121). In women, galactorrhea is usually present when prolactin levels reach 200 ng/ml but may occur at much lower levels. Galactor-

rhea rarely occurs in males even with very high prolactin levels (120). Although an association between the degree of hyperprolactinemia and the presence of a prolactinoma exists, tumors are found in patients with minimally elevated prolactin levels (124).

The diagnosis of idiopathic hyperprolactinemia was common in women with coexisting amenorrhea and galactorrhea prior to the advent of sensitive radiographic techniques for evaluating the sella turcica (4). Subsequent use of high-resolution computed tomography (CT) revealed occult pituitary tumors in many of these patients (124).

Hypothyroidism

Hyperprolactinemia, galactorrhea, and radiologic signs of pituitary enlargement may occur in association with primary hypothyroidism (125). The longer the duration of untreated hypothyroidism, the higher the prolactin levels and incidence of galactorrhea (126). Increased TRH secretion or an enhanced response of the lactotroph to TRH may lead to inappropriate prolactin secretion (127). Endocrine abnormalities, galactorrhea, and sellar abnormalities usually resolve with appropriate thyroid replacement therapy (128).

Although hypothyroidism is associated with galactorrhea, thyrotoxicosis rarely causes galactorrhea. When it does occur, prolactin levels may be normal. The pathophysiologic mechanism for galactorrhea in thyrotoxicosis is unknown, but an association appears to exist (129).

Adrenal Disorders

Amenorrhea and galactorrhea may occur in patients with adrenal insufficiency (Addison's disease), and symptoms resolve after treatment with glucocorticoids (130). Galactorrhea and elevated prolactin levels also occur in patients with Cushing's syndrome (131) and Cushing's disease (4). This is probably due to a direct effect of glucocorticoids on the breast, as corticotropin-releasing hormone does not stimulate prolactin secretion. The relationship between ACTH and prolactin is less clear, although occasional pituitary tumors secrete ACTH as well as prolactin.

Acromegaly

Galactorrhea is seen in approximately 20% of patients with acromegaly (132). In some patients with acromegaly the intrinsic lactogenic effect of growth hormone is responsible for galactorrhea (64), but about one-third of patients also have hyperprolactinemia (132). Histochemical study of pituitary tumors from patients with acromegaly reveals positive staining for prolactin in about 45% of cases (133).

Hyperprolactinemia may occur in the absence of prolactin staining, presumably due to pressure of the tumor on the pituitary stalk or hypothalamus and interference with dopaminergic inhibition of prolactin secretion.

Renal Failure

Hyperprolactinemia occurs in 20 to 37% of patients with renal disease and in nearly 80% of patients requiring hemodialysis (134). Reduced clearance of prolactin and increased pituitary prolactin secretion account for elevated prolactin levels in patients with renal failure.

Neurogenic

Chest wall and cervical spine lesions, mastectomy, and herpes zoster may result in hyperprolactinemia through stimulation of afferent neural pathways. Excessive stimulation of the nipple or areola may also result in hyperprolactinemia and galactorrhea in some women (55).

Ectopic Prolactin

Galactorrhea may be the first indication of an underlying carcinoma. Bronchogenic carcinomas and hypernephromas have been shown to secrete prolactin, and resolution of hyperprolactinemia occurs after therapy (135).

Idiopathic

A careful history, physical examination, and appropriate laboratory studies will reveal the etiology of galactorrhea in 50 to 70% of patients (86). However, approximately one-third will have no discernible cause for their galactorrhea, hence the classification of idiopathic. Long-term follow-up of patients with idiopathic hyperprolactinemia indicates either no change or a reduction in prolactin values in the majority of cases and a low incidence of tumor development (136).

Most patients with normal menstrual function and galactorrhea will have normal prolactin levels (4). The true prevalence of galactorrhea is unknown, because many women with mild galactorrhea do not seek a physician's care if there are no menstrual abnormalities. Furthermore, galactorrhea may be missed unless specifically looked for on physical examination.

Evaluation of Galactorrhea

The diagnostic approach to patients with galactorrhea is directed toward excluding both physiologic and pharmacologic causes of hyperprolactinemia. Physiologic considerations in hyperprolactinemia, including pregnancy, sleep, stress, exercise, and nipple stimulation, were mentioned previously. Serum prolactin should be measured in the fasting state and at least 2 hours after awakening to avoid the sleep-related increase in prolactin (119). A careful history will elicit use of pharmacologic agents that increase prolactin secretion. Drug-induced hyperprolactinemia is generally less than 100 ng/ml, and levels return to normal when the causative agent is discontinued.

Once physiologic and pharmacologic causes of galactorrhea and hyperprolactinemia are excluded, pathologic entities must be considered. Laboratory and radiologic studies are essential to identify the etiology. If prolactin levels are elevated, repeat serum prolactin values should be obtained under basal conditions to exclude laboratory error. A serum TSH measurement is essential to detect primary hypothyroidism. Treatment with thyroxine will lower TSH and prolactin values into the normal range. If prolactin remains elevated after 4 weeks of adequate thyroid hormone replacement, evaluation for a pituitary tumor should follow. Radiographs of the sella turcica are not indicated in the initial evaluation of patients with hypothyroidism, because pituitary enlargement will regress with appropriate replacement therapy.

Other endocrine studies of pituitary function are indicated, depending on clinical suspicion, and may include ACTH, growth hormone, and gonadotropin measurements. Ovulatory function should be evaluated in any patient with menstrual irregularity or infertility. Some studies have reported that dynamic stimulation tests of prolactin secretion will differentiate lactotroph hyperplasia from an occult prolactinoma (137). Despite intensive investigation, none of the stimulation tests are sensitive or specific enough for routine use. Basal serum prolactin levels are as useful as provocative tests.

A high-resolution CT scan of the sella turcica is recommended to detect a pituitary adenoma in patients with galactorrhea and elevated prolactin levels, regardless of associated menstrual abnormalities. Although serum prolactin levels are related to tumor size (121), there is a significant variability among patients, and normal or modestly elevated prolactin levels are found in patients with prolactinomas (124). Cone-down views and hypocycloidal tomography of the sella have been recommended to evaluate patients with modest hyperprolactinemia (138). However, small tumors may be missed, and variations in sellar architecture result in a high incidence of false-positive results, necessitating corroboration with CT scanning (121). CT scanning is more sensitive and specific than polytomography in the diagnosis of pituitary adenomas (139), and adequate baseline evaluation with CT scanning is necessary for patients with hyperprolactinemia, especially when they are contemplating pregnancy. Judicious use of sellar x-rays will prevent unnecessary irradiation to the optic chiasm. The role of nuclear magnetic imaging for prolactinomas is still being evaluated. Excellent anatomic visualization can be obtained in many cases without the side effects of radiation exposure (140). The sensitivity and specificity of the technique are still unknown (141), and the expense and relative unavailability of this procedure prevent its widespread use.

Treatment of Galactorrhea

Idiopathic

Patients with galactorrhea, in the absence of menstrual dysfunction or hyperprolactinemia, may be followed with reassurance and yearly prolactin determinations. If galactorrhea is severe or if fertility is the prime goal, reduction of prolactin with bromocriptine or other dopamine agonists is the treatment of choice.

Bromocriptine can induce ovulation in hyperprolactinemic anovulatory patients by reducing prolactin levels (142). Bromocriptine can also induce ovulation in some normoprolactinemic anovulatory patients, suggesting "latent" or intermittent hyperprolactinemia as the cause of anovulation (143). In one study, bromocriptine therapy also improved pregnancy rates in normoprolactinemic patients with unexplained infertility and galactorrhea (144). These patients may have subtle alterations of follicular development because of an increased sensitivity to endogenous prolactin, as suggested by the presence of breast secretions. In these cases, low-dose bromocriptine therapy (1.25 to 2.5 mg daily) may correct abnormalities in folliculogenesis and result in successful pregnancy.

Idiopathic hyperprolactinemia is defined as an elevated serum prolactin level in the absence of a demonstrable pituitary tumor, central nervous system disease, or other recognized causes of increased prolactin secretion (Table 3.2). A normal sella turcica CT scan excludes the presence of a microadenoma, although very small (<1 mm) adenomas may be missed. Long-term follow-up of patients with idopathic hyperprolactinemia has confirmed that eventual tumor development is unlikely (136, 145).

Pituitary Tumors

The goals of therapy for prolactin-secreting tumors include a reduction in tumor mass, preservation of normal pituitary function, restoration of fertility in anovulatory women, and elimination of troublesome lactation. Modes of therapy include irradiation, surgery, drug therapy, and close periodic observation.

Radiation therapy of prolactinomas usually consists of cobalt beam irradiation with a tumor dose of 4500 rads over a 4- to 5-week period. The eyes, optic chiasm, and hypothalamus may receive unwanted irradiahion, but this can be limited with careful technique. Limited data are available on the use of radiation therapy as primary treatment of pituitary tumors. Although radiotherapy was advocated prior to bromocriptine-induced pregnancy to prevent complications of tumor expansion (4), radiotherapy is rarely curative and may have other long-term risks such as hypopituitarism (146). Radiation therapy is not effective for prompt reduction of tumor size, and normalization of prolactin levels may take 5 years.

Prior to the availability of dopamine agonists and noninvasive methods of evaluating the sella turcica, surgery was often employed to diagnose and treat pituitary adenomas. Polytomography and CT scanning to diagnose prolactinomas and the use of bromocriptine to reverse tumor growth have replaced surgery for the treatment of pituitary adenomas in most patients.

Transsphenoidal surgery is the most widely used surgical approach for removal of prolactin-secreting tumors. When performed by an experienced neurosurgeon, tumors can be selectively removed with low morbidity (147). Complications include aseptic meningitis and the fairly common occurrence of diabetes insipidus, which usually resolves within 3 to 6 months (122).

Optimal results with surgical therapy are obtained with small pituitary tumors (microadenomas)—normalization of prolactin occurs in 50 to 100% of patients (147–149). The experience with macroadenomas is not as favorable—0 to 80% of patients have normal prolactin levels postoperatively (147–149). The preoperative prolactin level may predict the response to surgery, as therapeutic failures occur more often in patients with higher preoperative prolactin levels (122). In addition, the incidence of recurrent hyperprolactinemia in patients with microadenomas is 50% within 4 ± 1.3 years of surgery and 80% withing 2.5 ± 1.6 years of surgery in patients with macroadenomas (150). Finally, long-term follow-up of patients with untreated microprolactinomas has shown that only 10% have significant tumor growth, and spontaneous tumor regression may occur (148). Therefore, the risks of surgery do not appear to warrant early intervention.

Several dopamine agonists, including bromocriptine and pergolide, have proven useful in the treatment of hyperprolactinemia (112). Bromocriptine is used not only for treatment of idiopathic hyperprolactinemia and microadenomas but also for large macroprolactinomas and persistent postoperative hyperprolactinemia (151). Patients with large prolactinomas treated with bromocriptine therapy have significant reductions in prolactin levels. In one multicenter study, a reduction in tumor size of 50% or more was noted in 64% of cases (151). Tumor enlargement did not occur during medical therapy. Because of the excellent results with bromocriptine therapy in most patients with micro- and macroadenomas, and in view of the significant recurrence rate after surgery, bromocriptine should be used as primary therapy for all symptomatic pituitary adenomas. Neurosurgery and/or radiation therapy should be reserved for refractory cases or when tumor growth escapes medical suppression (112, 121, 151). The major hazard for asymptomatic patients who do not desire pregnancy is the risk of premature osteoporosis due to sustained hyperprolactinemia (152). The side effects of long-term dopaminergic agonist therapy must be balanced against the risks of long-standing hyperprolactinemia. Bromocriptine therapy must be considered suppressive, as hyperprolactinemia and tumor regrowth usually occur upon its discontinuation (112). No adverse effects have been reported with long-term therapy, but the occurrence of rare tumor growth during medical treatment emphasizes the need for close observation of these patients.

Long-term management of patients with prolactinomas includes a careful history, physical examination, and measurement of prolactin at least yearly. Periodic evaluation of sellar architecture by either polytomography or CT scanning is critical, as a rise in the prolactin level does not always antecede tumor growth (148). The frequency of testing must be individualized, depending on tumor size and previous therapy. For patients with an apparently stable microadenoma, yearly prolactin determinations and CT scans every 2 to 5 years are appropriate. Patients with macroadenomas require closer follow-up, with history, physical examination, and prolactin measurement every 6 months, and a yearly cone-down view of the sella. CT scans should be reserved for situations suggestive of tumor expansion (121). Patients treated with irradiation or surgery require long-term follow-up, because late complications or tumor regrowth may occur. For the patient on long-term medical suppression, a prolactin level should be obtained several weeks after discontinuing medication to identify the patient whose tumor has regressed following bromocriptine or radiation therapy. Tumor fibrosis has been noted after bromocriptine therapy (153) and may be responsible for remission of clinical symptoms and persistent normalization of prolactin levels seen after long-term therapy (154).

Treatment during Pregnancy

The outcome of pregnancy in hyperprolactinemic women is generally good, but controversy exists over optimal management. In women with idiopathic hyperprolactinemia, bromocriptine is the treatment of choice for restoring cyclic menses and fertility and is not associated with an increase in spontaneous abortions, congenital malformations, or premature births (155), even when administered throughout pregnancy (156). However, bromocriptine crosses the placenta and lowers fetal prolactin (157) and should be discontinued as soon as pregnancy is diagnosed.

For the woman with a microprolactinoma, there are three alternatives to restore fertility: bromocriptine alone, transsphenoidal surgery, or bromocriptine after radiation or surgery. Transsphenoidal surgery is successful in restoring regular menses and allowing conception in 50 to 60% of patients (122). As mentioned previously, radiotherapy prior to ovulation induction does not appear warranted, as the risk of tumor expansion without radiotherapy is low, and the long-term sequelae of radiation, e.g., panhypopituitarism, are significant (155). Conservative therapy is appropriate in patients with microadenomas because of the low incidence of symptomatic or asymptomatic tumor enlargement during pregnancy—1.6% and 4.5%, respectively (155). Despite the low incidence of complications, patients with microprolactinomas treated only with bromocriptine should be monitored carefully during pregnancy. Prolactin levels are not helpful because they are not predictive of tumor expansion. Routine visual field testing is of little benefit but should be performed in patients who become symptomatic. CT scanning should be reserved for patients with symptoms of tumor expansion during pregnancy and is useful postpartum to monitor asymptomatic tumor growth. When neurologic or visual symptoms occur during pregnancy, further evaluation is indicated, but bromocriptine may be prescribed immediately at doses of 5 to 7.5 mg daily and usually results in a rapid disappearance of symptoms.

The management of the pregnant woman with a macroadenoma has become more conservative. Surgical excision or irradiation of the tumor before allowing pregnancy are not justified in light of recent experience. The risk of symptomatic tumor enlargement ranges from 15 to 35%. Although this risk is considerably attenuated in patients who receive radiation or surgery (155), reduction of tumor size with bromocriptine also confers considerable protection against tumor expansion during pregnancy (146). When symptoms of tumor expansion occur during pregnancy, bromocriptine administration usually results in rapid remission of symptoms.

Continuous administration of bromocriptine throughout pregnancy has been recommended to prevent complications of tumor expansion (156). Symptomatic tumor expansion, however, is rare after adequate bromocriptine therapy. During treatment, the prolactinoma shrinks away from the walls of the pituitary fossa (146), thus allowing room for the pituitary expansion that occurs normally during pregnancy. Nevertheless, patients with macroadenomas require close observation during pregnancy. Routine assessment of visual fields or prolactin levels is of little benefit because tumor expansion can occur rapidly and may be missed with routine testing. In the event of headache or impaired vision, bromocriptine therapy will result in rapid improvement of symptoms. CT scanning either during pregnancy or postpartum will identify the effect of pregnancy on the prolactinoma: tumor enlargement, no change in tumor size, or tumor regression, possibly due to autoinfarction induced by pregnancy (158).

Breast-feeding may be encouraged and does not appear to increase the risk of tumor enlargement. Agalactia has been reported in some patients with surgically or radiation-treated prolactinomas, but lactation is usually normal and may occur even in patients treated with bromocriptine during the puerperium (95). In nonnursing mothers, inhibition of lactation is indicated. Bromocriptine in doses of 5 to 10 mg daily for 14 days followed by gradual tapering is generally adequate.

One month after delivery, all patients with adenomas should be evaluated with neurologic, ophthalmologic, and radiologic testing. Serum prolactin levels should also be obtained in nonnursing mothers. Long-term follow-up is the same as for nonpregnant patients. Resumption of ovarian function after delivery is common, especially in patients with idiopathic hyperprolactinemia or those on bromocriptine therapy (156), and appropriate contraception is indicated. The use of oral contraceptives is contraindicated because of the known stimulatory effects of estrogen on the pituitary; nonhormonal contraceptive methods are advised. Patients must understand the chronic nature of their disease and the importance of extended follow-up. In young women with hyperprolactinemia and amenorrhea, long-term bromocriptine therapy or estrogen replacement may be necessary to reduce the risk of osteoporosis.

REFERENCES

1. Lyons WR, Li CH, Johnson RE. The hormonal control of mammary growth and lactation. Recent Prog Horm Res 1958;14:219–250.
2. Topper YJ, Freeman CS. Multiple hormone interactions in the developmental biology of the mammary gland. Physiol Rev. 1980;60:1049–1106.
3. Hendrickson DA, Anderson WR. Diethylstilbestrol therapy. Gynecomastia. JAMA 1970;213:468.
4. Kleinberg DL, Noel GL, Frantz AG. Galactorrhea: A study of 235 cases, including 48 with pituitary tumors. N Engl J Med 1977;296:589–600.
5. Newton M. Breast-feeding by adoptive mother. JAMA 1970;212:1967.
6. Patten BM. Human embryology, 3rd ed. New York: McGraw-Hill, 1968:195–205.
7. Moore KL. The developing human. 2nd ed. Philadelphia: Saunders, 1977:376–386.
8. Salazar H, Tobon H. Morphologic changes of the mammary gland during development, pregnancy and lactation. In: Josimovich JB, Reynolds M, Cobo E, eds. Lactogenic hormones, fetal nutrition, and lactation. New York: Wiley, 1974:221–227.
9. Friesen HG. Human prolactin in clinical endocrinology: the impact of radioimmunoassays. Metabolism 1973;22:1039–1045.
10. Madlon-Kay DJ. Galactorrhea in the newborn. Am J Dis Child 1986;140:252–253.
11. Tho PT, McDonough PG. Gonadal dysgenesis and its variants. Pediatr Clin North Am 1981;28(2):309–329.
12. Cowie AT, Forsyth IA, Hart IC. Hormonal control of lactation. In: Monographs on endocrinology, vol 15. New York: Springer-Verlag, 1980.
13. Gould SF. Anatomy of the breast. In: Neville MC, Neifert MR, eds. Lactation: physiology, nutrition, and breast feeding. New York: Plenum Press, 1983:23–47.
14. Anderson RR. Endocrinological control. In: Larsen BL, Smith VR, eds. Lactation: a comprehensive treatise, vol 1. New York: Academic Press, 1974:3–40.
15. Tyson JE, Hwang P, Guyda H, Friesen HG. Studies of prolactin secretion in human pregnancy. Am J Obstet Gynecol 1972;113:14–20.
16. Kletzky OA, Rossman F, Bertolli SI, Platt LD, Mishell DR Jr. Dynamics of human chorionic gonadotropin, prolactin, and growth hormone in serum and amniotic fluid throughout normal human pregnancy. Am J Obstet Gynecol 1985;151:878–884.
17. Grumbach MM, Kaplan SJ, Sciarra JJ, Burr IM. Chorionic growth-hormone prolactin (CGP): secretion, disposition, biologic activity in man, and postulated function as the "growth hormone" of the second half of pregnancy. Ann NY Acad Sci 1968;148:501–531.
18. Spellacy WN, Buhi WC. Pituitary growth hormone and placental lactogen levels measured in normal term pregnancy and at the early and late postpartum periods. Am J Obstet Gynecol 1969;105:888–896.
19. Braunstein GD, Rasor JL, Engvall E, Wade ME. Interrelationships of human chorionic gonadotropin, human placental lactogen, and pregnancy-specific β_1-glycoprotein throughout normal human gestation. Am J Obstet Gynecol 1980;138:1205–1213.
20. Talwalker PK, Meites J. Mammary lobulo-alveolar growth induced by anterior pituitary hormones in adreno-ovariectomized-hypophy-

sectomized rats. Proc Soc Exp Biol Med 1961;107:880–883.

21. Topper YJ. Multiple hormone interactions in the development of mammary gland in vitro. Recent Prog Horm Res 1970;26:287–308.

22. Franks S, Kiwi R, Nabarro JDN. Pregnancy and lactation after pituitary surgery. Br Med J 1977;1:882.

23. Nielsen PV, Pedersen H, Kampmann E-M. Absence of human placental lactogen in an otherwise uneventful pregnancy. Am J Obstet Gynecol 1979;135:322–330.

24. Niall HD, Hogan ML, Sauer R, Rosenblum IY, Greenwood FC. Sequences of pituitary and placental lactogenic and growth hormones: evolution from a primordial peptide by gene reduplication. Proc Natl Acad Sci USA 1971;68:866–869.

25. Varma SK, Sonksen PH, Varma K, Soeldner JS, Selenkow HA, Emerson K Jr. Measurement of human growth hormone in pregnancy and correlation with human placental lactogen. J Clin Endocrinol Metabol 1971;32:328–332.

26. Rimoin DL, Holzman GB, Merimee TJ, et al. Lactation in the absence of human growth hormone. J Clin Endocrinol Metab 1968;28:1183–1188.

27. Tulchinsky D, Hobel CJ, Yeager E, Marshall JR. Plasma estrone, estradiol, estriol, progesterone, and 17-hydroxyprogesterone in human pregnancy. 1. Normal pregnancy. Am J Obstet Gynecol 1972;112:1095–1100.

28. Miller WL, Knight MM, Gorski J. Estrogen action in vitro: regulation of thyroid stimulating and other pituitary hormones in cell cultures. Endocrinology 1977;101:1455–1560.

29. Raymond V, Beaulieu M, Labrie F, Boissier J. Potent anti-dopaminergic activity of estradiol at the pituitary level on prolactin release. Science 1978;200:1173–1175.

30. Yen SSC, Ehara Y, Siler TM: Augmentation of prolactin secretion by estrogen in hypogonadal women. J Clin Invest 1974;53:652–655.

31. Vleugels MP, Eling WM, Rolland R, deGraaf R. Cortisol levels in human pregnancy in relation to parity and age. Am J Obstet Gynecol 1986;155:118–121.

32. Carr BR, Parker CR, Madden JD, MacDonald PC, Porter JC. Maternal plasma adrenocorticotropin and cortisol relationships throughout human pregnancy. Am J Obstet Gynecol 1981;139:416–422.

33. Rosenthal HE, Slaunwhite WR Jr, Sandberg AA. Transcortin: a corticosteroid-binding protein of plasma. X. Cortisol and progesterone interplay and unbound levels of these steroids in pregnancy. J Clin Endocrinol Metab 1969;29:352–357.

34. Vorherr H. Human lactation and breastfeeding. In: Larsen BL, ed. Lactation: a comprehensive treatise, vol 4. New York: Academic Press, 1978:181–280.

35. Tucker HA. Endocrinology of lactation. Semin Perinatol 1979;3:199–223.

36. Brodbeck U, Denton WL, Tanahashi N, Ebner KE. The isolation and identification of the B protein of lactose synthetase as α-lactalbumin. J Biol Chem 1967;242:1391–1397.

37. Martin RH, Glass MR, Chapman C, Wilson GD, Woods KL. Human α-lactalbumin and hormonal factors in pregnancy and lactation. Clin Endocrinol 1980;13:223–230.

38. Rigg LA, Yen SSC. Multiphasic prolactin secretion during parturition in human subjects. Am J Obstet Gynecol 1977;128:215–218.

39. Brun del Re R, del Pozo E, deGrandi P, Friesen H, Hinselmann M, Wyss H. Prolactin inhibition and suppression of puerperal lactation by a Br-ergocryptine (CB 154). A comparison with estrogen. Obstet Gynecol 1973;41:884–890.

40. Kuhn NJ. Lactogenesis: the search for trigger mechanisms in different species. Symp Zool Soc London 1977;41:165–192.

41. Neville MC, Berga SE. Cellular and molecular aspects of hormonal control. In: Neville MC, Neifert MR, eds. Lactation: physiology, nutrition, and breast feeding. New York: Plenum Press, 1983:141-177.

42. Kaplan NM. Successful pregnancy following hypophysectomy during the 12th week of gestation. J Clin Endocrinol Metab 1961;21:1139–1145.

43. Turkington RW. Phenothiazine stimulation test for prolactin reserve: the syndrome of isolated prolactin deficiency. J Clin Endocrinol Metab 1972;34:247–249.

44. Kauppila A, Chatelain P, Kirkinen P, Kivinen S, Ruokonen A. Isolated prolactin deficiency in a woman with puerperal alactogenesis. J Clin Endocrinol Metab 1987;64:309–312.

45. Lyons WR. Hormonal synergism in mammary growth. Proc Roy Soc Lond (Biol) 1958;149:303–325.

46. Rosen JM, Matusik RJ, Richards DA, Gupta P, Rodgers JR. Multihormonal regulation of casein gene expression at the transcriptional and posttranscriptional levels in the mammary gland. Recent Prog Horm Res 1980;36:157–193.

47. Shiu RPC, Friesen HG. Mechanism of action of prolactin in the control of mammary gland function. Annu Rev Physiol 1980;42:83–96.

48. Hwang P, Guyda H, Friesen H. A radioimmunoassay for human prolactin. Proc Natl Acad Sci USA 1971;68:1902–1906.

49. Jaffe RB, Yuen BH, Keye WR Jr, Midgley AR Jr. Physiologic and pathologic profiles of circulating human prolactin. Am J Obstet Gynecol 1973;117:757–773.

50. Bohnet HG, Gomez F, Friesen HG. Prolactin and estrogen binding sites in the mammary gland of the lactating and non-lactating rat. Endocrinology 1977;101:1111–1121.

51. Djiane J, Durand P. Prolactin-progesterone antagonism in self regulation of prolactin receptors in the mammary gland. Nature 1977;266:641–643.

52. Djiane J, Durand P, Kelly PA. Evaluation of prolactin receptors in rabbit mammary gland during pregnancy and lactation. Endocrinology 1977;100:1348–1356.

53. McNeilly AS, Robinson ICAF, Houston MJ, Howie PW. Release of oxytocin and prolactin in response to suckling. Br Med J 1983;286:257–259.

54. Johnston JM, Amico JA. A prospective longitudinal study of the release of oxytocin and prolactin in response to infant suckling in long-term lactation. J Clin Endocrinol Metab 1986;62:653–657.

55. Noel GL, Suh HK, Frantz AG. Prolactin release during nursing and breast stimulation in post-

partum and nonpostpartum subjects. J Clin Endocrinol Metab 1974;38:413–423.

56. Leake RD, Waters CB, Rubin RT, Buster JE, Fisher DA. Oxytocin and prolactin responses in long-term breast-feeding. Obstet Gynecol 1983;62:565–568.

57. Battin DA, Marrs RP, Fleiss PM, Mishell DR Jr. Effect of suckling on serum prolactin, luteinizing hormone, follicle-stimulating hormone, and estradiol during prolonged lactation. Obstet Gynecol 1985;65:785–788.

58. Rolland R, Lequin R, Schellekens LA, DeJong FH. The role of prolactin in the restoration of ovarian function during the early post-partum period in the human female. I. A study during physiological lactation. Clin Endocrinol 1975;4:15–25.

59. Delvoye P, Demaegd M, Uwayitu-Nyampeta, Robyn C. Serum prolactin, gonadotropins, and estradiol in menstruating and amenorrheic mothers during two years' lactation. Am J Obstet Gynecol 1978;130:635–639.

60. Gross BA, Eastman CJ. Prolactin secretion during prolonged lactational amenorrhea. Aust NZ J Obstet Gynaecol 1979;19:95–99.

61. Shani J, Goldhaber G, Sulman FG. Effect of antiserum to rat prolactin on milk yield and food intake in the rat. J Reprod Fertil 1975;43:571–573.

62. Taylor JC, Peaker M. The effects of bromocriptine on milk secretion in the rabbit. J Endocrinol 1975;67:313-314.

63. Benedek-Jaszmann LJ, Sternthal V. Late suppression of lactation with bromocriptine. Practitioner 1976;216:450–454.

64. Lyons WR, Li CH, Ahmad N, Rice-Wray E. Mammotrophic effects of human hypophysial growth hormone preparations in animals and man. Excerpta Med Int Congr Ser 1968;158:349–363.

65. Sciarra JJ, Sherwood LM, Varma AA, Lundberg WB. Human placental lactogen (HPL) and placental weight. Am J Obstet Gynecol 1968;101:413–416.

66. Vigneri R, Squatrito S, Pezzino V, Cinquerui E, Proto S, Montoneri C. Spontaneous fluctuations of human placental lactogen during normal pregnancy. J Clin Endocrinol Metab 1975;40:506-509.

67. Josimovich JB, Archer DF. The role of lactogenic hormones in the pregnant woman and the fetus. Am J Obstet Gynecol 1977;129:777–780.

68. Kaplan SL, Gurpide E, Sciarra JJ, Grumbach MM. Metabolic clearance rate and production rate of chorionic growth hormone-prolactin in late pregnancy. J Clin Endocrinol Metab 1968;28:1450–1460.

69. Tulchinsky D. The postpartum period. In: Maternal-fetal endocrinology. Philadelphia: Saunders, 1980:144–166.

70. Emane MN, DeLouis C, Kelly PA, Djiane J. Evolution of prolactin and placental lactogen receptors in ewes during pregnancy and lactation. Endocrinology 1986;118:695–700.

71. McGuire WL, Horwitz KB, Pearson OH, Segaloff A. Current status of estrogen and progesterone receptors in breast cancer. Cancer 1977;39:2934–2947.

72. Bohnet HG, McNeilly AS. Prolactin: assessment of its role in the human female. Horm Metab Res 1979;11:533–546.

73. Nathanielsz PW. Endocrine mechanisms of parturition. Annu Rev Physiol 1978;40:411–445.

74. Halban J. Die innere Secretion von Ovarium und Placenta und ihre Bedeutung für die Function der Milchdruse. Arch Gynaekol 1905;75:353–441.

75. Kuhn NJ. Progesterone withdrawal as the lactogenic trigger in the rat. J Endocrinol 1969;44:39–54.

76. Shyamala G, McBlain WA. Distinction between progestin- and glucocorticoid-binding sites in mammary glands. Biochem J 1979;178:345–352.

77. Davis JW, Liu TMY. The adrenal gland and lactogenesis. Endocrinology 1969;85:155–160.

78. Ganguly R, Ganguly N, Mehta NM, Banerjee MR. Absolute requirement of glucocorticoid for expression of the casein gene in the presence of prolactin. Proc Natl Acad Sci USA 1980;77:6003–6006.

79. Ganguly R, Majumder PK, Ganguly N, Banerjee MR. The mechanism of progesterone-glucocorticoid interaction in regulation of casein gene expression. J Biol Chem 1982;257:2182–2187.

80. Riskind PN, Millard WJ, Martin JB. Opiate modulation of the anterior pituitary hormone response during suckling in the rat. Endocrinology 1984;114:1232–1237.

81. Smith ID, Shearman RP, Korda AR. Lactation following therapeutic abortion with prostaglandin $F_{2\alpha}$. Nature 1972;240:411–412.

82. Camaniti F, DeMurtas M, Parodo G, Lecca U, Nasi A. Decrease in human plasma prolactin levels by oral prostaglandin E_2 in early puerperium. J Endocrinol 1980;87:333–337.

83. Tyson JE, Perez A, Zanartu J. Human lactational response to oral thyrotropin releasing hormone. J Clin Endocrinol Metab 1976;43:760-768.

84. Baldwin RL, Louis S. Hormonal actions on mammary metabolism. J Dairy Sci 1975;58:1033–1041.

85. Ances IG. Serum concentrations of epidermal growth factor in human pregnancy. Am J Obstet Gynecol 1973;115:357–362.

86. Aragona C, Friesen HG: Lactation and galactorrhea. In: De Groot LJ, Cashill GF Jr, Martini L, Nelson DH, Odell WD, Potts JT, eds. Endocrinology, vol III. New York: Grune & Stratton, 1979:1613–1627.

87. Brownstein MJ, Russell JT, Gainer H. Synthesis, transport and release of posterior pituitary hormones. Science 1980;207:373–378.

88. Weitzman RE, Leake RD, Rubin RT, Fisher DA. The effect of nursing on neurohypophyseal hormone and prolactin secretion in human subjects. J Clin Endocrinol Metab 1980;51:836–839.

89. Cobo E. Neuroendocrine control of milk ejection in women. In: Josimovich JB, Reynolds M, Cobo E, eds. Lactogenic hormones, fetal nutrition, and lactation. New York: Wiley, 1974:433–452.

90. Vorherr H. Hormonal and biochemical changes of pituitary and breast during pregnancy. Semin Perinatol 1979;3:193–198.

91. Richardson KC. Contractile tissues in the mammary gland, with special reference to myoepithelium in the goat. Proc Roy Soc Lond (Biol) 1949;136:30–45.

92. Aono T, Shioji T, Shoda T, Kurachi K. The initiation of human lactation and prolactin response to suckling. J Clin Endocrinol Metab 1977;44:1101–1106.
93. Aono T, Aki T, Koike K, Kurachi K. Effect of sulpiride on poor puerperal lactation. Am J Obstet Gynecol 1982;143:927–932.
94. Howie PW, McNeilly AS, McArdle T, Smart L, Houston M. The relationship between suckling-induced prolactin response and lactogenesis. J Clin Endocrinol Metab 1980;50:670–673.
95. Canales ES, Garcia IC, Ruiz JE, Zarate A. Bromocriptine as a prophylactic therapy in prolactinoma during pregnancy. Fertil Steril 1981;36:524–526.
96. Lumpkin, MD, Samson WK, McCann SM. Hypothalamic and pituitary sites of action of oxytocin to alter prolactin secretion in the rat. Endocrinology 1983;112:1711–1717.
97. Gibbs DM. High concentrations of oxytocin in hyphophysial portal plasma. Endocrinology 1984;114:1216–1217.
98. Samson WK, Lumpkin MD, McCann SM. Evidence for a physiological role for oxytocin in the control of prolactin secretion. Endocrinology 1986;119:554–560.
99. Noel GL, Dimond RC, Wartofsky L, Earll JM, Frantz AG. Studies of prolactin and TSH secretion by continuous infusion of small amounts of thyrotropin-releasing hormone (TRH). J Clin Endocrinol Metab 1974;39:6-17.
100. deGreef WJ, Voogt JL, Visser TJ, Lamberts SWJ, van der Schoot P. Control of prolactin release induced by suckling. Endocrinology 1987;121:316–322.
101. Riskind PN, Millard WJ, Martin JB. Evidence that thyrotropin-releasing hormone is not a major prolactin-releasing factor during suckling in the rat. Endocrinology 1984;115:312–316.
102. Cholst IN, Wardlaw SL, Newman CB, Frantz AG. Prolactin response to breast stimulation in lactating women is not mediated by endogenous opioids. Am J Obstet Gynecol 1984;150:558–561.
103. Farina MA, Newby BG, Alani HM. Innervation of the nipple areola complex. Plast Reconstr Surg 1980;66:497–501.
104. Neifert MR, Seacat JM, Jobe WE. Lactation failure due to insufficient glandular development of the breast. Pediatrics 1985;76:823–828.
105. Sheehan HL. Simmond's disease due to postpartum necrosis of the anterior pituitary. Q J Med 1939;8:277–309.
106. Brown RE. Relactation: an overview. Pediatrics 1977;60:116–120.
107. Kauppila A, Kivinen S, Ylikorkala O. A dose response relation between improved lactation and metoclopramide. Lancet 1981;1:1175–1177.
108. Lewis PJ, Devenish C, Kahn C. Controlled trial of metoclopramide in the initiation of breast feeding. Br J Clin Pharmacol 1980;9:217–219.
109. Kouchenour NK. Lactation suppression. Clin Obstet Gynecol 1980;23:1045–1059.
110. Croxatto HB, Díaz S, Peralta O, et al. Fertility regulation in nursing women. II. Comparative performance of progesterone implants versus placebo and copper T. Am J Obstet Gynecol 1982;144:201–208.
111. Jeffcoate TNA, Miller J, Roos RF, et al. Puerperal thromboembolism in relation to the inhibition of lactation by oestrogen therapy. Br Med J 1968;4:19–25.
112. Vance ML, Evans WS, Thorner MO. Diagnosis and treatment. Drugs five years later. Bromocriptine. Ann Intern Med 1984;100:78–91.
113. Varga L, Lutterbeck PM, Pryor JS, Wenner R, Erb H. Suppression of puerperal lactation with an ergot alkaloid: a double blind study. Br Med J 1972;2:743–744.
114. England MJ, Tjallinks A, Hofmeyr J, Harber J. Suppression of lactation. A comparison of bromocriptine and prostaglandin E₂. J Reprod Med 1988;33:630–632.
115. Sharp EA. Historical review of a syndrome embracing utero-ovarian atrophy with persistent lactation (Frommel's disease). Am J Obstet Gynecol 1935;30:411–414.
116. Argonz J, del Castillo EB. A syndrome characterized by estrogenic insufficiency, galactorrhea and decreased urinary gonadotropin. J Clin Endocrinol Metab 1953;13:79–87.
117. Forbes AP, Hennemen PH, Griswold GC, Albright FA. A syndrome, distinct from acromegaly, characterized by spontaneous lactation, amenorrhea, and low follicle-stimulating hormone excretion. J Clin Endocrinol 1951;11:749.
118. Archer DF. Current concepts of prolactin physiology in normal and abnormal conditions. Fertil Steril 1977;28:125–134.
119. Frantz AG. Prolactin. N Engl J Med 1978;298:201–207.
120. Frantz AG. Prolactin secretion in physiologic and pathologic human conditions measured by bioassay and radioimmunoassay. In: Josimovich JB, Reynolds M, Cobo E, eds. Lactogenic hormones, fetal nutrition, and lactation. New York: Wiley, 1974:379–412.
121. Blackwell RE. Diagnosis and management of prolactinomas. Fertil Steril 1985;43:5–16.
122. Schlechte J, Sherman B, Halmi N, et al. Prolactin-secreting pituitary tumors in amenorrheic women: a comprehensive study. Endocr Rev 1980;1:295–308.
123. Keye WR, Chang RJ, Wilson CB, Jaffe RB. Prolactin-secreting pituitary adenomas. III. Frequency and diagnosis in amenorrhea-galactorrhea. JAMA 1980;244:1329–1332.
124. Brenner SH, Lessing JB, Quagliarello J, Weiss G. Hyperprolactinemia and associated pituitary prolactinomas. Obstet Gynecol 1985;65:661–664.
125. Groff TR, Shulkin BL, Utiger RD, Talbert LM. Amenorrhea-galactorrhea, hyperprolactinemia, and supraseller pituitary enlargement as presenting features of primary hypothyroidism. Obstet Gynecol 1984;63:86S–89S.
126. Contreras P, Generini G, Michelsen H, Pumarino H, Campino C. Hyperprolactinemia and galactorrhea: spontaneous versus iatrogenic hypothyroidism. J Clin Endocrinol Metab 1981;53:1036–1039.
127. Onishi T, Miyai K, Anono T, et al. Primary hypothyroidism and galactorrhea. Am J Med 1977;63:373–377.
128. Tolis G, Hoyte K, McKenzie JM, Mason B, Robb P. Clinical, biochemical, and radiologic reversibility of hyperprolactinemic galactorrhea-

amenorrhea and abnormal sella by thyroxine in a patient with primary hypothyroidism. Am J Obstet Gynecol 1978;131:850–852.

129. Kapcala LP. Galactorrhea and thyrotoxicosis. Arch Intern Med 1984;144:2349–2350.

130. Kelver ME, Nagamani M. Hyperprolactinemia in primary adrenocortical insufficiency. 1985;44:423–425.

131. Mahesh VB, Dalla Pria S, Greenblatt RB: Abnormal lactation with Cushing's syndrome, a case report. J Clin Endocrinol Metab 1969;29:978–981.

132. Nabarro JDN. Acromegaly. Clin Endocrinol 1987;26:481–511.

133. Kanie N, Kageyama N, Kuwayama A, Nakane T, Watanabe M, Kawaoi A. Pituitary adenomas in acromegalic patients: an immunohistochemical and endocrinological study with special reference to prolactin-secreting adenoma. J Clin Endocrinol Metab 1983;57:1093–1101.

134. Sievertsen GD, Lim VS, Nakawatase C, Frohman LA. Metabolic clearance and secretion rates of human prolactin in normal subjects and in patients with chronic renal failure. J Clin Endocrinol Metab 1980;50:846–852.

135. Turkington RW. Ectopic production of prolactin. N Engl J Med 1971;285:1455–1458.

136. Martin TL, Kim M, Malarkey WB. The natural history of idiopathic hyperprolactinemia. J Clin Endocrinol Metab 1985;60:855–858.

137. Marrs RP, Bertolli SJ, Kletzky OA. The use of thyrotropin-releasing hormone in distinguishing prolactin-secreting pituitary adenoma. Am J Obstet Gynecol 1980;138:620–625.

138. Speroff L, Glass RH, Kase NG. Clinical gynecologic endocrinology and infertility, 3rd ed. Baltimore: Williams & Wilkins, 1983:141–184.

139. Syvertsen A, Haughton VM, Williams AL, Cusick JF. The computed tomographic appearance of the normal pituitary gland and pituitary microadenomas. Radiology 1979;133:385–391.

140. Kaufman B. Magnetic resonance imaging of the pituitary gland. Radiol Clin North Am 1984;22:795–803.

141. Davis PC, Hoffman JC, Spencer T, Tindall GT, Braun IF. MR imaging of pituitary adenoma: CT, clinical, and surgical correlation. AJR 1987;148:797–802.

142. Lloyd SJ, Josimovich JB, Archer DF. Amenorrhea and galactorrhea: results of therapy with 2-bromo-α-ergo-cryptine (CB-154). Am J Obstet Gynecol 1975;122:85–89.

143. Suginami H, Hamada K, Yano K, Kuroda G, Matsuura S. Ovulation induction with bromocriptine in nomoprolactinemic anovulatory women. J. Clin Endocrinol Metab 1986;62:899–903.

144. Devane GW, Guzick DS. Bromocriptine therapy in normoprolactinemic women with unexplained infertility and galactorrhea. Fetil Steril 1986;46:1026–1031.

145. March CM, Kletzky OA, Davajan V, et al. Longitudinal evaluation of patients with untreated prolactin-secreting pituitary adenomas. Am J Obstet Gynecol 1981;139:835–844.

146. Tan SL, Jacobs HS. Management of prolactinomas — 1986. Br J Obstet Gynecol 1986;93:1025–1029.

147. Post K, Biller B, Adelman L, Molitch M, Wolper S, Reichlin S. Selective transsphenoidal adenomectomy in women with galactorrhea-amenorrhea. JAMA 1979;242:158.

148. Weiss MH, Teal J, Gott P, et al. Natural history of microprolactinomas: six year follow-up. Neurosurgery 1983;12:180–183.

149. Chang RJ, Keye WR Jr, Young YR, Wilson CB, Jaffe RB. Detection, evaluation, and treatment of pituitary microadenomas in patients with galactorrhea and amenorrhea. Am J Obstet Gynecol 1977;128:356–363.

150. Serri O, Rasio E, Beauregard H, Hardy J, Somma M. Recurrence of hyperprolactinemia after selective transsphenoidal adenomectomy in women with prolactinoma. N Engl J Med 1983;309:280–283.

151. Molitch ME, Elton RL, Blackwell RE, et al. Bromocriptine as primary therapy for prolactin secreting macroadenomas: results of a prospective multicenter study. J Clin Endocrinol Metab 1985;60:698–705.

152. Klibanski A, Neer RM, Beitins IZ, Ridgway EC, Zervas NT, McArthur JW. Decreased bone density in hyperprolactinemic women. N Engl J Med 1980;303:1511–1514.

153. Esiri MM, Bevan JS, Burke CW, Adams CBT. Effect of bromocriptine treatment on the fibrous tissue content of prolactin-secreting and nonfunctioning macroadenomas of the pituitary gland. J Clin Endocrinol Metab 1986;63:383–388.

154. Moriondo P, Travaglini P, Nissim M, Conti A, Faglia G. Bromocriptine treatment of microprolactinomas: evidence of stable prolactin decrease after drug withdrawal. J Clin Endocrinol Metab 1985;60:764–772.

155. Molitch ME. Pregnancy and the hyperprolactinemic woman. N Engl J Med 1985;312:1364–1370.

156. Ruiz-Velasco F, Tolis G. Pregnancy in hyperprolactinemic women. Fertil Steril 1984;41:793–805.

157. Bigazzi M, Ronga R, Lancranjan I, et al. A pregnancy in an acromegalic woman during bromocriptine treatment: effects on growth hormone and prolactin in the maternal, fetal and amniotic compartments. J Clin Endocrinol Metab 1979;48:9–12.

158. Daya S, Shewchuk AB, Bryceland N. The effect of multiparity on intrasellar prolactinomas. Am J Obstet Gynecol 1984;148:512–515.

4

Lactation and Its Disorders

Edward R. Newton

Although 60% of new mothers breast-feed their babies, this basic act of reproduction is largely ignored by the obstetric community. In the last 10 years, there have been less than 20 publications, including case reports, concerning lactation in the *American Journal of Obstetrics and Gynecology* and *Obstetrics and Gynecology*. Most training programs in obstetrics and gynecology do not give residents direct exposure to lactating women after postpartum discharge, and their knowledge comes through reading or a limited number of didactic lectures. Although pediatric literature and training address lactation, their focus is on the growth and development of the child, not the physiology and disorders of lactation. The practicing pediatrician may not feel comfortable performing breast examinations and observing feeding techniques.

One purpose of this chapter is to begin the educational process through which obstetricians will adopt the lactating mother as their patient. The chapter will discuss the limitations of breast-feeding research, epidemiology, benefits, and physiology, as well as the management of lactation. Specific problems will be discussed, including breast pain, mastitis, drugs in breast milk, and medical diseases in the mother or infant that affect the process.

LIMITATIONS OF BREAST-FEEDING RESEARCH

Unfortunately, there have been major flaws in the designs and conclusions of epidemiologic research concerning breast-feeding (1–3). For example, only 6 of 20 studies concerning breast-feeding and childhood infection published in the English language between 1970 and 1984 met minimal statistical standards (1).

Controls are necessary to demonstrate significant sociodemographic differences between mothers choosing to breast-feed and those who do not (Table 4.1), and operational definitions should be clear. An examination of frequency,

Table 4.1. Epidemiology of Breast-Feeding at 1 Week (United States 1985)[a]

Characteristics	% Breast-Feeding
Ethnicity	
Black	33
White	65
Maternal age	
<20 years old	37
≥20 years old	65
Maternal education	
≤12 years	51
>12 years	78
Family income	
<$7,000 yearly	39
≥$25,000 yearly	72

[a]Data from Martinez GA, Krieger FW. 1984 Milk-feeding patterns in the United States. Pediatrics 1985;76:1004–1008.

duration, and exclusivity of breast-feeding is required. In a study concerning the mode of infant feeding and infection rates in the first year of life, Agre (4) concluded that the mode of feeding had no bearing on the frequency of infection, but his definition required exclusive breast-feeding for only the first 3 months. If an infant was weaned at 4 to 5 months of age and started bottle-feeding, an episode of gastroenteritis at 10 months would be misclassified as related to breast-feeding.

Most of the data concerning the mode of infant feeding relies on self-report and recall, usually long after the behavior has occurred. This introduces biases, such as combining events into convenient ages or socially acceptable times of weaning.

An unavoidable bias in breast-feeding research is due to self-selection. Intrinsic personality characteristics of mothers may be determinants of feeding choice. Women most likely to choose to breast-feed their infants are more mature, in a higher socioeconomic class, and more educated than women who do not not.

45

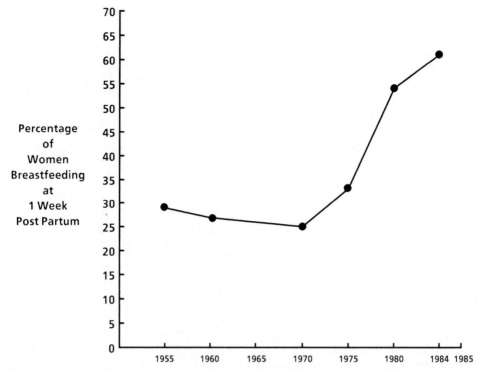

Figure 4.1. Incidence of at least partial breast-feeding at 7 days after birth, which has risen sharply since its nadir in 1970.

There is also evidence that women choosing to breast-feed exhibit more nurturant behavior (5–7). These intrinsic differences may explain some of the differences observed in the growth and development of breast-fed and bottle-fed infants.

EPIDEMIOLOGY OF BREAST-FEEDING

The incidence of at least partial breast-feeding at 7 days after birth has risen sharply since its nadir in 1970 (Fig. 4.1). Between 1970 and 1984, there has also been an increasing number (5.5% vs. 27.7%) of women still breast-feeding infants at 5 to 6 months of age (8). The reasons for the recent increase are largely speculative. A general increase in health consciousness and specific promotion of breast-feeding by the government and consumer groups may be factors.

Population data concerning the incidence of breast-feeding depend on marketing research by the formula companies, Ross Laboratories in particular. These studies are based on mailed questionnaires (8) that depend on the literacy, cooperation, understanding, and 6-month recall of the respondents. The large proportion of nonrespondents (34 to 46%) probably bias the data. Lower socioeconomic groups and non-English-speaking respondents are underrepresented. Statistical control for this bias was provided in the 1985 study by Martinez and Kreiger (8).

The decision to breastfeed is a composite of demographic, psychologic, and sociocultural-economic influences (9). Demographic factors are significant covariates in predicting the incidence (Table 4.1). A well-educated, upper income Anglo-American woman has a better than 70% chance of breast-feeding, but the incidence is as low as 21% among Mexican-Americans.

The psychologic makeup of the mother may affect the decision (6, 7, 9). Mothers who choose to breast-feed are more likely to perceive their marriages as having less conflict and their partners as more supportive (9). Mothers who have a positive reaction to the first sight of their baby are more likely to express a desire to breast-feed than those who have a neutral or negative reaction (10). In a review, Sauls concludes, "Breast feeding mothers reportedly have a more positive perception of themselves, may place more importance on affection, and are seen as more secure in their sexuality than bottle-feeding mothers" (2). They also exhibit more self-determination in their own health care (2), and are more likely to choose "natural" birth situations, with less anesthesia and less intervention. They are more conscious of nutrition and exercise, and less likely to smoke cigarettes, drink alcohol, or take illicit drugs.

Some of the sociocultural-economic factors affecting the incidence of breast-feeding include social networks, taboos, marketing of infant formula, cost of infant formula, and employment of the mother outside the home. The number of a mother's friends who breast-feed and her having been breast-fed herself may determine her choice. In developed countries, especially in the United States, the triple role of the female breasts, sexual, aesthetic, and nurturing, creates social paradoxes (see Chapter 5). On the one hand, there is a taboo against nursing or showing pictures of nursing babies in public, whereas advertisements are becoming more sexually explicit, and bottle-feeding in public and pictures of bottle-feeding babies are acceptable. Bottle-feeding mothers may be more susceptible to these social pressures. Jones and Beasley examined the attitudes of mothers who breast-fed or bottle-fed their infants and found that bottle-feeding mothers are more likely to disapprove of women breast-feeding in public (11).

Prenatal education by health care providers during pregnancy or in the early postpartum period might be expected to play a central role in the decision to breast-feed. However, for a majority of women, the decision is made outside of the provider-patient relationship. Forty to 60% of mothers report that it was made prior to conception, and less than 20%, after delivery. Only a minority, 2 to 38%, consult their obstetrician or pediatrician during the prenatal period concerning the choice. This low percentage may reflect either disinterest by the obstetrician or influences outside the provider-patient relationship. However, in urban, low-income families with a low prevalence of breast-feeding, prenatal promotion increases the incidence.

BENEFITS OF BREAST-FEEDING

Constructive counseling for the obstetric patient who is undecided about her method of infant feeding requires a clear understanding of the alternatives. The differences may be divided into four categories: nutritional, resistance to infection, psychologic, and prophylaxis against allergy.

Nutritional Differences

The differences in nutritional qualities between human milk and formulas are distinct. Most formulas are based on nonfat bovine milk. Supplementary fat, sugar, amino acids, vitamins, and minerals are added by the manufacturer. The fats are usually derived from plant sources, including coconut, soy bean, and/or corn oil. The addition of a constituent is based on the increased concentration of the nutrient in human milk, deficiency diseases noted in laboratory animals, and the taste or texture of the product. Table 4.2 depicts the major constituents of milk in several mammalian species as well as those of a representative bovine-milk-based formula. The respective neonatal growth rates of the respective mammals are shown. In general, the faster the doubling time of the birthweight, the richer the milk.

There are differences in the growth patterns of bottle-fed and breast-fed infants. The former have a higher weight-to-height ratio (5, 12), but overfeeding and early introduction of solids to the diet of bottle-fed babies may explain the increase. Breast-feeding seems to protect infants against adolescent obesity (13), but the literature contains many conflicting results concerning obesity and mode of feeding (5). Failure to define the duration and exclusivity of breast-feeding remains a major methodologic weakness in most studies.

The composition of lipids in human milk is different from that in infant formulas. The major lipids of human milk are oleic (40%), palmitic (23%), and linoleic (14%) (14). The average fat content of 240 pooled human milk samples varied between 2.1 and 3.3%. Average fat content changes little with additional dietary fat. The fatty acid composition of mature human milk is remarkably uniform unless the maternal diet is unusually bizarre. The ratio of unsaturated to saturated fats is 1.34. The level of cholesterol in human milk is 20 mg/dl and does not change with dietary manipulation. The major lipids of infant formula (average weight percent of regular formulas) are linoleic (39%), oleic (31%), and palmitic (11%) (15). The average fat content is constant at 5 to 6%. The fatty acid composition varies with the type of oil added to the bovine milk, and the ratio of unsaturated fats to saturated fats is about 2.8.

Casein, α-lactalbumin, β-lactoglobulin, immunoglobulins, and serum albumin are the major proteins of milk. Casein, or curd, is a group of milk-specific proteins characterized by ester-bond phosphate, high protein content, and low solubility at pHs of 4.0 to 5.0. Casein has a species-specific amino acid composition. The major difference between the

Table 4.2.   Growth Rates and Major Constituents of Milk in Various Mammals

Species	Days Required to Double Birthweight	Grams per 100 ml			
		Fat	Protein	Lactose	Ash
Human					
Milk	180	3.8	0.9	7.0	0.2
Formula	180	5.4	2.2	6.0	2.3
Cow	47	3.7	3.7	4.8	0.7
Sheep	10	7.4	5.5	4.8	1.0
Rat	6	15.0	12.0	3.0	2.0

proteins of bovine and human milk relate to sulfur-containing amino acids, cystine, methionine, and taurine, and the aromatic amino acids phenylalanine and tyrosine (15, 16). In human milk, the ratio of methionine to cystine is 1:1, which is unique for an animal protein. The methionine-cystine ratio for bovine milk is 2 to 3:1. The significance of the unusual methionine-cystine ratio in humans is unknown. Taurine is found in high concentrations in human milk while being virtually absent in bovine milk. Taurine is associated with bile acid conjugation and may play an important role in neural development and membrane stability (17). Recently, taurine has been added to formula. Human milk has one-half as much phenylalanine and tyrosine as bovine milk. The human newborn has low levels of the enzymes needed to metabolize them.

Whey proteins are contained in the supernatant after casein congeals to form curd. The ratio of whey proteins to casein is 1.5 for human milk and 0.2 for bovine milk. α-Lactalbumin and lactoferrin are the major constituents of whey proteins in human milk. α-Lactalbumin is a part of the enzyme lactose synthetase, and its high concentration parallels the increased concentration of lactose in human milk. Lactoferrin is an iron-binding protein that inhibits the growth of iron-dependent pathogenic bacteria in the gastrointestinal tract. β-lactoglobulin, the chief constituent of the whey proteins in bovine milk, is not measurable in human milk.

The predominant carbohydrate of human milk is lactose, a disaccharide compound of galactose and glucose. It is present in higher concentrations in human milk (7.0 g/dl) than in formula (5.0 to 7.0 g/dl). The total carbohydrate count (10.6 g/dl) is higher in formulas because of sugars, i.e., glucose, which have been added to the formula. In addition to being an important energy source, lactose enhances calcium absorption and provides the substrate galactose for the production of galactolipids, including cerebrosides, which are important compounds in neural development.

In general, there is an inverse relationship between the concentration of lactose and the total salt content of milk. This may relate to the growth rate and bony structure of a species. While all the minerals that appear in human milk are also present in bovine milk, human milk has one-third the total ash content of bovine milk. The osmolarity of human milk is similar to that of human serum (286 mosmol), whereas the osmolarity of bovine milk is 350 mosmol. The mean calcium concentration of human milk is 35 mg/100 ml, in bovine milk 130 mg/100 ml. The mean phosphorus concentration is also different; in human milk it is 15 mg/100 ml, in bovine milk 120 mg/ml. The increased total ash and protein content of formulas results in an excessive renal solute load; thus, the blood urea concentration of breastfed infants is about 22 mg/100 ml, for formula-fed infants 47 mg/100 ml.

Tables 4.3, 4.4, and 4.5 depict the vitamin and mineral content (per 100 ml) in various milk sources. In general, human milk contains smaller amounts of vitamins and minerals than bovine milk or formula. All of the vitamins are present in sufficient quantities to be associated with the good health and normal growth of the breast-fed infant in the first 4 to 6 months of life, but some pediatricians have recommended supplemental vitamin K for all newborns, even though vitamin K is synthesized by gut flora and absorbed by the infant. Bleeding from vitamin K deficiency is virtually unheard of among completely breast-fed infants. The changes in bowel flora associated with supplemental or total formula feeding may alter the production of vitamin K.

Each of the tables gives the published recommended daily allowance of vitamins and minerals (RDA) for infants 0 to 0.5 years old. These RDAs are higher than those a healthy neonate would receive in the normal volume of breast milk per day (500 to 1500 ml). RDAs are established by the Food and Nutrition Board, National Research Council, National Academy of Science, and are the standard used by formula companies to determine vitamin or mineral supplements. Caution is warranted in

Table 4.3. Comparison of Water-Soluble Vitamins in Various Milk Sources

	Vitamin Content per 100 ml			
	Mature Human Milk	Bovine Milk	Representative Formula	RDA (mg)[a]
Thiamine (μg)	14	43	58	0.3
Riboflavin (μg)	40	145	98	0.4
Niacin (μg)	160	82	735	6
B_6 (μg)	14	64	40	0.3
Pantothenic Acid (μg)	246	340	294	2
Biotin (μg)	0.6	2.8	2.2	35
Folic acid (μg)	0.14	0.13	10	30
B_{12} (μg)	0.1	0.6	15	0.6
Vitamin C (μg)	5.0	1.1	6	35

[a]1980 Recommended daily allowance for infants 0 to 0.5 years old.

Table 4.4. Comparison of Fat-Soluble Vitamins in Various Milk Sources

	Vitamin Content per 100 ml			
Vitamin	Mature Human Milk	Bovine Milk	Representative Formula	RDA (mg)[a]
A (μg)	75	41	53	420
D (μg)	1	0.5	1	10
E (μg)	0.25	0.07	0.004	3
K (μg)	1.5	6.0	5.3	12

[a]1980 Recommended daily allowance for infants 0 to 0.5 years old.

Table 4.5. Content of Selected Minerals in Various Milk Sources

	Mineral Content per 100 ml			
Mineral	Mature Human Milk	Bovine Milk	Representative Formula	RDA (mg)[a]
Calcium (mg)	35	130	46	360
Phosphorus (mg)	15	120	34	240
Sodium (mg)	15	58	21	250
Potassium (mg)	57	145	71	288
Zinc (mg)	0.2	0.4	0.5	3
Copper (μg)	3	3	59	6
Iron (μg)	70	100	120	10

[a]1980 Recommended daily allowance for infants 0 to 0.5 years.

the use of these standards. RDAs are estimates based on deficiency and toxicity studies in laboratory animals or weight-mediated fractions for preadolescent and adolescent children. Neither of these models adequately demonstrates the needs of a breast-fed 0 to 0.5-year-old infant.

Additionally, the RDAs incorrectly assume equivalent bioavailability and absorption of nutrients from various milk sources. The bioavailability and absorption of vitamins and minerals is greater in human milk than in bovine milk or formula. The vitamins and minerals known to have improved bioavailability and absorption in human milk include vitamin D, vitamin E, calcium, iron, and zinc. For example, iron absorption from human milk is 49%, from bovine milk 10%, and only 4% is absorbed from iron-fortified formulas.

Many hormones are present in human milk but not in pasteurized bovine milk or formula. Hormones of smaller molecular size would be expected to appear in the milk by passive diffusion from maternal serum. The hormones identified, so far, include gonadotropin-releasing hormone, thyroid-releasing hormone, thyroid-stimulating hormone, estrogen, progesterone, luteinizing hormone, follicle-stimulating hormone, oxytocin, prostaglandins, and prolactin. The exact role of these hormones is not understood, but it is thought that some control the gastrointestinal function of the neonate. The basal levels and response to insulin, motilin, enteroglucagon, neurotensin, and pancreatic polypeptide are higher in formula-fed than in breast-fed infants (18).

Prostaglandins are found in breast milk at concentrations 100 times their concentration in adult plasma (19), but none is found in formula. Prostaglandins are thought to play a role in gastrointestinal mobility and partially explain the increased stool frequency in breast-fed, as compared with formula-fed, infants. However, prostaglandins are a heterogeneous class of hormones, and their ultimate role in the physiology of infants is yet to be determined.

Human milk is digested twice as fast as bovine milk or formula; stomach emptying time is 1.5 to 2 hr with human milk and 3 to 4 hr with formula. The improved digestibility of human milk relates to mechanical properties, the character of some constituents, and the presence of active enzymes. Human milk fat and protein are contained in smaller, more easily digested packets. The emulsion of fat in human milk is less than in bovine milk, and human milk forms a flocculent suspension with little curd tension. The biochemical formula of human lipids allows for more efficient absorption. For example, palmitic acid in human milk is primarily in the number 2 position and is absorbed quickly as a 2-monoglyceride. On the other hand, palmitic acid in bovine milk or formula is more often in the 1 and 3 positions, resulting in the production of more free palmitic acid, which binds calcium and inhibits the absorption of both nutrients.

Human milk contains more than 20 active enzymes (20). While many passively diffuse from higher concentrations in maternal serum and many are at least partially inactivated by gastric acid and enzymes in the infant's gastrointestinal tract, several are synthesized by the breast and play an important role in digestion. The milk enzymes of possible importance are amylase, diastase, lactose synthetase, lactic and malic acid dehydrogenase, lipase, protease, and lysozyme. The amylases, lipase, and protease have pancreatic analogues. Lactose synthetase is related to the high concentrations of lactose in human milk. Lysozyme has a very important antibacterial activity, and its content is 300 times greater than in bovine milk.

Host Resistance Factors

At birth, the fetus enters an unsterile world, and the immune system has not experienced antigenic challenges. Full development of the immune system may take 6 to 9 months. During the first year, the infant is at serious risk from infection, the third leading cause of postnatal death in the United States. The infant derives some protection in the first 3 to 4 months through maternal IgG antibodies passed prenatally through the placenta. However, major factors in the prevention of infection are the host resistance factors in breast milk. These consist of leukocytes, antibodies, antibacterial products, and competitive inhibition. The first, and perhaps the most important, component is cellular, which is completely eliminated by pasteurization or freezing. Raw breast milk contains 4000 cell/cu mm; 90% macrophages, 5% T lymphocytes, 3% B lymphocytes, and 2% plasma cells or neutrophils. The concentration of these cells is higher in the first week of breast-feeding. Later, the concentration decreases, but the change in the absolute number is not dramatic.

Cellular components enhance the infant's resistance to infection by direct antibacterial action (phagocytosis), the production of antibodies (secretory immunoglobulin A [SIgA]), the secretion of antibacterial products (complement, lysozyme), and stimulation of the infant's immune system.

A critical event in host resistance is the recognition of pathogenic agents in the environment. The infant is at risk for infection by the same organism likely to infect the mother. Through breast milk, the neonate takes advantage of the maternal recognition of these infectious agents. This important mechanism is depicted in Figure 4.2 and is reviewed by Slade and Schwartz (21). An antigen or infective agent (virus, bacteria, fungus, protozoa) stimulates the activity of local white blood cells in the gastrointestinal or respiratory tract of the mother. Lymphocytes travel to the nearest lymph node and stimulate lymphoblasts to develop cytotoxic T cells, helper T cells, and plasma cells programmed to destroy the initiating antigen through phagocytosis or immunoglobulins produced by the plasma cells. This effect in the local lymphnodes is amplified by the migration of helper lymphocytes to other sites of white blood cell production, the bone marrow and spleen. The newly programmed white blood cells go back through the circulation to the site of the original infection. Some also travel to the breast in lactating women. Here, they may migrate into the milk (macrophages) or locally produce immunoglobulins (plasma cells). Both are uniquely programmed to fight the specific infectious agent challenging the mother.

Immunoglobulins form a sizable portion of the protein content of the early milk (colostrum) for the first 2 to 4 days (Table 4.6). In serum, the concentration of monomeric IgA is only one-fifth the concentration of the major immunoglobulin (IgG). In human breast milk the ratio is reversed. During the first day of lactation, the various concentrations of immunoglobulin are IgA 600 mg%, IgG 80 mg%, and immunoglobulin class M (IgM) 125 mg%. By

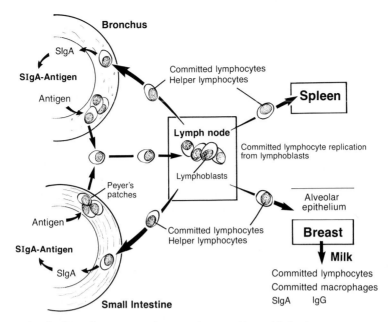

Figure 4.2. Beneficial effects for neonate if maternal recognition of infectious agents transmitted through breast milk.

Table 4.6. Comparison of Colostrum (Day 1) and Mature Milk (Day 6)[a]

Constituent per kg Infant Weight	Colostrum (Day 1)	Mature Milk (Day 6)
Volume (g)	13±16	155±29
Energy (kcal)	12±12	100±20
Protein (g)	0.7±0.6	2.4±0.5
Lactose (g)	0.7±0.7	8.9±2.1
Calcium (mg)	3.4±4.2	52±16

[a]Data from Casey CE, Meifert MR, Seacat JM, et al. Nutrient intake by breast-fed infants during the first five days after birth. Am J Dis Child 1986;140:933–936.

day 4, the concentration has fallen fourfold to a steady level; IgA 80 mg%, IgG 16 mg%I, IgM 30 mg%. The other classes of immunoglobulins, such as IgD and IgE, are represented only in small quantities. The source, variation, and importance of class D and E immunoglobulins in breast milk are not understood.

Whereas serum IgA is monomeric, the IgA in breast milk is dimeric or polymeric and is termed secretory IgA (SIgA). Polymerization improves transport through the mucous membrane and protects the protein from proteolysis in the infant's gut. Human SIgA is produced locally in the mucosa rather than concentrated and filtered from the serum.

This has been confirmed by immunohistochemical staining for intracytoplasmic immunoglobulins. IgA-producing plasma cells account for 49 to 84% of the white blood cells in the submucosa (21).

The antibody activity of SIgA is different from IgG or IgM. SIgA does not activate complement or promote opsonic complement subfragments. As a consequence SIgA is not bactericidal. It appears that SIgA acts by blocking adhesion of potential pathogens to the mucosal epithelial cells. The virulence of enteric bacteria is related to their ability to elaborate special adhesive structures (adhesins) capable of interacting with complementary epithelial cell-surface receptors. When the adhesin-specific SIgA attaches, the pathogen is effectively neutralized. Secretory IgA may also increase host resistance through stimulation of macrophages or neutralization of bacterial toxins. However, these mechanisms are less well defined than those of IgG and IgM.

Studies of the immune response in breast-fed babies demonstrate that cellular or humoral components in human milk activate and stimulate the infant's immune system. After control for transplacental transmission of immunity, a significant number (8/13) of infants born to women with a positive skin reaction to tuberculin had tuberculin-reactive peripheral blood T cells after 4 weeks of breast-feeding, compared with those of bottle-fed infants (1/13) of positive mothers or breast-fed infants (0/9) of negative mothers (22). Likewise, human milk has been shown to stimulate B cell proliferation and immunoglobulin production (23). This stimulation results in higher levels of IgA and IgM in the nasopharyngeal secretions of breast-fed versus bottle-fed neonates. The difference is most prominent at less than 6 weeks of age (24). The mechanism by which the activation and stimulation occurs is not well understood, but some communication between the maternal cellular or humoral components in breast milk and the infants uncommitted lymphoblasts must occur.

Human breast milk contains several compounds that are bactericidal or bacteriostatic. They include lysozyme, complement, lipids (resistance factor), and interferon. Lysozyme is a bacteriostatic, thermostable, and acid-stable enzyme. Lysozyme levels increase during lactation and show minimal change with variation in nutritional status (25). The level in human milk (30 to 40 mg/dl) is 300 times the level in bovine milk, or formula. Complement is an important part of the bactericidal cascade involving IgG and IgM antibody fractions. Activated C_3 also has a role in opsonization and chemotaxis. Lipids, especially unsaturated fatty acids and monoglycerides, have important antiviral properties. Milk lipids reduce the in vitro and in vivo infectivity of lipid-coated flavoviruses, α-viruses, and herpesviruses, such as cytomegalovirus. A free fatty acid in the phosphide fraction, probably $C_{18:2}$, distinct from linoleic acid, has been shown to have antistaphylococcal properties. This resistance factor is nondialyzable and thermostable. Cellular elements of human milk also produce an interferon-like substance with strong antiviral activities.

The fourth major component of host resistance associated with human milk is a combination of factors that allows the growth of nonpathogenic species of bacteria, i.e., *Bifidobacterium bifidum*, over more pathogenic enterobacteria, i.e., *Escherichia coli*. The stool flora of breast-fed infants has *Bifidobacterium* species as the predominant organism, with a ratio of 1000:1, compared with that of enterobacteria. On the other hand, in the stool flora of formula-fed infants enterobactereae and *Bacteroides* species are more common than *Bifidobacteria* species in a ratio of 10:1 (26).

Three factors in human milk support the predominance of *Bifidobacterium* species. First, bifidus factor present only in human milk is growth-promoting for *B. bifidum*. It is as a thermostable, dialyzable, nitrogen-containing carbohydrate with no amino acids. Second, *Bifidobacterium* species metabolizes milk saccharides to create organic acids, such as acetic and lactic acid. Human milk has a reduced buffer capacity when compared with formula, and the pH of the stool in breast-feeding infants is lower than the stool of bottle-fed infants (5.1 vs. 6.5). This lower pH subsequently inhibits the growth of pathogenic organisms. Finally, human milk contains compounds that compete for the essential nutriments needed by pathogenic bacteria. Two of these compounds are vitamin B_{12} binding protein and lactoferrin. Unsaturated B_{12}-binding protein is found in very high levels in human milk, and the stool of breast-fed infants relative to the low or nonexistent levels in formula or the stool of formula-fed infants. Enterobactereae and *Bacteroides* species require vitamin B_{12} for growth; binding with the protein renders the vitamin unusable for these bacteria.

Lactoferrin binds exogenous iron in a similar fashion. This property has a strong bacteriostatic action against staphylococci, *E. coli* and, perhaps, *Candida albicans*. Lactoferrin has a concentration of 480 mg/dl in colostrum and 260 mg/dl in mature milk (25). Bovine milk and formula do not contain lactoferrin. Additional iron in the diet has a minimal effect on the bacteriostatic properties of lactoferrin.

Given the presence of host resistance factors in breast milk and none in formula, does their presence reflect differences in morbidity and mortality between breast-fed and bottle-fed infants, especially in developed countries? Jason et al. (27), and Kovar et al. 1984 (5), have recently reviewed this question. Several observations can be made from this large volume of data.

1. Important methodological details of the study design are frequently lacking, such as: (a) control for those factors other than feeding method that could affect outcome; (b) clear descriptions of what constituted a clinical diagnosis; (c) control for surveillance bias, i.e., the likelihood of hospitalization; (d) documentation of the duration and exclusivity of breast-feeding; and (e) control for the one way flow of infants from the breast-feeding group to the bottle-feeding group.

2. In developing countries, prolonged exclusive breast-feeding is associated with significant reductions in mortality. This observation holds true even when important confounding epidemiologic factors are controlled, such as early neonatal mortality, birth intervals, and duration of breast-feeding.

3. In developing countries, as with overall mortality, studies on diarrheal illness suggest that breast-feeding is inversely associated with disease incidence and severity.

The reduction of disease associated with specific bacteria, such as *Salmonella, Shigella,* and *Vibrium cholerae,* in breast-fed infants corroborates the prior observation.

4. In developing countries there is an inverse dose-response relationship with breast milk and the incidence of infection; the more and longer infants are breast-fed, the lower the rate of infection.

5. In developed countries the data suffer from many methodologic flaws, and studies require a much larger sample size because of the lower overall prevalence of infection. As a result of small sample size, no study has demonstrated a significant decrease in infant mortality associated with breast-feeding in a developed country. Most studies in developed countries have focused on the incidence of severity of disease.

6. In developed countries the association between lower infection rates and breast-feeding is strongest for gastrointestinal disease. This protective effect has persisted in prospective longitudinal studies where demographic variables have been controlled (5, 27). A possible reduction in the incidence of otitis media associated with breast-feeding has been contraverted by the observation that the practice of bottle-feeding in a supine position increases the risk of otitis media. The data on respiratory illness are incomplete and does not allow a clear judgment concerning the effect of breast-feeding on the incidence or severity of disease.

Some of the strongest evidence supporting the benefits of host resistance factors in breast milk come from studies in which maternal feeding choice and nursing behavior are eliminated as covariables. In these studies, high-risk neonates are artificially fed formula, breast milk, or a combination, and the incidence and severity of neonatal infection is analyzed in these groups. For example, Narayanan et al. (28) demonstrate that, when artifically fed to high-risk neonates, breast milk offers protection against gastrointestinal disease, lower respiratory tract disease, and sepsis in general.

Psychologic Benefits

The frequent and intense physical contact in the breast-feeding dyad, where behavior is triggered by physiologic cues, such as hunger in the infant or breast engorgement in the mother, would seem to predict differences in behavior later in life. The study of this phenomenon is difficult. Newton (6, 7), in her classic reviews, has outlined the salient problems with the study of the psychologic differences

between breast- and bottle-fed infants and mothers. She points out that the preexisting psychology of the breast-feeding mother is likely to be different from that of the bottle-feeding mother and that the bottle-feeding mother does not have the psychophysic changes that are associated with unrestricted breast-feeding.

For years, psychologic research has examined the differences in "maternal behavior" between breast-feeding and bottle-feeding mothers. Several researchers have observed more maternal behavior among mothers who chose to breast-feed (5). However, preexisting psychology was not eliminated as a covariate in those studies.

Animal studies can be controlled for social and psychologic variables and have demonstrated that breast-feeding improves maternal behavior and that oxytocin, and perhaps prolactin, are the physiologic mediators of maternal behavior. In a carefully controlled behavioral study in the mouse model, Newton demonstrated significantly more maternal behavior in nursing mice than in controls (29). Oxytocin applied locally to the central nervous system of animals results in more maternal behavior than other compounds or a placebo (30).

Prophylaxis Against Allergy

Allergy is a major cause of morbidity and increased health care costs in children. There has been a 10-fold increase in the number of allergy-related diseases in the last 20 years. The increase has been attributed to better recognition of allergy-related diseases and increased incidence of exposure to allergens. Neonatal exposure to bovine milk or formula has played an important part in this. Allergic syndromes associated with bovine milk include gastroenteropathy, atopic dermatitis, rhinitis, and asthma. Approximately 20% of pediatric allergy conditions are related to bovine milk, but the incidence is only 1% in infants exclusively fed formula, since the species-specific proteins are denatured during the manufacturing process. However, formula-fed infants often receive bovine milk products as a supplement.

Breast milk protects the infant by SIgA, which is directed against allergens recognized by the mother. The "sensitized" SIgA binds the allergen and confines the antigen to the gut. Absorption is delayed, which allows proteolysis and reduced risk of sensitization. The formula-fed infant does not benefit from SIgA, and the small intestine of the neonate absorbs the macromolecule.

The mother's prior response to an allergen is the key to understanding the role of heredity in atopy. Approximately 50% of children of two atopic parents and 25% of those with one atopic parent will develop atopy, but only 14% will if both parents are unsensitized. Since sensitized mothers produce sensitized SIgA in their breast milk, breast-feeding protects the infant during the critical first several weeks when macromolecular allergens are more easily absorbed through the small intestine.

The effectiveness of early neonatal dietary manipulation on the incidence of atopy has been reviewed by Businco (31). Breast-feeding has been shown to reduce allergic disease in infants. The positive effects can be intensified by the identification of infants at risk, reduction of maternal allergen intake during the last trimester and the puerperium, and exclusive breast-feeding.

PHYSIOLOGY OF LACTATION

Many hormones, including insulin, growth hormone, corticosteroids, thyroxine, and human placental lactogen, play important supportive roles in breast development and lactation, but nipple stimulation, feedback release of prolactin and oxytocin, and relief of alveolar duct distension are essential for milk production. Failure in any of these categories may be the basis for lactation failure. The same mechanisms are utilized in the most common methods of lactation suppression; pharmacologic doses of estrogens suppress prolactin secretion; bromocriptine stimulates the dopamine pathways in the hypothalamus that inhibit prolactin production; and binders cause reduced stimulation and alveolar distension to disrupt the secretory activity of the alveolar epithelium.

The complex neuroendocrine feedback loop, the letdown reflex, is described in Chapter 3. In summary, the central focus is direct stimulation of the nipple and areola. In late pregnancy and early puerperium there is a threefold increase in the tactile sensitivity of the nipple and areola (32). With adequate nursing stimulus, impulses travel through the mammary afferent nerve fibers to the hypothalamus and the intraventricular and supraoptic nuclei. Prolactin and oxytocin secretion are efferent responses from the anterior and posterior pituitary, respectively. Simultaneously, the autonomic nervous system increases cardiac output by 5 to 10% and blood flow to the mammary glands by 20 to 40% (33). Prolactin stimulates lactogenesis in the alveolar epithelium, and oxytocin initiates contraction of the myoepithelial cells, which have greatly increased sensitivity in pregnant women. The major determinant of the initiation and maintenance of lactation is the frequency and intensity of nipple stimulation (34–36).

There appears to be a critical period just after birth when imprinting occurs. Randomized trials of early nursing vs. delayed nursing have demonstrated that early nursing is associated with a higher incidence of subsequent breast-feeding. This observation is significant when controlled for the variable of early, close contact without nursing (37).

During the first week after birth there is considerable change in the volume and character of breast milk (Table 4.6). While the concentration of protein is less in colostrum than in mature milk, the quality may be more suited to the needs of the neonate (38). The colostrum contains proportionally higher amounts of immunoglobulin, which help the neonate meet the challenges of a new, unsterile environment. The hormonal control of milk constituents is discussed in Chapter 3.

The increased blood flow to the breast, the stimulation of milk production by prolactin, and the ejection of milk by oxytocin results in 40 to 80 ml of milk per feeding episode. Initially, the average volume is 0.14 ml per suck, which decreases at the end of the feed. Approximately 80% of the volume is consumed in the first 4 minutes of nursing at each breast. The volume and concentration of constituents vary during the day. The volume increases by 10 to 15% in the late afternoon and evening. Nitrogen peaks at 160 mg% in the late afternoon and falls to a nadir 145 mg/ml at 0500. Fat concentration peaks in the early morning at 2.50 g/100 ml and reaches a nadir of 2.25 g/100 ml at 2100. Lactose stays relatively stable between 7.7 and 8.0 g/100 ml.

There are also within feed and between breast differences in nutriments (39). During a feeding episode, the lipid content rises by more than two- to three-fold (1 to 2% to 4 to 5%) with a corresponding 5% fall in lactose concentration. The protein concentration remains the same. At the extreme, there can be a 30 to 40% difference in the volume of milk obtained from each breast. Likewise, there are some intraindividual variations in lipid and lactose concentration, but this must be viewed with caution, as prior feeding experience and the completeness of drainage at the previous feeding can affect results.

The inhibition of the letdown reflex, faulty sucking behavior, and subsequent alveolar distension play major roles in lactational failure. In a series of experiments, Newton's studies demonstrated that noxious physical stimuli, emotional disturbance, and maternal attitudes reduced milk production by as much as 40 to 50% (10, 40–42). This inhibition was reversed

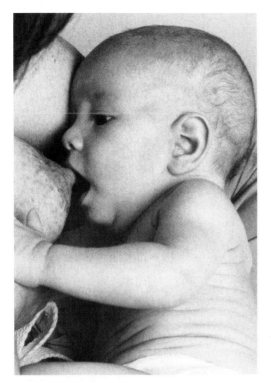

Figure 4.3. Appropriate infant sucking behavior. Infant reflexively turns its head and opens its mouth, as in a yawn, after light stimulation of his cheek.

by the administration of oxytocin and not by placebo (40).

Appropriate sucking behavior is critically important to the development and maintenance of the letdown reflex and subsequent complete emptying of the alveoli and ducts. Like many infant behaviors, sucking is a combination of inherent reflexes and learned behavior. The importance of learning is illustrated by nipple confusion when the infant is presented both the breast and rubber nipples. The sucking action on a human nipple has been described using radiologic and real-time ultrasound techniques (43, 44). As shown in Figure 4.3, the infant reflexively turns its head and opens its mouth, as in a yawn, after light stimulation of the cheek. The nipple and areola are drawn into the mouth as far as the areola-breast line (Fig. 4.4). The areola and nipple are held in place against the hard palate by cheek muscles and slight negative pressure (Fig. 4.4**A**). The tongue then strips the milk from the milk ducts in a stroking fashion (Fig. 4.4**B**).

Sucking on a rubber nipple is quite different (Fig. 4.5); the relatively inflexible nipple resists the milking motion of the tongue. Since rapid

flow from the bottle can gag the infant, it quickly learns to use the tongue to regulate the flow, but this may adversely affect breast-feeding; tongue action may force the soft human nipple out of the mouth and abrade the tip of the nipple. The resulting pain inhibits the letdown reflex. As bottle-fed infants learn to hold the bottle in place with their gums, the learned tongue action from bottle-feeding may cause them to lose their grip on the mother's nipple.

Inhibition of the letdown reflex and failure to empty the breast completely leads to engorgement. Ductal and parenchymal swelling further compromise sucking (Fig. 4.6). Hard periareolar tissue makes it difficult for the infant to pull the areola into its mouth. In addition, the widened base of the areola disrupts the milking motion and allows the tongue to abrade the nipple tip. Without intervention, lactation will cease.

Distension of the alveoli by retained milk causes a rapid (6- to 12-hr) decrease in milk secretion and enzyme activity by the alveolar epithelium. In rats, unilateral ductal ligation, with continued nursing on both ligated and unligated teats, causes involution on the ligated side (45). In goats, distension of the alveoli by infusing isotonic sucrose through the ducts causes a rapid decrease in milk secretion and enzyme activity (46). These experiments prove that distension of the alveoli inhibits secretion directly rather than indirectly by a decrease in nutriment or hormonal access, or by an inhibitor in the retained milk.

SUCCESSFUL MANAGEMENT OF LACTATION

The goal of successful management of lactation is to create a supportive environment that encourages good maternal behavior and allows breast-feeding to be directed by infant cues. The infant should be exclusively breast-fed until it shows a desire to feed itself. This generally occurs between 4 and 7 months and is manifested by the baby's desire and ability to put food into its mouth. Even after the introduction of solids, the breast-fed infant on a "demand feeding" schedule will receive most of its nutrition through breast milk for the next year. The physical security of nursing provides critical psychologic support for the child.

Unrestricted breast-feeding occurs out of necessity in primitive cultures and among self-selected groups in developed countries. Cable and Rothenberger (47) described unrestricted breast-feeding behavior patterns among 24 La Leche League mothers in North Carolina. The mean age of the group was 29.5 years; 62% had a college or postgraduate degree; and 96%

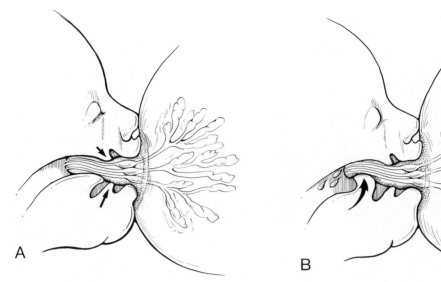

Figure 4.4. Appropriate infant sucking behavior. Nipple and areola are drawn into the mouth as far as areolo-breast line. **A**, Areola and nipple are held in place against hard palate by cheek muscles and slight negative pressure, **B**, Tongue strips milk from milk ducts in a stroking fashion.

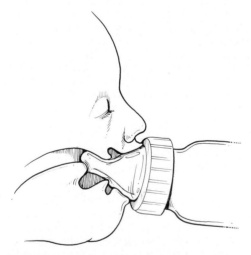

Figure 4.5. Infant sucking on a rubber nipple. Relatively inflexible nipple resists milking motion of tongue. Infant uses tongue to regulate flow of milk so as to avoid gag reflex.

were married. The mothers averaged 15±8.5 sucking episodes/day. Fifty-eight percent of the mothers nursed their infants an average of 55% of nights. Only 12% indicated that they did not sleep with their children. The average number of days in which a 6-hour lapse occurred between nursing episodes during the recording period was 29 of 60 days. The frequency of nursing had a profound effect on menstruation. Ninety-two percent of mothers with infants between 5 and 16 months of age were amenorrheic. Twenty-two percent of the mothers relied on lactation alone for contraception.

A wide variety of influences can affect the ultimate success of lactation (Fig. 4.7). The provider needs to ask: What is inhibiting the let-

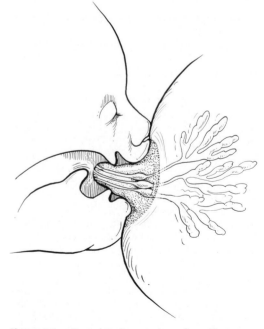

Figure 4.6. Ductal and parenchymal swelling compromise sucking. Hard periareolar tissue makes it difficult for infant to pull areola into its mouth.

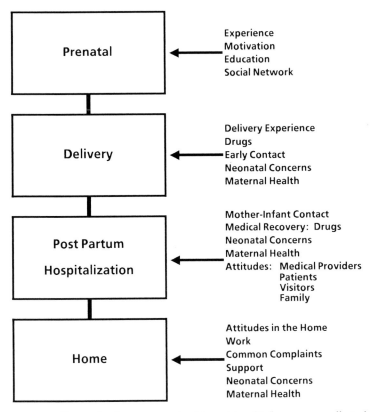

Figure 4.7. Components of breast feeding success. A wide variety of influences can affect ultimate success of lactation.

down reflex and the frequency and effectiveness of the sucking? Intervention in the antepartum, peripartum, and postpartum time periods will identify and minimize the common problems of lactation.

Antepartum Management

The goal of the antepartum period is education and preparation. In the first trimester, the choice of infant feeding should be addressed during the routine breast examination, and the benefits of breast-feeding discussed. In the second trimester, the patient should be taught the essentials of the physiology of lactation, with focus on the letdown reflex, early and frequent stimulation, and correct nursing technique. Books are useful resources for the prospective mother. (See Torgus, J (ed). *The womanly art of breast-feeding*, ed. 4. Franklin Park IL, La Leche League International, 1987; Sears W (ed): *Creative parenting*. New York, Dodd, Mead, 1983; Huggins K, (ed): *The nursing mother's companion*. Boston, Harvard Common Press, 1986.)

In the third trimester, discussion should focus on the management of lactation and breast anatomy. During the examination at 36 weeks, self-

doubt concerning the size or shape of breasts should be addressed, and the patient should be reassured that less than 5% of lactational failures are caused by faulty anatomy. Augmentation mammoplasty usually does not affect lactation, but reduction mammoplasty usually makes it impossible. The texture of the breast and tethering of the nipple are also assessed. An inelastic breast gives the impression that the skin is fixed to dense underlying tissue whereas the elastic breast allows elevation of the skin and subcutaneous tissue from the parenchyma. Lack of elasticity may complicate nursing because of increased rigidity with engorgement. Massage of the periareolar tissue 4 times/day for 10 minutes is recommended. Engorgement should be assiduously avoided in the postpartum period by early, frequent nursing.

Congenital tethering of the nipple to underlying fascia is diagnosed by squeezing the outer edge of the areola (Fig. 4.8); normally the nipple will protrude (Fig. 4.8A), but a tethered nipple will retract (Fig. 4.8B). Severe tethering is manifested by an inverted nipple. Flat or inverted nipples do not preclude breast-feeding. Three methods of helpful intervention have

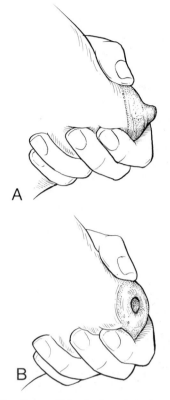

Figure 4.8. Congenital tethering of nipple to underlying fascia is diagnosed by squeezing outer edge of areola; normally, nipple will protrude (**A**), but tethered nipple will retract (**B**).

been described. The breast is supported by a cupped hand while the thumb and index finger grasp the flat nipple, draw it out to the point of discomfort, not pain, and release it. This is repeated 5 to 6 times several times per day. The effectiveness of this technique has not been documented, and occasionally (5%) nipple stimulation will stimulate uterine contractions lasting longer than 2 minutes. A fetal heart rate deceleration may accompany these contractions. Although this may not be detrimental to the fetus, the technique is not recommended for pregnancies complicated by premature labor or uteroplacental insufficiency.

A second method, the Hoffman exercise, was designed to evert severely tethered nipples. The technique involves placing the thumbs or forefingers opposite each other on the outer third of the areola and gently pulling laterally (Fig. 4.9). This is done in four quadrants. The previously mentioned contraindications apply to Hoffman exercises as well.

The final method is to use a nipple cup (shield) (48). A hard plastic or glass (not rubber) tent (Fig. 4.10) is placed around and over the nipple and areola and held in place by a tight-fitting brassiere. The nipple and areola are everted through the center hole by the circumferential pressure. This therapy may be started as soon as a flat or inverted nipple is identified. Initially, the cup should be worn for only 3 to 4 hrs/day. As the breasts adjust, the duration should be increased. Since nipple cups may retain moisture, ventilation holes and frequent rest periods for drying are important.

Modern clothing, especially protective brassieres, prevent friction, which toughens the skin and helps protect the nipple from cracking during early lactation. In the second half of pregnancy, nipple skin may be toughened by wearing a nursing brassiere with the flaps open. However, washing with harsh soaps, buffing the nipple with a towel, and using alcohol, benzoin, or other drying agents are not helpful and may increase the incidence of cracking. Normally the breast is washed with clean water and should be left to air dry. A cautiously used sunlamp or hair dryer may facilitate drying. Trials involving nipple rolling, application of breast cream, or expression of colostrum have not shown a reduction in nipple trauma or sensitivity, when compared to those with untreated nipples.

Peripartum Management

The peripartum period is critical for achieving successful lactation. Nursing should be initiated soon after birth, preferably in the delivery room. Contraindications include (*a*) a heavily medicated mother; (*b*) an infant with a 5-minute Apgar test result less than 6; (*c*) a premature infant at less than 36 weeks' gestation. If there has been polyhydramnios, or the neonate has excess secretions, a tracheoesophageal abnormality must be ruled out. In such cases, a small nasogastric catheter should be passed into the stomach to make sure the esophagus is patent and the risk of aspiration is small. Glucose solutions or formula are very irritating if aspirated and, as many babies are bottle-fed, a delay in feeding has become standard. However, colostrum is not so irritating and is readily absorbed.

The instructor should pay special attention to the mother's position during the first feeding; she should be in a related, comfortable position. With skin-to-skin contact, the infant is presented to the breast with his ventral surface to the mother's ventral surface. A supported sitting position (Fig. 4.11) or a side-ly-

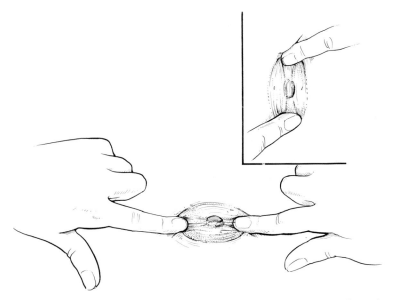

Figure 4.9. Hoffman exercise. Technique was designed to evert severely tethered nipples and involves placing thumbs or forefingers opposite each other on outer third of areola and gently pulling laterally.

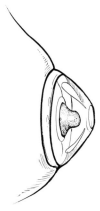

Figure 4.10. Diagnosis of tethering of nipples by use of a nipple cup shield. A hard plastic or glass (not rubber) tent is placed around and over nipple and areola is held in place by a tight-fitting brassiere.

Routine neonatal examinations and interventions can be performed at the bedside. This al-

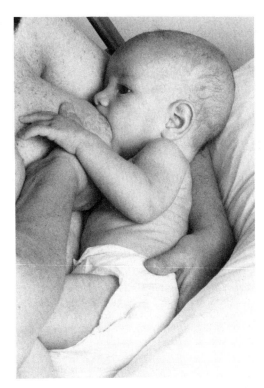

Figure 4.11. A comfortable, convenient position for breast-feeding that allows appropriate mouth-areola attachment.

ing position (Fig. 4.12) is convenient. A dry neonate, skin-to-skin contact, and supplemental radiant heating will prevent neonatal cold stress. Routine eye treatment should be delayed, as it may disrupt the important family bonding process.

In the recovery room and on the ward, the best place for the neonate is with the mother. This maximizes mother-infant bonding and allows "on demand" feeding every 1 to 2 hours.

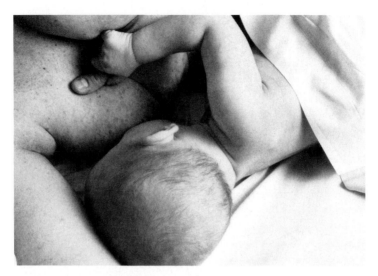

Figure 4.12. In cesarean section patients in whom pressure on the abdomen is uncomfortable, a "side-lying" hold may be efficient for breast-feeding.

lows the mother to participate in the care and gives her an opportunity to ask questions. The mother should be encouraged to sleep when the neonate sleeps. Since the hospital runs on an adult diurnal pattern, the patient should be discharged early in order to get her rest.

The frequency of early feeding is proportional to milk production and weight gain in neonates (34, 35). Therefore, supplementation with glucose or formula should be discouraged. Supplementation decreases milk production through a reduction in nursing frequency by satiation of the neonate and slower digestion of formula. Supplementation also undermines the mother's confidence by undermining her confidence about her lactational adequacy. The measured effects of supplemental feeding on breast-feeding success are mixed. Some studies show a clear detrimental effect (49, 50), and others show no differences (51, 52). A randomized trial of giving or withholding free formula samples at the time of discharge demonstrated a significantly reduced incidence of breast-feeding at 1 month and an increased likelihood of solid food introduction by the mothers given the formula samples (49). This was most significant in high-risk groups: those less educated, primiparas, and those reporting illness since leaving the hospital.

Other factors influencing the success of lactation are improper positioning and nursing technique, which can lead to increased nipple trauma and incomplete emptying. In the early postpartum period, nursing technique should be evaluated in three areas; presentation and latching on, maternal-infant positioning, and breaking of the suction. The infant should not

have to turn its head to nurse. A ventral surface to ventral surface presentation is necessary. When latching on to the nipple, the neonate should take as much of the areola as possible into its mouth. This is facilitated by gently stimulating the baby's cheek to elicit a yawn-like opening of its mouth and rapid placement of the breast into it (Fig. 4.3). A supporting hand on the breast helps; the "C" hold involves four fingers cupping and supporting the weight of the breast, which is especially important in the weak or premature neonate whose lower jaw may be depressed by the weight of the breast. The thumb rests above and 1 to 2 cm away from the areolar edge and points the nipple downward. Retraction by the thumb will pull the areola away from the mouth and cause an incorrect placement.

Any position that is comfortable and convenient, while allowing the appropriate mouth-areolar attachment, should be encouraged; the sitting position is the most common (Fig. 4.11). In cesarean section patients in whom pressure on the abdomen is uncomfortable a "side-lying" (Fig. 4.12) or "football hold" (Fig. 4.13) may be better. A rotation of positions is recommended to reduce focal pressure on the nipple and to ensure complete emptying.

Removal of the nursing infant can be a problem; suction by the neonate can injure the nipple if it is not broken prior to disengagement. A finger inserted between the baby's lips and the breast will break the suction (Fig. 4.14).

The single most difficult management issue is the control of routines and hospital attitudes detrimental to lactation. Winikoff et al. (3) studied how feeding patterns are affected by

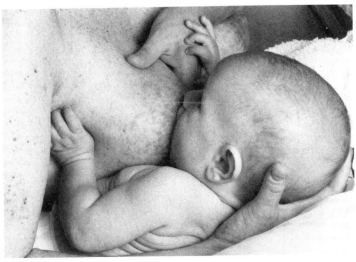

Figure 4.13. For the same type of patient mentioned in Figure 4.11, a "football hold" may be efficient for breast-feeding.

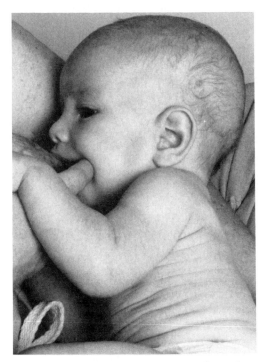

Figure 4.14. Removal of nursing infant can be a problem; suction by the neonate can injure the nipple if it is not broken prior to disengagement. A finger inserted between baby's lips and mother's breast will break the suction.

routine procedures in a New York City hospital with 2000 deliveries a year and a residency training program. Policies that worked against the physiology of lactation included formula distribution and supplementation unless otherwise ordered, constant questioning of the mother about breast-feeding, preprinted orders for lactation suppression medication, pediatric clearance prior to the first feeding, limited maternal access to the infant and little educational material for new mothers or staff. In a correlated study of professional knowledge, a large number of staff personnel were found to have inadequate information about lactation (Table 4.7) (3).

When mothers were interviewed at least 24 hours postpartum, 51% planned to breast-feed, but only 16% were breast-feeding when discharged. Supplemental formula was given to 9% of the infants. One-half of those who discontinued breast-feeding stated that the reason was "insufficient milk." Thirty-two percent felt that the hospital preferred combined breast- and bottle-feeding; 13% felt that the hospital preferred bottle-feeding alone (3).

These problems are common to many hospitals (3, 50, 53); hospitals are paternalistic, and when providers are ignorant or apathetic about lactation, success of lactation is unlikely. This theme underscores the role of the physician in educating patients, nursing staff, and support personnel about the physiology and benefits of lactation.

Postpartum Management

The first few weeks after discharge are most important (50, 53). Twenty to 50% of women will stop breast-feeding, and an additional 20%

Table 4.7. Lack of Professional Knowledge About Breast-Feeding[a]

	Physicians		Nursing Staff	
Misconceptions	Pediatricians (%)	Obstetricians (%)	Pediatrics (%)	Obstetrics (%)
Colostrum should not be fed to a baby	0	27	15	26
Some babies are allergic to human milk and should be bottle-fed	50	64	46	61
Breast-feeding mothers should supplement with formula routinely in infants under 3 months	33	36	32	48
A baby with diarrhea should be taken off the breast for at least 24°	33	73	72	77

[a]Data from Winikoff B, Laukaran VH, Myers D, et al. Dynamics of infant feeding: mothers, professionals, and the institutional context in a large urban hospital. Pediatrics 1986;77:357–365.

will start supplementation. The majority (64%) start formula feedings without medical consultation. Patterns developed in the hospital predict early termination (<8 weeks) of breast-feeding (50). Nursing staff ratings of infants for excessive crying, demanding personality, or trouble with feeding predicted 60 to 83% of cases of early termination and were identified in 7 to 18% of breast-feeding mothers. The reasons cited by mothers who terminated early were "insufficient milk" (45%), anticipation of work (20%), maternal or infant illness (21%), nipple problems (5%), other problems (9%) (50). The lessons learned from these studies are that hospital routines and attitudes have long-lasting effects on lactational success and that building the confidence of the mother is an essential component of postpartum management.

The new mother also needs a supportive environment at home and an interested and readily available resource for practical information. Prior to discharge, a family meeting concerning the early postpartum period and lactation is essential. The meeting should include the father, other children, and any significant other. The dialogue should review the physiology of lactation, the importance of unrestricted nursing, the negative influences on lactation, and the need to avoid fatigue. The importance of adequate nutrition and fluids should be stressed and reassurance given that the learning process will produce good results.

These latter points are reinforced at the first office visit. New maternal concerns, the interaction in the dyad, and the physical health of the mother and infant are assessed. The observation of a nursing episode may give clues to defective functioning.

For a new mother, contact with a mother experienced in long-term breast-feeding is helpful, and regular contacts with this person provide ongoing support. Local, national, and international groups provide breast-feeding information and support. Local groups are also available for this purpose. The best-known international group is La Leche League International, an organization of women with nursing experience and dedication to the importance of lactation. Their leaders are instructed not to interfere with the doctor-patient relationship and not to give medical advice. Local physicians provide medical expertise in situations in which medical intervention is necessary. The address of the organization is:

La Leche League International
9616 Minneapolis Ave.
Franklin Park, IL 60131

COMMON CONCERNS IN LACTATION

Common concerns related to breast-feeding include diet, drugs in breast milk, pain and nipple trauma, mastitis, infant growth and development, jaundice in the newborn, return to work, and complicating medical diseases. The reader is referred to texts included in the references for more detailed information (54–57).

Maternal Nutrition during Lactation

Maternal requirements for nutrients during lactation are functions of the maternal and infant's basal metabolic rates, the efficiency of conversion of maternal foodstuffs into milk, and the degree of stored energy used to produce milk. The metabolic needs of mothers are greater among teenagers and in those recovering from cesarean section or medical complica-

Table 4.8. Energy and Protein Requirements in Nonpregnant, Pregnant, and Lactating Women

Requirements per kg Body Weight	Physiologic States			Lactating Teenager
	Nonpregnant	Pregnant	Lactation	
Energy (kcal)	36	41	45	58
Protein (g)	0.84	1.38	1.16	1.43

tions. Likewise, size, age, and health determine the metabolic needs of the infant. A daily consumption of 1000 ml of breast milk supplies the energy requirements of a 3 month old in the 95th percentile for weight and a 9 month old in the 5th percentile (58). Infection and other medical diseases increase the metabolic needs of the infant.

The efficiency of conversion of maternal foodstuff to milk is about 80 to 90%. If the average milk volume per day is 900 ml, and milk has an average energy content of 75 kcal/dl, the mother must consume an extra 794 kcal/day, unless stored energy is used.

During pregnancy most women store an extra 2 to 5 kg (19,000 to 48,000 kcal) in tissue, mainly fat, in physiologic preparation for lactation. These calories and nutrients supplement the maternal diet during lactation. As a result, dietary increases are easily attainable in healthy mothers and infants. Table 4.8 depicts the energy and protein requirements in a variety of physiologic states.

In lactation, most vitamins and minerals should be increased 20 to 30% over nonpregnant requirements. Folic acid should be doubled. Calcium, phosphorus, and magnesium should be increased by 40 to 50%, especially in the teenager who is lactating. In practical terms, these needs can be supplied by the following additions to the diet: 2 cups of 2% milk, 2 oz of meat or peanut butter, a slice of enriched or whole wheat bread, a citrus fruit, a salad, and an extra helping (½ to ¾ cup) of a dark green or yellow vegetable. The appropriate intake of vitamins can be ensured by continuing prenatal vitamins with 1 mg of folic acid through the lactational period. The mother should drink at least 1 extra liter of fluid per day to make up for the fluid loss through milk.

Vegetarianism has become increasingly more common, and if this is the case, dietary deficiencies may include B vitamins (especially B12, total protein, and the full complement of essential amino acids. The recommendation should be to take a good dietary history with the focus on protein, iron, calcium, and vitamins D and B; supplement with soy flour, molasses, or nuts; use complementary vegetable protein combinations; and avoid excess phytates and bran.

Many women are concerned about losing weight postpartum. If 700 to 1200 kcal are used daily to nourish an infant, a mother could lose weight by not increasing her caloric intake, but a thoughtful selection of food groups and the elimination of "empty calories" are necessary. A reduction of total calories (<25 kcal/kg) and total protein (<0.6 g/kg) may reduce the daily milk volume by 20 to 30%, but not the milk quality, unless the mother is more than 10% below her ideal body weight. Since dieting mobilizes fat stores that may contain environmental toxins, such as DDT, women with high exposure to such toxins should not lose weight during lactation.

Drugs in Breast Milk

Most medications taken by the mother will appear in breast milk, but the calculated dose consumed by the nursing infant ranges from 0.001 to 5% of the standard therapeutic doses tolerated by infants without toxicity (59). Table 4.9 lists common drugs used in obstetrics that are considered compatible with lactation (59, 60), but this list is not exhaustive. Very few drugs are absolutely contraindicated. These include anticancer agents, radioactive materials, lithium, chloramphenicol, phenylbutazone, atropine, and the ergot alkaloids.

When the literature does not reveal the concentration of a drug in breast milk, an approximation can be derived. First, the apparent volume in which the drug is distributed is calculated as $V_d = dose/Cp0$, where V_d is the apparent volume of distribution (liters per kilogram), dose is the quantity (milligrams per kilogram) administered to the mother, and Cp0 is the drug concentration in the plasma at zero time. Cp0 is a derived value reflecting the concentration in maternal plasma, if instantaneous distribution of the drug had taken place prior to metabolism and elimination from the body; it is the plasma concentration predicted from extrapolation of the elimination phase to time 0. The Cp0 is available for most drugs given to nonpregnant patients. In the first 2 to 3 weeks postpartum, the literature values for Cp0 may be unreliable because of differences in the physiology of postpartum women: greater blood volume, decreased serum albumin, and increased renal clearance.

Table 4.9.   Common Drugs Compatible with Lactation

Analgesics
  Acetaminophen, aspirin, codeine, meperidine, morphine
Anticonvulsants
  Carbamazepine, phenytoin, magnesium sulphate
Antihistamine
  Diphenhydramine, brompheniramine
Anti-infective agents
  Aminoglycosides, cephalosporins, penicillins, nitrofurantoin, clindamycin, isoniazid
Cardiovascular drugs
  Atenolol, propranolol, methyldopa, captopril, digoxin, hydrochlorothiazide
Gastrointestinal cathartics
  Milk of magnesia, mineral oil, bulk-forming laxatives
Hormones
  Insulin, heparin, epinephrine, liothyronine, thyroxine, prednisone
Antithyroid medications
  Propylthiouracil
Psychotropic drugs
  Phenothiazine, tricyclic antidepressants
Narcotics
  Codeine, meperidine, methadone, morphine
Antiasthma medication
  Terbutaline, theophylline

Once the volume of distribution is known, the concentration of the drug in breast milk can be calculated as $C_B = \text{dose}/V_d$, in which C_B is the concentration (milligrams per liter) of drug in breast milk, V_d is the volume of distribution in liters per kilogram, and dose in milligrams per kilogram is the amount delivered to the maternal systemic circulation.

In general, the maternal serum concentration of unbound drug determines the amount excreted in breast milk. Drug characteristics that predict a higher breast milk concentration are low molecular weight, high lipid solubility, low protein binding, small volume of distribution, and long half-life. Drugs that are prescribed in megadoses and those prescribed for chronic conditions have higher concentrations in breast milk.

The risk of a drug to the infant is related to the dose consumed, the oral bioavailability, and the elimination. Solubility, gastrointestinal pH, gastric emptying time, interaction with food constituents, and gastrointestinal membrane permeability determine absorption of drugs, and each of these characteristics is affected by the infant's age. For example, in the first several weeks of life, low gastric acid secretion enhances the absorption of drugs unstable in acid, such as penicillin, and the neonate's gastrointestinal tract is more permeable

to these macromolecules. On the other hand, gastric emptying time is prolonged for 6 to 8 months and may decrease drug absorption.

There are several differences between infants and adults that affect the elimination of drugs. Extracellular fluid volume falls from 50% of the total fluid volume to 25% after 1 year of age. Water-soluble drugs are distributed freely into this compartment, thus reducing and delaying the elimination of "free" drug. The total body fat content varies with age: 3% in the preterm neonate, 12% at full term, and 30% at 1 year. Highly lipid-soluble drugs are more likely to affect the neonatal brain because of fewer fat storage sites. Neonates have decreased protein binding because of lower albumin concentrations and affinity, which results in more free drug, greater drug metabolism, and more drug displacement of unconjugated bilirubin. Neonates also have deficient mechanisms for drug metabolism and elimination because of hepatic enzymatic deficiencies and renal immaturity; the half-lives of many drugs in neonates are 2 to 10 times longer than those in adults.

Given the complexities of drug transfer to breast milk, neonatal tolerance, and the lack of data regarding to specific drugs, the following guidelines are helpful:

1. Evaluate the therapeutic benefit of medication. Diuretics given for ankle swelling provide very different benefits from those for congestive heart failure. Are drugs really necessary, and are there safer alternatives?
2. Choose drugs most widely tested and with the lowest milk-plasma ratio.
3. Choose drugs with the lowest oral bioavailability.
4. Select the least toxic drug with the shortest half-life.
5. Avoid long-acting forms. Usually, these drugs are detoxified by the liver or bound to protein.
6. Schedule doses so that the least amount gets into the milk. The rate of maternal absorption and the peak maternal serum concentration are helpful in scheduling dosage. Usually, it is best for the mother to take the medication immediately after a feeding.
7. Monitor the infant during the course of therapy. Many pharmacologic agents for maternal use are also used for infants. This implies the availability of knowledge about therapeutic doses and the signs and symptoms of toxicity. Toxic effects include sedation, anorexia, diarrhea, rash, and hyperkinesis. In most cases, the dose received by the infant is less than the therapeutic dose. The dose can be calculated as follows:

$$\text{Dose/24 hr} = C_B \times \text{weight} \times \text{volume of milk,}$$

Where C_B is the concentration of the drug in milk, weight is the infant weight in milligrams, and volume is the amount of milk consumed in milligrams per kilogram per 24 hours.

Breast Pain

Breast or nipple pain is one of the most frequent complaints of lactating mothers. The frequency is related to failures in the initial management of lactation: late first feed, decreased frequency of feedings, poor nipple grasp, and/or poor positioning. The differential diagnosis of breast pain includes problems with latching-on, engorgement, nipple trauma, mastitis and, occasionally, the letdown reflex.

Symptoms assist with the differential. One type of problem with latching-on is the anxious, vigorous infant who sucks strongly against empty ducts until the letdown occurs. The other is the nipple-confused infant who chews on the nipple and abrades the tip with his tongue (Fig. 4.5). In these cases, the nipple and breast pain starts with latching-on and diminishes with letdown. Contact pain suggests nipple trauma and may persist as long as the nipple is manipulated. Engorgement causes a dull, generalized discomfort in the whole breast, worse just before a feed and relieved by it. Localized, unilateral, and continuous pain in the breast may be due to mastitis. Occasionally, women describe the letdown reflex as painful; this occurs after the first minute of sucking and usually lasts only a minute or two as the ductal swelling is relieved by nursing.

A physical examination and observation of nursing technique can confirm the impression left by a good history. Through observation of a nursing episode, an infant's personality and nursing technique can be assessed. The whole of the nipple and much of the areola should be included in the infant's mouth. An examination of the nipple may reveal a fissure or blood blister. Bilateral breast firmness and tenderness may indicate engorgement. Engorgement may be peripheral, periareolar, or both. Mastitis is characterized by localized erythema, heat, tenderness, and induration.

The management of breast pain consists of general, as well as specific, steps. Prevention is a key component. Appropriate nursing technique and positioning will prevent, or significantly decrease, the incidence of nipple trauma, engorgement, and mastitis. Rotation of nursing position will reduce the suction pressure on the same part of the nipple, as well as ensuring complete emptying of all lobes of the breast. Frequent nursing will reduce engorgement and milk stasis. The use of soaps, alcohol, and other drying agents on the nipples tends to increase nipple trauma and pain (61). The nipples should be air dried for a few minutes after each feed, and clean water is sufficient to cleanse the breast, if necessary.

Stimulating a letdown and manual expression of milk are useful in the management of many breast problems. The flow of milk can be improved by placing the mother in a quiet, relaxed environment. The breast is massaged in a spiral fashion, starting at the top and moving toward areola; the fingers are moved in circular fashion from one spot to another, much like a breast examination. After the massage, the breast is stroked from the top of the breast to the nipple with a light stroke and shaken, while the woman leans forward. Once milk starts to flow manual expression is begun.

This technique is performed by holding the thumb and first two fingers on either side of the areola, in a half circle, but the breast should not be cupped. The hand pushes the breast straight into the chest wall, as the thumbs and fingers are rolled forward. Large, pendulous breasts may need lifting prior to this. The maneuver is repeated in all four quadrants of the areola to drain as many reservoirs as possible. The procedure is repeated rhythmically and gently since squeezing, sliding, or pulling may injure the breast. The technique is illustrated in Figure 4.15.

The sequence of massage, stroke, shake, and express is useful in providing milk immediately for the vigorous infant, in allowing an improved latch-on by reducing periareolar engorgement, and in reducing high suction pressures on a traumatized nipple. The letdown produced by manual expression is never as complete as a normally elicited one. An effective letdown can be elicited by initiating nursing on the side without nipple trauma or mastitis. This will effectively reduce breast pain.

In the first 5 days after birth, about 35% of the nipples of breast-feeding mothers show damage, and 69% of mothers have nipple pain (61). The management of painful, tender, or injured nipples includes prefeeding manual expression, correction of latching-on, rotation of positions, and initiation of nursing on the less painful side first, with the affected side exposed to air. It may be helpful to apply expressed milk to nipples and let it dry between feedings. Drying is facilitated by the application of dry heat, hair dryer on low setting, for 20 minutes four times per day. Aspirin or codeine (15 to 30 mg) given ½ hour before nursing may be helpful in severe cases. Engorgement can be avoided, but if it occurs, feeding

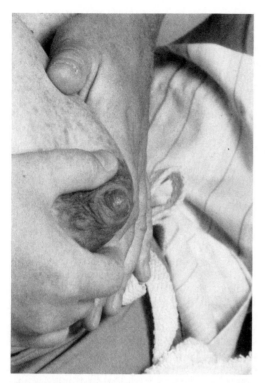

Figure 4.15. Manual expression of milk in management of breast problems.

frequency should be maintained or increased. A wide variety of preparations have been applied to traumatized nipples, including alcohol, soap, lanolin, A & D ointment, white petrolatum, antibiotics, vitamin E oil, and used tea bags, but none of these has been evaluated scientifically. Soap and alcohol have been shown to injure nipples (61). Until therapies have been tested, it is best to avoid those with theoretic concerns; white petrolatum retains moisture; antibiotics are passed to the infant. Nipple shields should be used only as a last resort because of a 20 to 60% reduction in milk consumption. Thin latex shields may be better than the traditional red rubber ones, although milk flow is still reduced by 22% (62).

Engorgement of the breast occurs when there is inadequate drainage of milk (63). Swollen, firm, and tender breasts are caused by distension of the ducts and increased extravascular fluid. Aside from the discomfort, engorgement leads to dysfunctional nursing behavior and nipple trauma (Fig. 4.6). The firm breast tissue pushes the infants face away from the nipple. The widened base of the nipple disrupts the attachment, and the infant's thrusting tongue abrades the tip. This leads to further engorgement, decreased milk production

and, in some cases, early termination of breast-feeding.

The best treatment is prevention, but when this has not occurred, management is centered on symptomatic support and relief of distension. Proper elevation of the breasts is important. The mother should wear a firm-fitting nursing brassiere, with neither thin straps nor plastic lining. Occasionally, aspirin, Tylenol, or codeine may be necessary. A warm shower or bath, with prefeed manual expression, is effective. Frequent suckling (every 1 to 2 hours), is the most effective mechanism to relieve engorgement. In selected cases, intranasal oxytocin may be given just prior to each feed if let down seems to be inhibited.

Mastitis

Mastitis is an infectious process of the breast characterized by high fever (39 to 40°C), localized erythema, tenderness, induration, and heat. Often these signs are associated with nausea, vomiting, malaise, and other flu-like symptoms. Mastitis occurs most frequently in the first 2 to 4 weeks and at times of marked reduction in nursing frequency. Risk factors include maternal fatigue, poor nursing technique, nipple trauma, and epidemic *Staphylococcus aureus*. The most common organisms associated with mastitis are *S. aureus, S. epidermis*, streptococci and, occasionally, gram-negative rods. The incidence of sporadic mastitis is 2 to 5% in lactating and <1% in nonlactating mothers. During epidemics involving *S. aureus*, 10 to 20% of lactating mothers may develop mastitis.

Until recently, the management of mastitis has been directed by retrospective clinical reviews of experience. In most cases, this consisted of bed rest, continued lactation, and antibiotics, with an 80 to 90% cure rate, a 10% abscess rate, a 10% recurrence rate, and a 50% cessation of breast-feeding. Starting in 1982, Thomsen et al. published four important articles concerning pathophysiology, diagnosis, and treatment of mastitis (64–67). He demonstrated that the diagnosis and prognosis of inflammatory symptoms of the breast are best established by counts of leukocytes and bacteria in breast milk. This is obtained after careful washing of the mother's hands and breasts with a mild soap. The milk is manually expressed, and the first 3 ml discarded. When the leukocyte count was greater than 10^6/ml, and the bacterial count less than 10^3 bacteria/ml, the diagnosis was noninfectious inflammation of the breast. With no treatment the inflammatory symptoms lasted 7 days; 50% developed mastitis, and only 21% returned to normal lactation.

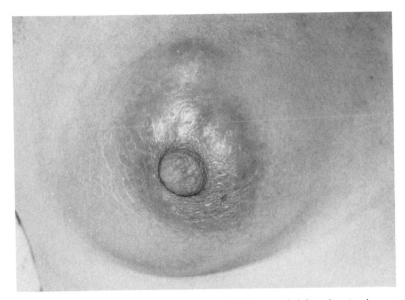

Figure 4.16. Breast abscesses as a result of lactational failure and delayed or inadequate therapy.

When the breast was emptied frequently by continued lactation, the symptoms lasted 3 days, and 96% returned to normal lactation.

If the breast milk showed greater than 10^6 leukocytes/ml and greater than 10^3 bacteria/ml, the diagnosis was mastitis. Delay in therapy resulted in abscess formation in 11%, and only 15% returned to normal lactation. Frequent emptying of the infected breast by continued nursing eliminated abscess formation, but only 51% returned to normal lactation. Additional antibiotic therapy increased the return to normal lactation in 97% with resolution of symptoms in 2.1 days.

In summary, the management of mastitis includes the following: (a) bed rest; (b) breast support; (c) fluids; (d) assessment of nursing technique; (e) nursing initiated on the uninfected side first to establish letdown; (f) the infected side emptied by nursing with each feed (occasionally, a breast pump helps to ensure complete drainage); and (g) dicloxacillin, 250 to 500 mg every 6 hours for 10 days. Erythromycin may be used in patients allergic to penicillin. It is important to continue antibiotics for a full 10 days since abscess formation is more likely with shorter courses. Hand washing before each feed and by nursing staff reduces nosocomial infection rates. Rooming-in does not reduce the acquisition of hospital strains of S. aureus nor infection rates. During epidemics, early discharge may reduce infection rates. Monilial infection of the nipple is a painful complication of antibiotic therapy. Therapy consists of rubbing a small amount of antifungal cream into the nipple after each feed.

Breast abscesses are usually the result of lactational failure and delayed or inadequate therapy (Fig. 4.16) (68). The signs include a high fever (39 to 40°C), and a localized area of erythema, tenderness, and induration. In the center a fluctuant area may be difficult to palpate. The patient feels sick. Abscesses usually occur in the upper outer quadrants and S. aureus is usually cultured from the abscess cavity.

The management of breast abscess is similar to that for mastitis, except that, (a) surgical drainage is indicated and (b) breast-feeding should be limited to the uninvolved side during the initial therapy. The infected breast should be mechanically pumped (Egnell pump) every 2 hours and with every letdown. The skin incision should be made over the fluctuant area in a manner parallel to and as far as possible from the areolar edge. While the skin incision follows skin lines, the deeper extension should be made bluntly in a radial direction. Sharp dissection perpendicular to the lactational ducts increases blood loss, the risk of a fistula, and the risk of ductal occlusion. Once the abscess cavity is entered, all loculations are bluntly reduced, and the cavity irrigated with saline. American surgeons pack the wound open for drainage and secondary closure. British surgeons advocate removal of the abscess wall and primary closure (69). In either case, wide closure sutures should be avoided, as they may compromise the ducts. Patients have a protracted recovery of 18 to 32 days and recurrent abscess formation is 9 to 15% of cases. Breast-feeding from the involved side may be resumed, if skin erythema and underlying cellulitis have resolved, which may occur in 4 to 7 days.

Infant Growth and Development

When is an exclusive diet of breast milk insufficient to supply the nutritional needs of the growing infant? Women who wean in the first 8 weeks most often say that insufficient milk is the reason for quitting, and well-meaning family members often ask, "When are you going to start feeding your child real food?"

Correct answers are not readily available (58, 70). Many nondietary factors affect the growth of infants, including high birth order, lower maternal age, low maternal weight, poor maternal nutrition during pregnancy, birth interval, birth weight less than 2.4 kg, multiple gestation, infection, death of either parent, or a broken marriage.

In addition, there are inconsistencies in the standard reference charts for growth or nutritional needs. Most growth charts are based on formula-fed infants, who often receive solid food supplementation earlier and in greater proportion than comparable breast-fed infants. Reference charts with sufficiently large numbers of exclusively breast-fed infants from developed countries are lacking. As milk volume is a quantitative measure of nutrition, variations in volume and concentrations of constituents caused by individual variation and different methods of collection compound the interpretation.

One method of evaluating nutritional adequacy is to calculate the energy requirements for normal growth and compare them to milk volumes, which are assumed to contain about 70 to 75 kcal/dl. Whitehead (58) has effectively argued that the 1973 FAO/WHO estimates for mean energy requirements in the first year are 15 to 20% too high. He calculates that infant needs are 100 kcal/kg at 3 months, 90 kcal/kg at 6 months, and 102 kcal/kg at 12 months. The adequacy of breast milk to supply these needs depends on the volume of milk. Unfortunately, differences between individuals, between populations, and between methods of collection can be as much as 200 to 500 ml daily. In addition, a severely malnourished mother may have the fat content of her milk reduced by 20 to 30%. As the fat content is the major source of energy in milk, the available energy per unit volume drops in a like fashion.

Despite the latter concerns, it is apparent that a healthy and successfully breast-feeding mother can supply enough nutrition through breast milk alone for 4 to 6 months. The clinical markers for adequate breast milk volume, regardless of the speed of infant growth, include

Table 4.10. Expected Weight Gain in Normal Term Neonates

Age (Months)	Males		Females	
	Mean (kg)	10th Percentile (kg)	Mean (kg)	10th Percentile (kg)
0–3	2.8	2.03	2.4	1.76
3–6	1.9	1.26	1.9	1.26
6–9	1.4	0.89	1.4	0.76
9–12	1.1	0.33	1.0	0.49

an alert, healthy appearance of the infant, good muscle tone, good skin turgor, six wet diapers per day, eight or more nursing episodes/day, frequent loose stools, consistent evidence of a letdown with operant conditioning, and a slow but consistent gain in weight.

The term, failure to thrive, has been used loosely to include all infants who show any degree of growth failure. For the breast-feeding mother, it may just be a matter of comparing the growth of her infant to growth charts compiled from formula-fed infants. The loosely applied term can seriously undermine the mother's confidence, and ill-advised supplementation further compromises milk volume and may mask other important underlying causes. The infant should be evaluated for failure to thrive or slowed growth if (*a*) it continues to lose weight after 10 days of life; (*b*) does not regain birth weight by 3 to 4 weeks; or (*c*) gains weight at a rate below the 10th percentile beyond the first month of age. Table 4.10 gives the expected gains for normal term neonates. If the infant is premature, ill, or small for gestational age, weight, height, and skin fold thickness can be used to define adequate growth. The cause of failue to thrive is often complex and is beyond the scope of this chapter. In general, the diagnosis follows the scheme shown in Figure 4.17.

Jaundice in the Newborn

Twenty-five percent of neonates will have jaundice defined by a serum bilirubin greater than 10 mg/dl in term infants and greater than 12 mg/dl in preterm infants. Pediatric concerns include hemolysis, liver disease, or infection as underlying causes, and kernicterus as a consequence. Unconjugated serum bilirubin greater than 20 mg/dl is considered the critical level for the development of kernicterus in term infants. Prematurity, hypoxia, acidosis, low serum albumin, lack of carbohydrates, low stooling rate, and medication may promote greater bilirubin movement into the tissue and lower the critical threshold for kernicterus. When the se-

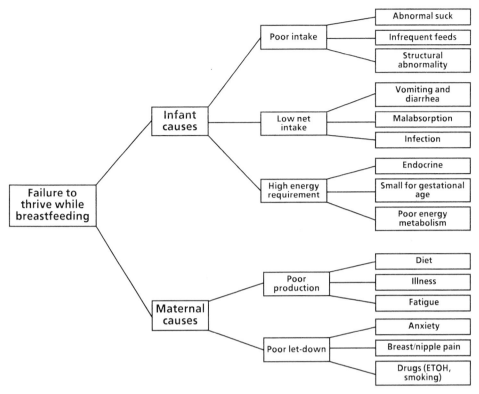

Figure 4.17. Diagnosis of infant's failure to thrive and factors causing and accompanying the condition. *ETOH*, alcohol.

rum bilirubin is greater than 5 mg/dl in the first 24 hours, a serious disease process (hemolysis) may be present, and intervention is appropriate.

The focus on breast-feeding as related to neonatal jaundice results from the characterization of two syndromes, breast-feeding jaundice syndrome and breast milk jaundice syndrome (71). In the early 1960s, 5 to 10% of lactating women were found to have a steroid metabolite of progesterone, 5β pregane-3 (α), 20 (β)-diol, in their icterogenic milk, but the compound was not found in the milk of women whose infants were normal (breast-milk jaundice syndrome). This metabolite is associated with an inhibition of gluconyl transferase in the liver, differences in the metabolism of long-chain unsaturated fatty acids, and/or increased resorption of bile acids in jaundiced infants.

In breast milk jaundice syndrome, the neonates are healthy and active. The hyperbilirubinemia develops after the fourth day of life and may last several months, with a gradual fall in level. When breast-feeding is stopped for 24 to 48 hr, there is a 30 to 50% decline in bilirubin levels. With resumption of nursing, serum levels will rise slightly (1 to 2 mg/100 ml), pla-

teau, and then start to fall slowly, regardless of feeding method. After excluding other causes of jaundice, and with careful monitoring of serum bilirubin, breast-feeding can continue.

Unfortunately, the focus on rare breast-milk jaundice cases, the concern about kernicterus, and the increased bilirubin in many breast-fed neonates between days 2 and 7 old led to routine supplementation of infants with water, glucose, and formula, even when bilirubin concentrations were in the moderate range of 8 to 12 mg/dl. These interventions have led to the breast-feeding jaundice syndrome, or starvation jaundice. The cause of the elevated bilirubin, reduced feeding frequency, is often unrecognized. It has been clearly demonstrated that feeding frequency greater than eight feedings per 24 hours is associated with lower bilirubin levels (72). Likewise, water supplementation studied in a controlled fashion, does not decrease the peak serum bilirubin (73).

Management consists of prevention by improvement in the quality and frequency of nursing. Rooming-in and night feedings should be encouraged. Additional or replacement feedings with water, glucose, or formula should be used only as a last resort. Additional fluid should be supplied, using a Lact-Aid nursing device rather than a bottle (48). This device delivers fluid through a soft plastic tube placed beside the nipple. The infant sucks the tip of the nursing tube and the nipple at the same time, which allows the stimulation needed to maintain the milk supply.

Working and Breast-Feeding

In 1984, approximately 26% of new mothers had full-time employment, and an additional 15% had part-time employment (8). At 5 or 6 months postpartum, 12.3% of full-time employees were breast-feeding, as were 29% of part-time employees or unemployed mothers. Two-thirds of the working mothers were supplementing their infants with formula.

The separation between mother and infant adversely affects the psychology and physiology of lactation through a decrease in the frequency of nursing, breast engorgement, and unsatisfied needs of the baby. The anxiety and fatigue associated with the combination of employment and lactation inhibits the letdown reflex, weakens maternal host defenses, and disrupts family dynamics. The infant must adapt to another caregiver, a new sucking technique, and unfamiliar infectious agents found in day-care settings. Therefore, it is not surprising that formula feeding is viewed as an improvement in mothers' lives, but it does create feelings of inadequacy and guilt in some women.

Breast-feeding during employment is both possible and fulfilling (74). Preparation, milk storage, and choice of child care are the cornerstones to easy adaptation to employment. Preparation involves preemployment change in life-style to accommodate the increased stresses. Lactation should be well-established with frequent nursing (10 to 14 times/day) and no complementation of supplementation prior to return to work. Return to full-time work prior to 4 months has a greater negative impact than return to work after 4 months (74). Part-time work lessens the impact. About 2 weeks prior to work, the mother should change her nursing schedule at home. During the workday, she should express or pump her breasts 2 or 3 times, while increasing her nursing with short, frequent feeds before and after work times. The infant is fed the bottles of stored breast milk by a different person in a different place to allow it to adapt more easily.

During the 2 weeks prior to employment, the day-care arrangements should be carefully selected and observed. In addition to references, several questions are pertinent to the selection of the day-care setting. Is the sitter a mother herself, and does the sitter have experience with nursing babies? Is the mother welcome to use the child care site for a midday nursing? Does the day care center provide in-arm feeding, or does it use high chairs and propped bottle-feedings? Is the time and activity of the center highly structured and rigid, or is it flexible to mother or infant needs and requests? Does the staff treat the parents and children with respect? Many of these questions can be answered by an extended (1- to 2 hours) observation of the center and its children.

Fatigue is the number one enemy of the working mother. Emotional and physical support of the mother is critical. Some helpful suggestions include (a) bringing the infant's bed into the parents' room. The construction of a temporary extension to the parents' bed may be helpful. Cofamily sleeping is another option. (b) Labor saving devices, division of domestic chores, and the elimination of less important household chores to reduce the workload. (c) Naps and frequent rest periods to conserve energy.

Continued stimulation of the breast during working hours is important. Not only does this improve milk supply, but also it supplies human milk for the infant. Manual expression and/or mechanical pumping should be performed more frequently (2 to 3 times) in the first 6 months postpartum. After 6 months, the frequency can be reduced and eliminated as the infant is supplemented by fluids or solids during the day.

The collection of breast milk has become simple with the wide variety of mechanical pumps available in the market (48, 75). Mechanical pumps that employ a bulb syringe produce the least amount of milk and have the highest rate of bacterial contamination (76, 77). Cyclic electric pumps produce the most milk with the least amount of nipple trauma. Water-driven pumps are both cheap and relatively effective (75).

The concern about bacterial growth in expressed and stored milk has been alleviated by recent studies showing that bacterial contamination does not increase significantly for up to 6 hours after expression, when the milk is stored at room temperature, nor were there differences in bacterial counts between specimens stored at room temperature and those stored under refrigeration for 10 hr (48, 78). However, it is prudent to store milk under refrigeration if possible. Freshly refrigerated milk should be used within 2 days.

Four to 6 oz of human milk can be frozen in partially filled ziplock plastic bags. When human milk is frozen, it should be cooled briefly prior to transfer to the freezer. The milk will keep for 2 to 4 weeks in the refrigerator freezer and up to 6 months in a freezer set at 0°F. The milk should be stored in layers and thawed quickly in warm tap water. After it is thawed it should be used within 6 to 8 hours.

Maternal Disease

Often, the management of lactating mothers with intercurrent disease is complex, time-consuming, and inconvenient. In the vast majority of cases, there is no medical reason to stop breast-feeding. However, appropriate management requires individualizing the care of the nursing dyad in order to preserve the supply and demand relationship of lactation. For example, a hospitalized nursing mother should have her nursing baby with her in the hospital for on-demand feedings. This situation stretches the flexibility of hospital administrators and nursing services, but the problem can be overcome by education. As it is rare for young, lactating women to be ill, the physician must educate himself and his staff about the effect of lactation on the disease, the effect of the disease on lactation, the effects of therapy on lactation, and the basic physiology of lactation.

If the physician, staff, or hospital administration feel that breast-feeding and bottle-feeding are equivalent, then cessation of breast-feeding will be viewed as the easy way out, an attitude that fails to take into account the value of lactation to both mother and infant. However, if critical evaluation of current information shows that the breast-feeding risks outweigh the benefits, the clinician and patient may have to make the necessary decision to stop breast-feeding.

As there are a wide variety of diseases and therapies, this review is necessarily brief and will consider the basic principles of management as illustrated by specific diseases or situations. The first principle is to maintain the normal physiology of lactation. An acute hospitalization for a surgical procedure is a common complication. If breast milk was the neonate's only source of nutrition, an acute reduction in nursing may lead to breast engorgement, confusing postoperative fever, and mastitis. The infant should be put to the breast just before premedication, and the breasts should be emptied in the recovery room. The most effective way is to have the mother nurse. Although some anesthetic may be present in the milk, most are compatible with lactation (73). If there is legitimate concern or if the mother cannot communicate, the breasts should be pumped mechanically and subsequently emptied every 2 to 3 hours by nursing or pumping.

The second principle is to adjust for the special nutritional requirements of nursing mothers. This principle is especially pertinent when intake is restricted postoperatively and when maternal diet must be manipulated, as in diabetes. In the postoperative period, the surgeon must account for the drain of lactation. Until oral intake is established, a lactating mother needs an additional 500 to 1000 ml of fluid per day. Early return to a balanced diet is essential to offset the additional energy and protein requirements of lactation and wound healing.

In many patients, the propensity for glucose intolerance is unmasked by pregnancy. While the gestational diabetic's glucose intolerance may resolve postpartum, she is at risk for developing diabetes later in life. As many of these women are obese, strict diets are prescribed to reduce this risk. The insulin-dependent diabetic may also have a restricted diet if she is overweight; if not, a lower calorie diet is often prescribed to standardize the carbohydrate load and reduce insulin requirements. In either case, the standard ADA diet may conflict with lactation. Normal milk volume and normal constituents of milk require minimum total calorie count of 30 to 35 kcal/kg, based on preconceptual body weight, and a protein intake of 1 g/kg body weight (79). Even this diet may be too restrictive during lactation, as the relationship between diet, maternal food stores, and infant growth are incompletely understood. Luckily, obese diabetic women may lose weight on well-balanced higher calorie diets because of the daily utilization of 800 to 1200 cal to produce milk and the increased insulin sensitivity and responsiveness of lactating women. Glucose control is best monitored by blood glucose levels rather than urine testing. The excretion of lactose in the urine of lactating women makes testing for reducing substances unreliable.

The third principle is to ensure that the maternal disease will not harm the infant. This is most pertinent with infectious disease, but it is equally important in cases where a mother's judgment is in question, such as severe mental disease, substance abuse, or a history of physical abuse. The benefits of breast-feeding in the latter situations must be carefully evaluated, using the resources of the patient, her family and social services.

Infectious disease is the most common area where breast-feeding is questioned. Table 4.11 gives recommendations as to the isolation of the mother and infant and the compatibility of breast-feeding. In general, the necessary exposure of the infant to the mother in day-to-day care is such that breast-feeding does not add

Table 4.11.   Infectious Disease and Breast-Feeding

Infection	Isolate Baby from Mother	Isolate Mother and Baby	Breast-Feed	Comment
Endometritis	No	No	Yes	
Chorioamnionitis	No	No	Yes	
Urinary tract infection	No	No	Yes	
Mastitis	No	No	Yes	
Wound infection	No	No	Yes	Cover wound
Group A streptococcus	No	Yes	Yes	
Group B streptococcus	No	No	Yes	
Staphylococcus	No	No[a]	Yes	[a]Isolate for methicillin resistance organisms
Salmonella/shigella	No	Yes	Yes	
Gonorrhea	No	No	Yes	
Syphilis	No	No	Yes	
Active tuberculosis	Yes	Yes	No	Untreated
Inactive tuberculosis	No	No	Yes	
Hepatitis A	No	Yes	Yes	
Hepatitis B	No	Yes	Yes	
Cytomegalovirus	No	No	Yes	
Herpes simplex	Isolate lesions	No	Yes[b]	[b]Except for breast lesions
Varicella-zoster	No	Yes	Yes	
Human immunodeficiency virus	No	Yes	No	
Toxoplasmosis	No	No	Yes	

much to the risk. This recommendation assumes that appropriate therapy is being given to both mother and infant. Isolation of infected areas should still be practiced, such as a mask in the case of respiratory infection and lesion isolation in herpes. The three acute infections in which breast-feeding is contraindicated are herpes simplex lesions of the breast, untreated tuberculosis, and human immunodeficiency viral (HIV) disease.

Most antibiotics are compatible with pregnancy. Many have no oral bioavailability, i.e., aminoglycosides, and others are present in such small amounts that the infant dose is 0.5 to 5% of the therapeutic dose for infants. However, chloramphenicol, tetracycline, and metronidazole should be avoided, if possible. Metronidazole may be given as a 2-g dose for vaginal trichomoniasis, while breast-feeding is withheld for 12 to 18 hours. The breasts should be manually expressed or pumped during this period. Sulfa drugs and erythromycin should be used with caution as they may displace bilirubin and cause jaundice in infants less than 1 month old.

The fourth principle is to evaluate adequately the need and type of medication used for therapy. The drug management of chronic hypertension illustrates this principle. First, the need for medication must be scrutinized. There is considerable controversy in the literature as to whether or not to treat patients with mild chronic hypertension (diastolic blood pressure 90 to 100 mm Hg). The desire of a mother with mild hypertension to breast-feed may change the risk-benefit ratio so that antihypertensive drug therapy should be delayed until after lactation. Second, the medication should be evaluated for its effect on milk production. In the first 3 to 4 months of therapy, diuretics reduce intravascular volume and, subsequently, milk volume. On the other hand, if a patient has been on low doses of thiazide diuretics for more than 6 months, the effect on milk volume is minimal as long as adequate oral intake is maintained. Methyldopa appears only in small amounts in breast milk, but it suppresses prolactin production. Third, the medication should be evaluated for its secretion in breast milk and its possible effects on the infant. Reserpine is not recommended during lactation, since it is present in breast milk in amounts large enough to cause nasal congestion, tachypnea, and bradycardia. Thiazide diuretics, ethacrynic acid, and furosemide also cross into breast milk in small amounts. These agents have the potential to displace bilirubin, and their use during lactation is of concern when the infant is less than 1 month old or is jaundiced. In general, most other antihypertensive drugs are compatible with breast-feeding. These include propranolol, atenolol, metropolol, nadolol, and captopril. Although new and similar drugs come onto the market frequently, it is wise to use drugs that have had a long history of clinical use.

REFERENCES

1. Bauchner H, Leventhal JM, Shapiro EO. Studies of breast-feeding and infections. How good is the evidence? JAMA 1986;256:887–892.
2. Sauls HS. Potential effect of demographic and other variables in studies comparing morbidity of breast-fed and bottle-fed infants. Pediatrics 1979;64:523–527.
3. Winikoff B, Laukaran VH, Myers D, et al. Dynamics of infant feeding: mothers, professionals, and the institutional context in a large urban hospital. Pediatrics 1986;77:357–365.
4. Agre F. The relationship of mode of infant feeding and location of care to frequency of infection. Am J Dis Child 1985;139:809–811.
5. Kovar MG, Serdula MK, Marks JS, et al. Review of the epidemiologic evidence for an association between infant feeding and infant health. Pediatrics 1984;74(S):615–638.
6. Newton N. Key psychological issues in human lactation. In: Waletzky LR (ed). Symposium on Human Lactation. GPO, 1979; DHEW publications No. (HSA) 79–5107.
7. Newton N, Newton M. Psychologic aspects of lactation. N Engl J Med 1967;277:1179–1188.
8. Martinez GA, Krieger FW. 1984 milk-feeding patterns in the United States. Pediatrics 1985;76:1004–1008.
9. Simopoulos AP, Grave GD. Factors associated with the choice and duration of infant-feeding practice. Pediatrics 1984;74(S):603–614.
10. Newton N, Newton M. Relationship of ability to breast-feed and maternal attitudes toward breast-feeding. Pediatr 1950:5:869–875.
11. Jones RAK, Beasly EM. Breast-feeding in an inner London borough: a study of cultural factors. Soc Sci Med 1977;11:175–179.
12. Fomon SJ. Infant nutrition, 2nd ed. Philadelphia, Saunders, 1974.
13. Kramer MS. Do breast-feeding and delayed introduction of solid foods protect against subsequent obesity? J Pediatr 1981;98:883–887.
14. Jensen RG, Clark RM, Ferris AM. Composition of the lipids in human milk: a review. Lipids 1980;15:345–355.
15. Hambraeus L. Proprietary milk versus human breast milk in infant feeding. Pediatr Clin North Am 1977;24:17–36.
16. Janas LM, Picciano MF. Quantities of amino acids ingested by human milk-fed infants. J Pediatr 1986;109:802–807.
17. Sturman JA, Rassin DK, Gaull GE. Taurine in development. Life Sci 1977;21:1–22.
18. Lucas A. Blackburn AM, Aynsley-Green A, et al. Breast vs bottle: endocrine responses are different with formula feeding. Lancet 1980;1:1267–1269.
19. Lucas A, Mitchell MD. Prostaglandins in human milk. Arch Dis Child 1977;52:800–802.
20. Shahani KM, Kwan AJ, Friend BA. Role and significance of enzymes in human milk. Am J Clin Nutr 1980;33:1861–1869.
21. Slade HB, Schwartz SA. Mucosal immunity: the immunology of breast milk. J Allergy Clin Immunol 1987;80:346–356.

22. Schlesinger JJ, Covelli HD. Evidence for transmission of lymphocyte responses to tuberculin by breast-feeding. Lancet 1977;2:529–533.
23. Juto P., Human milk stimulates B cell function. Arch Dis Child 1985;60:610–613.
24. Stephens S. Development of secretory immunity in breast-fed and bottle-fed infants. Arch Dis Child 1986;61:263–269.
25. Reddy V, Bhaskaram C, Raghuramuhr N, et al. Antimicrobial factors in human milk. Acta Paediatr Scand 1977;66:229–232.
26. Yoshioka H, Iseki K, Fujita K. Development and differences of intestinal flora in the neonatal period in breast-fed and bottle-fed infants. Pediatrics 1983;72:317–321.
27. Jason JM, Nieburg P, Marks JS. Mortality and infectious disease associated with infant-feeding practices in developing countries. Pediatrics 1984;74(S):702–726.
28. Narayanan I, Murthy NS, Prakash K, et al. Randomized controlled trial of effect of raw and holder pasteurized human milk and of formula supplements on incidence of neonatal infection. Lancet 1984;2:1111–1113.
29. Newton N, Peeler D, Rawlins C. Effect of lactation on maternal behavior in mice with comparative data on humans. J Reprod Med 1968;1:257–262.
30. Pedersen CA, Prange AJ. Oxytocin and mothering behavior in the rat. Pharmac Ther 1985;28:287–302.
31. Businco L. Prevention of atopic disease in "at-risk newborns" by prolonged breast-feeding. Ann Allergy 1983;51:691–698.
32. Robinson JE, Short RV. Changes in breast sensitivity at puberty, during the menstrual cycle, and at parturition. Br Med J 1977;1:1188–1191.
33. Katz M, Creasy RK. Mammary blood flow regulation in the nursing rabbit. Am J Obstet Gynecol 1984;150:497–500.
34. Anderson AN, Schioler V. Influence of breast-feeding pattern on the pituitary-ovarin axis of a woman in an industrialized country. Am J Obstet Gynecol 1982;143:673–675.
35. Egli GE, Egli NS, Newton M. The influence of the number of breast-feedings on milk production. Pediatrics 1961;27:314–317.
36. Short RV. Breast-feeding. Sci Am 1984;250:183–189.
37. Taylor M, Maloni JA, Brown DR. Early suckling and prolonged breast-feeding. Am J Dis Child 1986;140:151–154.
38. Casey CE, Neifert MR, Seacat JM, et al. Nutrient intake by breast-fed infants during the first five days after birth. Am J Dis Child 1986;140:933–936.
39. Neville MC, Keller RP, Seacat J, et al. Studies on human lactation. 1. Within-feed and between-breast variation in selected components of human milk. Am J Clin Nutr 1984;40:635–646.
40. Newton M, Egli GE. The effect of intranasal administration of oxytocin on the let-down of milk in lactating women. Am J Obstet Gynecol 1958;76:103–107.
41. Newton M, Newton NR. The let-down reflex in human lactation. J Pediatr 1948;33:698–704.

42. Newton N, Newton M. Relation of the let-down reflex to the ability to breast-feed. Pediatrics 1950;5:726–733.

43. Ardran GM, Kemp FH, Lind J. A cineradiographic study of bottle feeding. Br J Radiol 1958;31:11–12.

44. Ardran GM, Kemp FH, Lind J. A cineradiographic study of breast feeding. Br J Radiol 1958;31:156–162.

45. Hanwell A, Linzell JL. The effects of engorgement with milk and of suckling on mammary blood flows in the rat. J Physiol (Lond) 1973;233:111–125.

46. Peaker M. The effect of raised intramammary pressure on mammary function in the goat in relation to the cessation of lactation. J Physiol (Lond) 1980;301;415–428.

47. Cable TA, Rothenberger MA. Breast-feeding behavioral pattern among La Leche League mothers: a descriptive survey. Pediatrics 1984;73:830–835.

48. Auerbach KG. Breast-feeding techniques and devices. Lactation Consultant Series. Garden City Park, NY, Avery Pub Group, 1987.

49. Bergevin Y, Dougherty C, Kramer MS. Do infant formula samples shorten the duration of breast-feeding? Lancet 1983;1:1148–1151.

50. Feinstein JM, Berkelhamer JE, Gruszka ME, et al. Factors related to early termination of breast-feeding in an urban population. Pediatrics 1986;78:210–215.

51. Gray-Donald K, Kramer MS, Munday S, et al. Effect of formula supplementation in the hospital on the duration of breast-feeding: a controlled clinical trial. Pediatrics 1985;75:514–518.

52. Schutzman DL, Hervads AR, Branca PA. Effect of water supplementation of full-term newborns on arrival of milk in the nursing mother. Clin Pediatr 1986;25:78–80.

53. Loughlin HH, Clapp-Channing NE, Gehlbach SH, et al. Early termination of breast-feeding: identifying those as risk. Pediatrics 1985;75:508–513.

54. Lawrence RA. Breast-Feeding: A Guide for the Medical Profession, 3rd ed. St. Louis, CV Mosby, 1989.

55. Lawrence RA (ed). Breastfeeding. Clin Perinatol 1985;14:1.

56. Neville MC, Neifert MR (eds). Lactation: Physiology, Nutrition, and Breast-Feeding. New York, Plenum Press, 1983.

57. Riordan J. A Practical Guide to Breast-Feeding. St. Louis, CV Mosby, 1985.

58. Whithead RG. Infant physiology, nutritional requirements, and lactational adequacy. Am J Clin Nutr 1985;41:447–458.

59. Rivera-Calimlim L. The significance of drugs in breast milk. Clin Perinatol 1987;14:51–71.

60. Committee on Drugs, American Academy of Pediatrics. The transfer of drugs and other chemicals into human breast milk. Pediatrics 1983;72:375–384.

61. Newton N. Nipple pain and nipple damage: problems in the management of breast-feeding. J Pediatr 1952;41:411–423.

62. Woolridge MW, Baum JD, Drewett RF. Effect of a lactational and of a new nipple shield on sucking patterns and milk flow. Early Hum Dev 1980;4:357–361.

63. Newton M, Newton NR. Postpartum engorgement of the breast. Am J Obstet Gynecol 1951;61;664–667.

64. Thomsen AC. Infectious mastitis and the occurrence of antibody-coated bacteria in milk. Am J Obstet Gynecol 1982;144:350–351.

65. Thomsen AC, Espersen T, Maigaard S. Course and treatment of milk stasis, non-infectious inflammation of the breast, and infectious mastitis in nursing women. Am J Obstet Gynecol 1984;149:492–495.

66. Thomsen AC, Hansen KPB, Moller BR. Leukocyte counts and microbiological cultivation in the diagnosis of puerperal mastitis. Am J Obstet Gynecol 1983;146:938–940.

67. Thomsen AC, Mogensen SC, Jepsen FL. Experimental mastitis in mice induced by coagulase-negative staphylococcus isolated from cases of mastitis in nursing women. Acta Obstet Gynecol Scand 1985;64;163–166.

68. Newton M, Newton NR. Breast abscess: a result of lactation failure. Surg Gynecol Obstet 1950;91:651–655.

69. Benson EA, Goodman MA. Incision with primary suture in the treatment of acute puerperal breast abscess. Br J Surg 1970;57:55–58.

70. Seward JF, Serdula MK. Infant feeding and infant growth. Pediatrics 1984;74(S):728–761.

71. Auerbach KG, Gartner LM. Breast-feeding and human milk: their association with jaundice in the neonate. Clin Perinatol 1987;14:89–105.

72. DeCarvalho M, Klaus MH, Merkatz RB. Frequency of breast-feeding and serum bilirubin concentration. Am J Dis Child 1982;136:737–738.

73. DeCarvalho M, Hall M, Harvey D. Effects of water supplementation on physiological jaundice in breast-feeding babies. Arch Dis Child 1981;56:568–569.

74. Auerbach KG, Guss E. Maternal employment and breast-feeding. Am J Dis Child 1984;138:958–960.

75. Johnson CA. An evaluation of breast pumps currently available on the American market. Clin Pediatry 1983;22:40–45.

76. Green D., Moye L, Schreiner R, et al. The relative efficacy of four methods of human milk expression. Early Hum Dev 1982;6:1530–1539.

77. Liebhaber M, Lewiston N, Asquith MT, et al. Comparison of bacterial contamination with two methods of human milk collection. Pediatrics 1978;92:236–237.

78. Barger J, Bull P. A comparison of the bacterial composition of breast milk stored at room temperature and stored in the refrigerator. Int J Childbirth Educ 1987;2:78–79.

79. Ferris AM, Dalindoqitz CK, Ingardia CM, et al. Lactation outcome in insulin-dependent diabetic women. Am Diabetic Assoc 1988;88:314–319.

5

Psychology and Psychopathology in Breast Disorders

Elizabeth Small

THE FEMALE BREASTS: SYMBOLS AND ORGANS

Psychosocial Aspects and Attitudes Toward Female Breasts

Anthropologists have observed that there is no society more obsessed with the female breast than the American. Interest in women's breasts is universal but, in the United States, the female breast has become so idealized that it is the primary focus of identification with the female role. Images of breasts convey delight to viewers, and the methods of display have included compression, uplifting, reshaping, enlarging, and diminishing. The whims and values of each era have determined image, so that "every delicate detail of the female body may of course be reinterpreted by the culture" (1).

Although the breasts are not primarily sexual organs, it is customary in American culture to eroticize breasts, and this obscures the fundamental anatomic and physiologic functions. Medical definitions usually describe breasts as bilateral hemispheric projections overlying the fascia of the pectoralis major muscle on either side of the anterior thorax and as the mammary glands, the organs of milk secretion. Essentially, breasts are designed for feeding mammalian young, but psychosocial descriptions include: (a) Breasts as milk-bearing organs representing nurturance and offering both physical and emotional gratification to baby and mother; (b) Breasts as symbols of femininity and sexual desirability. Because cultural values are fundamentally involved, understanding their importance is essential in the management of patients with breast disorders.

Due to a confusing information base, there is a lack of clarity in the separation of the sexual and the reproductive-nurturing functions of the breast. The overemphasis of sexual function by equating the male penis with the breast in psychoanalytic literature has contributed to the haze. This inaccurate analogy is clarified in studies that assign the clitoris as the homologue of the penis (2). Furthermore, if only from the point of view of structure as bilateral pendants, breasts would be better compared with testes and would have a reproductive rather than a sexual status.

Although breasts are capable of vascular engorgement, data regarding the role of breasts in sexual response is inconclusive. Studies generally agree that breast eroticism is potentially present, but not all women find their breasts to be of sexual importance (3, 4). The wide range of female responses to breast stimulation suggests that reactivity may be acquired by sociophysiologic learning as well as by physiology. Sexual values are acquired from culture through the influence of art, advertisements, cinema, theater, television, and literature. Individuals are subjected to overt and covert stimuli idealizing the female breasts. Displays of naked breasts are present in erotic publications hidden under counters and on the covers of women's magazines, sports magazines, and general periodicals sold above counters in supermarkets and stores throughout the country.

A curious feature is the sociopolitical assignment of the female breasts in the 1960s. Associated with the women's liberation movement,

75

the burning of brassieres was construed as a symbolic gesture of freedom from the constraints of male domination. During this phase, the wearing of a bra was equated with submission. Improvement in social and economic opportunities for women has reinstated the value of a brassiere as a natural support, rather than a binder, so that wearing a bra is no longer a stigma.

Cultural attitudes also affect developing children. For the girl, there is an early awareness that the appearance of her breasts is a criterion of her desirability and acceptability as a woman and necessitates constant attention to that part of her anatomy. She feels that her value as a person may be measured by the size and shape of her breasts so that, whatever their actual physical state, she will subliminally interpret her development in terms of societal expectations. When large breasts are equated with greater femininity, she will be unhappy with small ones. Recently, the movement toward physical fitness and exercise has emphasized smaller breasts, and women who are more heavily endowed may be made to feel less adequate.

A widely read popular magazine recently published a tongue-in-cheek article in praise of smaller breasts, which discussed breasts in terms of a "critical erotic mass." It further assigned positive human values to small breasts, while pointing out negative values in women with large breasts (5). Dissatisfaction with breast contours supports a large industry that alters breast size or shape, with plastic surgery as the ultimate resort.

The American male is subject to the same stimuli. How much of his interest in the female breast is biologically, and how much is psychosocially, determined is unclear. The sight of female breasts is often thought to be more of a sexual stimulus than that of female genitalia. Sexual responses developed through psychosocial learning can explain a range of behaviors. Thus, if a man places a high sexual value on his female partner's breasts, the threat of a loss of a breast is a serious deprivation for him as well as for her.

BREAST-FEEDING

In contrast to the fascination with the sexualized breast, there is a fairly prevalent distaste and lack of interest and support for the nursing mother. In an advice-on-etiquette column in a popular magazine, a hostess who had been uneasy about a dinner guest who was nursing her infant was advised to avoid entertaining the woman until she had weaned the child (6). Breast-feeding was common in early American history, and wealthy families hired "wet nurses" to suckle their young. This practice became less common in the industrialized era, when women sought work outside the home. With the decrease in the pattern of breast-feeding came a commensurate increase in the use and sale of proprietary infant formulas, and for decades the sight of an American mother suckling her baby was rare.

There is no longer much doubt that the breast is best. Although there are minimal risks of pathogens and pollutants transmitted through breast milk, and some nutritional deficiency states resulting from poor maternal instruction and support, human milk provides distinct nutritional immunologic and metabolic advantages over bottle-feeding (7–11) (see Chapter 4). Medical approval of breast-feeding has tended to be lukewarm in its support and ill-informed as to the psychoneurophysiology of lactation and the properties of human milk. However, the infant formula industry has filled the gap with media saturation in both the medical and public sectors, extending its market to Third World countries. Evidence from World Fertility Surveys and secondary sources notes that in these countries, although breast-feeding is still nearly universal, particularly in Asia and Africa, in Latin America earlier weaning has become more common. The economic and social consequence of these changes in breast-feeding affects not only the provision of superior nutritional and immunologic protection but also control of fertility through prolongation of the amenorheic phase (12, 13).

Bottle-feeding and breast-feeding cannot be considered interchangeable phenomena either emotionally or psychophysiologically. The interaction between mother and infant in each situation is different. Neonatal-maternal bonding has been shown to relate to that sensitive period during the first day of life and proceeds to a mutually reinforcing reflex behavior, particularly during biologic breast-feeding. "Disorders of mothering," including child abuse and psychosocial maladjustments in childhood, are considered more prevalent in situations of bonding failure. The neonatal somatosensory stimulations and the maternal hormonal status in breast-feeding result in a quality of contact that is more biologically intimate and direct. Serious consideration must be given to the consequences of Western-style neonatal practices of separating the mother and the newborn and the use of bottle-feeding in the development of psychosocial maladaptations (14, 15).

Sexualization of the breasts contributes directly to resistance to breast-feeding. Guilt, shame, repugnance, and male resentment stem from the sexual role. Exposure of the breast is thought to be an abandonment of modesty. The paradox is that in a society where little in women's attire is left to the imagination, hostility is directed toward a public display of nursing. There is embarrassment when exposure reveals breasts that do not conform to the current ideal. The possibility that breast-feeding may cause disfigurement is also a matter of concern.

Physiologic factors also affect resistance to breast-feed. In the sexual response cycle, vascular engorgement, as a reflex associated with pelvic congestion involving the clitoris and vagina, will occur with or without direct breast stimulation. As the cycle proceeds, breast changes occur, with enlargement, nipple erection, and areolar and skin hyperemia. In the resolution phase, vascular decongestion occurs with a gradual return of the breast to the normal state (16).

Men are less well-informed than women about breast feeding and are often inherently opposed to the process. The analytical explanation is competition with the infant for exclusive possession of the woman's breast. Fathers who have not been breast-fed may feel the competition more intensely. Fear that the breasts may lose their erotically arousing shape and reduce sexual pleasure may cause some men to refuse to allow breast-feeding. Usually such negative feelings are not directly expressed, because they may be unconscious or embarrassing. In such cases, a woman who would like to breast-feed cannot fully communicate her feelings to her partner.

Lack of cultural support is the reason that many American women do not know how to breast-feed. Inadequate preparation, lack of permission, and lack of role models and support systems giving the required emotional and social support can result in the "anxiety-nursing failure syndrome" (7). Studies of the prevalence of breast-feeding in Western countries have identified some general features that apply to Americans. Women who choose to breast-feed have made the decision before pregnancy and delivery and are likely to be better educated and relatively more affluent. They are more likely to have been breast-fed themselves and to have watched a mother breast-feed, and they usually have thought about the process and studied in prenatal courses (12, 17). The complex variables affecting a woman's attitude toward nursing include early life experiences, feelings about one's body and nudity, sexuality, the pregnancy, the relationship with the infant's biologic father, the quality and quantity of contact with her mother, the resolution of her developmental

crises, and the availability of support systems. The period in history, and the geographic location, are also determinants of breast-feeding patterns.

SEXUAL CONCERNS IN PATIENT MANAGEMENT

Although the teaching of human sexuality is still not universally considered a legitimate medical concern, the sexual significance of the breast affects medical management. The importance of a sexual history as an integral part of the general medical history must be emphasized, since omission of relevant sexual data leaves the physician with an incomplete data base upon which to arrive at a diagnosis and plan treatment. With an attitude of serious professional concern, the physician should tactfully and candidly question the patient about her sexual concerns and practices in relation to the presenting problem. Successful data gathering depends on a nonjudgmental attitude about sexual issues and skill in integrating the information into the treatment plan and management.

When a woman presents with a breast problem, the sexual factors can easily be assessed by questions such as "Do you understand the implications of the problem?" "Has it affected your sexual functioning?" How does your partner feel about the problem (or the proposed treatment)?" "How will the proposed treatment affect your life?"

Explicit sexual detail may not always be necessary, but basic information is essential, such as "Are you sexually active?" "Are there any problems in your sexual functioning?" "Sexual activity" does not specify heterosexual, homosexual or self-stimulatory behavior, which may not be relevant, depending on the presenting problem. However, specific behaviors should be explored if pathology and treatment might be related to them. When this is the case, not only is a detailed history necessary, but also the physician is responsible for preparing the patient for the possibility of a change in her activities, which may require sexual counseling, either by the physician or a trained sex therapist.

Any planned change in the appearance of the breast caused by invasive techniques (biopsy, mastectomy, plastic procedures, radiation) necessitates information from the couple on how breasts are perceived and their role in the couple's sexual practices and relationship. Fondling, caressing, and suckling female breasts as a sexual stimulus may not always be important, but the partner's needs must be considered. If he has learned that breast stimulation is part of the masculine role and is aroused and gratified by breast petting, his concerns must be addressed as part of the management.

The resistance to breast self-examination is a curious phenomenon that may also be associated with the sexualization of the breasts. The monthly breast self-examination has been an accepted aspect of early screening for breast cancer for many years, but studies consistently reveal that too low a percentage of American women actually examine themselves. Women who had a family history of breast cancer are more likely to practice self-examination. No association of self-examination with educational level, intelligence, or other health practices was demonstrated (18).

Breast self-examination is an intimate experience. It is not only anxiety-provoking because of its association with cancer, pain, and death but also because of its sexual inference. It can be compared to the testicular self-examination, in which an emotionally charged organ may be associated with a life-threatening disease. There is a need to touch oneself slowly and carefully. In both instances, touching can initiate anxiety about masturbation. In cultures that discourage autoarousal, self-examination of erogenous zones is unacceptable, even for health reasons. The physician can educate the patient and give authoritative permission to feel these areas by a supportive and positive attitude.

BREAST PATHOLOGY

Benign Disease

Breast pain is occasionally associated with benign breast disease, but cyclic symptoms of swelling, soreness, and lumpiness occur in at least 90% of women during their reproductive lifetimes and may be considered normal unless intolerably severe. These hormonally induced variants may occur in the presence of palpable thickening in the breasts, especially in the upper outer quadrants, often referred to as fibrocystic change, or even "disease." Since the microscopic form of this process is almost universally present in women, reassurance that it is not generally precancerous is essential (see Chapter 6, Pathology of Benign Breast Disease). Nevertheless, the monthly symptoms have an adverse effect on female sexual function since touch or contact may be painful and may initiate a negative response to sexual overtures. Alleviation of pain and discomfort is the obvious goal in the treatment of mastalgia. In the past, treatment consisted of surgery and analgesics, but present management techniques include many pharmaceutical and dietary remedies, but especially explanation and reassurance. The patient must be made aware that the side effects of some of these drugs can affect sexuality.

Unexplained breast pain is often considered to be a psychosomatic complaint and should be so judged in some cases. A history of sexual abuse as a child or an adult sometimes explains the focus of pain in the breasts or other parts of the body, as a manifestation of the assault, in direct or symbolic fashion. For such patients, psychotherapeutic treatment is indicated, as for any posttraumatic stress disorder. However, recent studies of women with breast pain do not show a greater incidence of neurotic or personality disorder. If the complaint persists and is debilitative, psychiatric consultation may be helpful to clarify the etiologic factors.

Malignant Disease

Studies by the National Cancer Institute and the National Institutes of Health reveal that the greatest health concern of women is breast cancer and that many women would like to play a more active role in their health care and not rely solely on physicians for decision-making and information. When found to have breast cancer, most women request a second medical opinion, with preference for a two-step surgical procedure, if mastectomy is necessary. Most women believe that unnecessary mastectomies are performed. Although nearly all the women had heard of breast self-examination, and a majority felt they were more likely to discover a breast lump before their physicians, fewer reported that they had examined their breasts in the past year, and only 29% said that they had actually performed monthly examinations. Most were aware of the increased risk of breast cancer in families with positive histories. A third were aware of the increased risk of advanced age and late parity (19) (see Chapter 18, Epidemiology of Breast Cancer).

Persistent misconceptions regarding the etiology of breast cancer were reported. Half believed that bumping or bruising of the breasts causes cancer. Black and Hispanic women were more likely to think that caressing or fondling breasts could cause cancer. Although nearly all realized that lumps in the breast might signal cancer, there was less awareness of the significance of nipple changes or breast appearance. There was little information regarding the diagnostic procedures available, and few realized that there are treatment options for breast cancer other than surgery (19).

Breast cancer was generally seen as a medical rather than a social or emotional issue, although Hispanic women tended to focus on the emotional aspect. While 75% of the women discussed surgery, only 15% mentioned mastectomy specifically, and the major concern was whether the cancer could be totally removed and whether there was risk of recurrence. They were more worried about medical costs than physical changes in appearance. Only 2 in 10 were aware of the availability of breast reconstruction in the event of mastectomy, and only 1 in 10 would want reconstruction in order to improve self-esteem and appearance (19).

It is necessary at all levels of management to include the partner and family of a patient with breast cancer in the discussion and counseling, since they play an important role in emotional and physical support during rehabilitation. Anxieties in the patient and her family can be dealt with simultaneously, since the disease and its sequelae affect not only the patient but also those closest to her. The implications of the diagnosis and preparation for the planned workup and treatment must be explained.

Severe anxiety is created by the fear of imminent death associated with the term "cancer." This should be dispelled immediately by verbal assurance that she will "not die tomorrow" and that curative treatment is available. Reduction in anxiety and tension at the outset is important, as fear of death may be so consuming and disabling that treatment may be hindered by helplessness, hopelessness, and noncompliance. When a physician uses the terms "cancer" and "death," it must be in a context that provides a sense of reassurance and hope, not rejection and fear. Truth is of the utmost importance but must not be expressed too boldly. The physician is expected to be someone who understands the medical issues and the human issues as well and can communicate encouragingly with all of those involved.

Additional fears result from lack of knowledge about anatomy and physiology and lack of understanding of hospital procedures. A common misconception is that the breast is like an orange pressed into the chest wall and, if removed, would leave a concavity. Simple descriptions of thoracic anatomy and the axilla, incorporating a discussion of preliminary tests and modalities of treatment, is very reassuring. Visual aids are helpful in giving the patient and partner an understanding of what anatomic or functional changes are expected. If mastectomy is planned, simple line drawings of the surgical approach and resultant scar will prepare the couple for the postoperative body image change. A full discussion of the risks and benefits of the various treatment options is required

in some states to fulfill the legal obligation of informed consent.

Deemphasis of the breast as an overvalued sex or maternal symbol is necessary in the early diagnostic phase to prepare the patient to accept the possible loss of her breast. At this stage, the breast should be perceived as a diseased organ that is a threat to life and is no longer essential. The devaluation of the organ and its separation from the former sexualized valuation may be the first therapeutic step in helping the couple to give it up. Emphasis on the lifesaving aspect may not be heard initially because of the concern about defeminization and disfigurement. Revaluation of the postoperative site as healthy, with replacement of the breast by a well-healed scar and reassurance that the woman is a "whole" woman, with or without a breast, aids the acceptance of the change.

Other myths which require early clarification are: (a) cancer always recurs or kills; (b) the patient may spread the disease because cancer is communicable; (c) the patient has caused the cancer by some past sin of omission or commission; and (d) the patient will lose sexual interest or desirability.

The most stressful time in the whole treatment period is felt by many women to be the time between biopsy of the discovered lesion and the definitive diagnosis. This waiting period can offer a time for reorganizing and reviewing the priorities of living, because of the awareness of the immediate reality of death, which often has been denied.

If diagnosis leads to mastectomy, adaptation to hospitalization, prospective loss of a body part and restoration of physical function become the primary concerns. Response to body change is often associated with a depressed, postoperative "fatigue" state, usually occurring within the first week after surgery (20). Symptoms include lassitude, anxiety, irritability, anorexia, insomnia, feelings of worthlessness, and shame. These symptoms usually appear on about the 4th postoperative day and should not persist beyond a month. If they last longer, factors other than breast loss and physiologic stress may be present, and psychiatric consultation is indicated.

Restoration of body image and functioning should be encouraged soon after surgery. The patient can be assured that although her body has changed, her self-worth has not, and she can be invited to see the scar at the time of the first dressing change, with the surgeon or nurse as support persons. If the patient is too emotionally unstable to look at the wound, time should be allowed for adaptation, and she should be encouraged to look at a later time.

The first view of the site of excision commonly produces a sense of the reality of the situation. Tears and anxiety are a normal part of the grief reaction. Women who refuse to look by the time of discharge may be a high risk for problems in adjustment to the change and may require further surveillance for maladaptive responses.

Tactile changes are part of the adaptation process experienced by the patient and her partner. When the wound is healed, both are encouraged to touch the unaffected side, then gently move the fingers over the affected area to learn subjective and objective sensations. Changes in skin sensations, such as numbness and paresthesias, are noted, and the patient can be reassured as to whether these are to be expected and as to whether they are likely to be permanent. Recognizing that women are often too inhibited to touch their bodies, the physician may have to give permission and encouragement for her to do this.

Resumption of sexual activity should be encouraged. This reestablishes a sense of body integrity and reintegrates the feminine sexual identity.

Symmetry and balance are of concern. The option to use a prosthetic cotton puff in the bra should be encouraged prior to discharge from the hospital. The Reach for Recovery volunteer group of postmastectomized women sponsored by the American Cancer Society can be helpful by providing counsel on dress, appearance, and the return to family and community. They also offer a role model for successful adaptation to mastectomy.

The phantom breast syndrome has been reported to occur among many mastectomy patients. Depending on the study, the range of occurrence is from one-quarter to one-half of such women. Symptoms range from awareness of a breast that does not exist to itching, aching, tightness, numbness, burning, tingling, and heaviness. There is no set pattern of onset or relationship to fatigue, mood, sexual state, or looking at the operative site. Some studies suggest that psychological factors, such as sexual attitudes toward the breast or maternal identification, are relevant, while others do not (21–23). These symptoms have varying effects on rehabilitation. The high-risk group appears to be associated with youth, premenopausal women subject to postoperative depression and women who felt they had a poor relationship with their partners or their surgeons. This points to the significant role of the physician in the education and support of the patient in the preoperative and rehabilitation phases.

Breast cancer in pregnancy presents particular problems. The difficulty of managing a potentially lethal, hormonally sensitive tumor in a host undergoing complex, progressive, and possibly adverse endocrine change is obvious. The reproductive issue may supersede the woman's concern about the threat to her own life or to the loss of a breast. Ambivalent feelings about the pregnancy may give rise to anger and guilt, anger at the fetus for causing the cancer or negative feelings that she is being punished for getting pregnant. Carrying the pregnancy to term is a stress state, since the mother and her family are concerned with the health and status of the fetus, the effect of the mother's treatment on fetal health, and whether the mother will live long enough to raise the child to adulthood. Further concerns will be whether further pregnancies should be avoided or, if they should occur, whether they should be terminated (24).

For many women, external prostheses are inadequate. They are psychologically crippled by a sense of deformity, and replacement by breast reconstruction is essential. In such cases, it is necessary to set realistic goals; a normal appearance can be realized when clothed, but perfect replacement may not be possible, nor can scars be entirely obliterated. Women who cannot clearly specify what they want may need further evaluation to rule out other serious emotional conflicts associated with reconstructive surgery.

When the primary treatment is radiotherapy, the sequelae are not so obvious as with breast loss, but harder consistency, loss of sensation, skin changes, and fear of local recurrence bring their own set of problems to the recovering patient. The effect on sexual function is less direct, but response to radiotherapy also includes a depressive component and fatigue.

Chemotherapy involves not only the physiologic response to the chemotherapeutic agent but also the side effects of gastrointestinal upset, fatigue, debilitation, depression, and decreased libido. Symptomatic treatment and support to increase physical strength (including attention to adequate nutrition) are essential to a sense of power, control and self-esteem which, in turn, may enhance the sexual component.

The debilitating effects of surgery, irradiation, and adjuvant chemotherapy inevitably inhibit sexual function. Nevertheless, it should be recommended that, when the patient is emotionally and physically ready, a return to sexual function is important, and there should be no alteration in capacity. Studies of male response to mastectomy reveal that it often is less of a problem than expected and that communication and love are more important in sexual rehabilitation. Partners are encouraged to be openly expressive of love and desire and to reassure the patient of continuing support. Inability to return to sexual activity when there is a concerned, caring, and willing partner suggests serious psychologic conflict and may require therapeutic attention (25).

The rhetorical question as to whether the female breasts are either symbols or organs can be answered simply: they are both. The awareness of the cultural and emotional attitudes towards the breasts is necessarily a medical/surgical responsibility for those caring for patients with breast disorders.

REFERENCES

1. Mead M. Male and female. New York, Morrow, 1975:231.
2. Lowry TP, Lowry TS. The clitoris. St. Louis: Green, 1976:9–86.
3. Kinsey AC, Pomeroy WB, Martin CE. Sexual behavior in the human female. Philadelphia: Saunders, 1953.
4. Pion RJ, Reich LA. Role of the breast in female sexual response. Med Aspects Hum Sex 1975;9:103–109.
5. Leonard A. In praise of small breasts. Forum 1983;12:27–37.
6. Post EL. Etiquette for everyday: the new Emily Post. Good Housekeeping June 1978;198:70.
7. Jelliffe DB, Jeliffe EFP. Breast is best, modern meanings. N Engl J Med 1977;297:912–915.
8. Glass RI, Svennerholm AM, Stoll BJ, et al. Protection against cholera in breast-fed children by antibodies in breast milk. N Engl J Med 1983;308:1389–1392.
9. Hambraeus L. Proprietary milk versus human breast milk in infant feeding. Pediatr Clin North Am 1977;24:17–36.
10. Rogan WJ, Bagniewska A, Damstra T. Pollutants in breast milk. N Engl J Med 1980;302:1450–1453.
11. Stagno S, Reynolds DW, Pass RF, Alford CA. Breast milk and the risk of cytomegalovirus infection. N Engl J Med 1980;302:1073–1076.
12. Martinez GA, Dodd DA. 1981 milk feeding patterns in the U.S. during the first twelve months of life. Pediatrics 1983;71:166–170.
13. Popkin BM, Bilsborrow RE, Akin JS. Breast feeding patterns in low income countries. Science 1982;218:1088–1093.
14. Cole JP. Breast feeding in the Boston suburbs in relation to personal-social factors. Clin Pediatr 1977;16:352–356.
15. Lynch MA. Ill health and child abuse. Lancet 1975;2:317–319.
16. Masters WH, Johnson VE. Human sexual response. Boston: Little, Brown, 1966;224–226.
17. Lewellyn-Jones D. The psychosocial aspects of breast feeding. In: Dennerstein L, Burrows GD, eds. Proceedings of the Ninth Annual Congress of the Australian Society for Psychosomatic Obstetrics/Gynecology. Victoria, Australia: York Press Property, 1982:67–82.
18. Baker LH. Breast Cancer Demonstration Project: five-year summary report. Cancer 1982;32:194–225.
19. National Institutes of Health: National survey on breast cancer. NIH Publication No. 84-2306 1984:1–30.
20. Rose EA, King TC. Understanding postoperative fatigue. Surg Gynecol Obstet 1978;147:97-102.
21. Jamison E, Wellisch DK, Katz RL, Pasnau RO. Phantom breast syndrome. Arch Surg 1979;114:93–95.
22. Ackerly W, Lhamon W, Fitts WT Jr. Phantom breast. J Nerv Ment Dis 1955;121:177–178.
23. Jarvis JH. Post-mastectomy breast phantoms. J Nerv Ment Dis 1967;144:266–272.
24. Donegan WL. Breast cancer and pregnancy. Obstet Gynecol 1977;50:244–252.
25. Frank D, Dornbush RL, Webster SK, Kolodny RC. Mastectomy and sexual behavior: a pilot study. Sex Disabil 1978;1:16–26.

6

Pathology of Benign Breast Disease

Ibrahim Ramzy

Many women seek medical advice because of breast masses. The breast responds to the presence or absence of estrogens, progesterone, prolactin, cortisol, and other substances by proliferation, secretion, involution, and fibrosis. This may be associated with the development of "lumps," which are a source of concern, since breast carcinoma is the most common cancer in women and, with the exception of lung carcinoma, has the highest mortality rate in the Western world. In this chapter, the gross morphology and histopathology of benign breast disease are considered. The discussion will include inflammatory and reactive conditions, hyperplastic and benign neoplastic lesions, and the role of cytology in diagnosis.

CONGENITAL ANOMALIES

Congenital anomalies of the breast are rare. The terms *athelia* and *amastia* signify the absence of the nipple or breast, respectively, and may be unilateral or bilateral. Polythelia denotes the presence of a supernumerary nipple, while polymastia indicates the presence of accessory breast glandular tissue. Both conditions can occur along the milk line, which extends from the axilla to the vulva.

INFLAMMATORY LESIONS

Acute Mastitis

Inflammatory conditions of the breast may be acute or chronic and may be caused by a variety of factors, including infectious agents, foreign bodies, or trauma. Acute mastitis is usually the result of spread of microorganisms from the nipple, particularly during lactation or when there is a disruption of the skin surface. Most cases are caused by *Staphylococcus aureus*,

while a few cases are due to streptococci and other organisms.

Gross Features

The breast shows the usual features of acute inflammation, with swelling, edema, congestion and, occasionally, nipple discharge. An abscess may form in the subareolar or deep glandular tissues. It contains an inflammatory exudate, and although these cases present little diagnostic difficulty, aspiration may be necessary to drain the abscess cavity, to obtain material for culture, or to exclude an "inflammatory" carcinoma. Diffuse cellulitis occasionally develops as a result of spread of infection along the ducts into the soft tissues without localization of the infection. Acute mastitis usually resolves following proper treatment, but fibrosis may develop, and fistula formation is rare.

Microscopic Features

In the early phases, there is edema of the periductal and interlobular stroma, with congestion and infiltration by acute inflammatory cells. The ducts are often distended due to accumulation of neutrophils and retained secretions. When an abscess is formed, a central area of necrosis with fibrin and bacterial colonies appears, surrounded by an intense accumulation of neutrophils (Fig. 6.1). Aspirates from such areas produce an abundance of neutrophils with debris.

Chronic Mastitis

This term should be limited to true inflammatory conditions of the breast. It should not be used to indicate fibrocystic and hyperplastic lesions, which are often associated with some

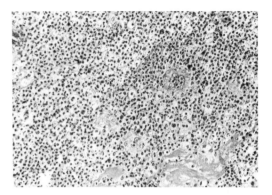

Figure 6.1. Acute breast abscess. The center of an abscess showing dense infiltrate of neutrophils and fibrinous exudate around degenerating small ducts.

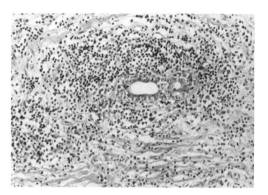

Figure 6.2. Chronic mastitis. The periductal inflammatory infiltrate consists of lymphocytes, plasma cells, and some histiocytes.

lymphocytic infiltrate but are not inflammatory in origin. Chronic mastitis may follow acute mastitis or may be of insidious onset. The causative organisms are similar to those responsible for acute mastitis. In addition to these "nonspecific" types, a granulomatous subgroup may be encountered and is discussed separately.

Gross Features

Chronic inflammation may result in a clinical and gross picture that mimics carcinoma, presenting as a slowly growing, nontender hard mass. Occasionally, abscess formation is encountered. The abscess has a poorly defined fibrous wall; its cavity contains a variable amount of creamy-yellowish debris, and the surrounding fibrosis may cause nipple retraction, adding to the risk of confusion with malignancy.

Microscopic Features

The wall of the abscess consists of fibrous tissue, which is heavily infiltrated by lymphocytes, plasma cells, and histiocytes (Fig. 6.2). A variable number of neutrophils is also seen, particularly when there is exacerbation of the acute phase. The inflammatory exudate extends into the breast tissue surrounding the abscess cavity, and the epithelial cells may show degenerative changes. Aspiration can establish the inflammatory nature of the lesion, provided that multiple samplings are performed in order to exclude the possibility of aspirating the necrotic center of a carcinoma.

Granulomas

Tuberculosis, actinomycosis, blastomycosis, cryptococcosis, and other granulomatous diseases rarely involve the breast. This is usually secondary to disease in other organs, and the accompanying inflammatory response in the breast is similar to that observed in these organs. Fistulas and abscesses may develop, and the resulting mass of scar tissue may be associated with nipple retraction, thus mimicking cancer. The diagnosis can be established by the demonstration of organisms using special stains and culture. Rare cases of sarcoidosis have been reported in the breast and in the regional nodes, but sarcoid-type reaction may also accompany carcinomas.

Foreign Body Mastitis

The introduction of synthetic material during mammoplasty, particularly silicone, may be followed by chronic inflammation. Rupture of the device or the development of leaks induces fibrosis and foreign body reaction, and patients may become apprehensive about the resulting ill-defined areas of induration around the prosthesis.

Microscopic Features

Intense infiltration by chronic inflammatory cells is seen, particularly in the early phases. Lymphocytes and histiocytes are prominent, as well as multinucleated foreign body giant cells. Globules of opaque refractile foreign material or crystals are seen within the giant cells as well as free in the stroma. Fat necrosis is not uncommon around such areas, and extensive fibrosis develops eventually (Fig. 6.3). If aspirated, the aspirate is comprised of lymphocytes, histiocytes, and plasma cells, together with ductal cells. A few atypical ductal cells may be encountered in such aspirates.

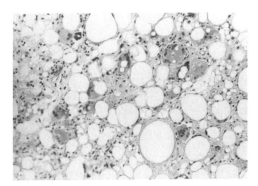

Figure 6.3. Foreign body reaction to silicone. The cytoplasmic vacuoles are distended with grayish foreign material. The fat cells exhibit variation in their size, and some (*at right*) have opaque cytoplasm. Note fibroblastic proliferation and multinucleated giant cells.

Plasma Cell Mastitis

This condition, often referred to as duct ectasia, affects older women and is characterized by dilatation of the mammary ducts, destruction of the lining epithelium, and chronic inflammation. Whether the dilatation appears first, followed by inflammation, or the inflammatory process destroys the epithelium, causing the dilatation, is not known.

Gross Features

The major ducts in the subareolar region are dilated, and a thick creamy white or greenish exudate may be seen in their lumen. Longstanding cases may be associated with extensive fibrosis, resulting in nipple retraction similar to that with cancer. The picture may be confused further by the appearance of a bloody discharge or the development of skin reaction around the nipple, suggesting Paget's disease.

Microscopic Features

The lumen of the dilated ducts is increasingly distended due to accumulation of granular lipid and proteinaceous secretions, crystalloid debris, ceroid-containing histiocytes, plasma cells, and lymphocytes. The lining epithelium is eventually replaced by a thin layer of epithelium or is completely destroyed, with fibrosis of the duct wall. The periductal breast tissue is infiltrated by similar chronic inflammatory exudate that is rich in histiocytes and plasma cells. Foreign body reaction to the contents of the lactiferous ducts is evident, and the elastic fibers may be increased in the surrounding stroma, which is similar to the response to infiltrating carcinoma cells (1).

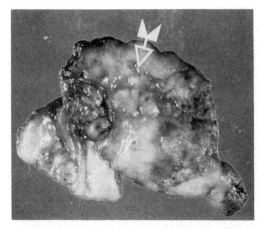

Figure 6.4. Fat necrosis. This hard mass was resected from the breast of a patient who had no definite history of trauma. Note necrotic calcified foci at *arrow*.

NECROSIS AND VASCULAR DISORDERS

Fat Necrosis

Necrosis of adipose tissue within the breast may follow trauma or augmentation mammoplasty using silicone or other injections. It may also be associated with necrosis developing in malignant neoplasms (2). A history of trauma with ecchymosis and pain is only elicited in about half the cases.

Gross Features

Fat necrosis presents as a small firm or hard nodular mass of insidious onset. The consistency, adhesion to skin, lack of pain, and yellowish-white color, as well as the presence of calcific deposits on mammography, add to the confusion with carcinoma. The involved area may show evidence of recent or old hemorrhage in the form of pigmentation. Older lesions for cystic spaces filled with altered liquefied fat, which is eventually replaced by fibrous tissue with calcific deposits (Fig. 6.4).

Microscopic Features

The adipose tissue is altered; the normally clear cytoplasm of the fat cells becomes opaque, homogeneous, or granular. It may stain pale blue or red in routine hematoxylin and eosin sections, and the damaged cells coalesce, forming larger spaces. Abundant histiocytic foam cells, occasionally with mitotic figures and nuclear pleomorphism, are seen. The necrotic fat induces a foreign body inflammatory response of lymphocytes, plasma cells, multinucleated histiocytes, and a few neutrophils. Repair is associated with the appearance of fibroblasts and young lipoblasts, the latter showing small cytoplasmic vacuoles. In chronic cases, extensive fibrosis is seen, and the fibroblasts may have atypical nuclear features. Although the histologic picture is characteristic, careful sampling of different areas of the lesion is necessary since malignant tumors may be associated with foci of fat necrosis.

Massive Necrosis and Infarction

Massive necrosis has been reported with the use of anticoagulants, while infarcts can occur during pregnancy or lactation, as well as in association with atherosclerosis in older patients.

HYPERPLASTIC, FIBROTIC, AND CYSTIC DISORDERS

The cyclic changes of breast tissue, under the influence of hormones, induces epithelial and stromal changes. In about 50% of women, areas of fibrosis and/or cyst formation develop. Several terms, such as mammary dysplasia, benign mastopathy, epithelial and fibrocystic mastopathy, fibrocystic disease, Schimmelbusch's disease, and chronic cystic mastitis, were previously used to encompass this broad group of morphologic changes. The condition affects women between 20 and 45 years of age, frequently presenting as a bilateral irregular induration that may be associated with pain and tenderness, particularly around menses.

Although the pathogenesis is not clear, it appears that an imbalance in the levels of estrogen and progesterone, or an altered target tissue sensitivity to these hormones may be the major factor responsible for the epithelial and stromal changes (3, 4). Oral contraceptives reduce the incidence of changes with minimal epithelial atypia but have no effect on those with marked epithelial atypias (5). Genetic makeup, age, parity, and lactational history, as well as psychosomatic factors, may also play a role. The epithelial hyperplasia and metaplasia are often associated with desquamation of the cells, blockage of some ducts, and the formation of cysts. The latter may also develop independent of any significant hyperplasia. Variable degrees of fibrosis and chronic inflammatory cell infiltrate are seen in the stroma.

While the majority of these changes are not premalignant, some may have a precancerous potential, particularly the atypical ductal hyperplasia (6) (Table 6.1). It is now generally accepted that a diagnosis of "fibrocystic disease" is not a complete one and should be qualified by indicating the type of changes present and whether or not epithelial atypia is seen. More than one type is usually encountered in the same breast, often intermixed within the same microscopic field. These types include cysts, fibrosis, apocrine metaplasia, and epithelial hyperplasia. The latter may be in the form of adenosis, sclerosing adenosis, intraductal hyperplasia with or without atypia, and papillomatosis. In addition to these, it seems appropriate to discuss other hypertrophic and cystic lesions, including juvenile hypertrophy and galactocele at this point.

Cysts

Cysts of variable sizes are found in the breasts of more than 50% of women (7). They occur in clusters, with the majority being a few millimeters in diameter while some may reach 1 to 4 cm. Microcysts, which can only be appreciated on microscopic examination, may represent involution of small ducts and lobules. Most small cysts have a firm, "shotty" consistency due to distension. They contain clear serous or straw-colored fluid and appear pale blue (blue-domed cysts). Larger cysts form fluctuant lesions that may contain brown fluid due to hemorrhage and have a fibrous wall (Fig. 6.5).

Microscopic Features

Blue-domed cysts are originally lined by the usual two layers of cuboidal to low columnar epithelium and myoepithelium. When obstruction ensues, the lining cells become flattened and may be disrupted in some areas. Cysts are often lined by apocrine metaplastic epithelium.

In some cysts the contents appear as homogeneous or granular eosinophilic material. In others, the lumen is filled with foam cells and occasionally cholesterol crystals, as a result of hemorrhage or accumulation of lipid secretions. When the cyst contents leak into the surrounding stroma following thinning and rupture of the wall, an inflammatory reaction is induced. This consists of lymphocytes, plasma cells, and histiocytes and some multinucleated foreign body giant cells.

Apocrine Metaplasia

This is characterized by a morphologic change in the epithelium lining the ducts and cysts. Apocrine metaplasia may appear as small brown foci on gross examination but may be intimately mingled within foci of fibrosis and hyperplasia.

Table 6.1. Fibrocystic Changes and Risk of Invasive Cancer[a]

No Increase	Slight Increase (1.5–2×)	Moderate Increase (5×)
Adenosis, sclerosing or florid	Hyperplasia	Atypical hyperplasia
Apocrine metaplasia	moderate or florid[b]	ductal
Cysts	solid or papillary	lobular
Duct ectasia	Papilloma with fibrovascular core	
Fibroadenoma		
Fibrosis		
Mastitis, inflammatory		
Mastitis, periductal		
Squamous metaplasia		
Hyperplasia, mild[c]		

[a]Based on biopsy examination; patients compared with women who have had no biopsy (Consensus report, College of American Pathologists, 1985).
[b]More than four epithelial cells in depth.
[c]Three to four epithelial cells in depth.

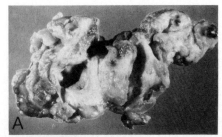

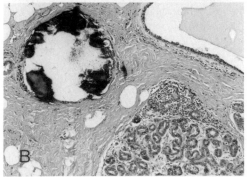

Figure 6.5. Breast cysts. (A) A firm breast mass with calcific deposits on mammography. Several "blue-dnmed" cysts surrounded by pale fibrous tissue are evident. (B) Histologic section showing epithelial hyperplasia and a cyst lined by a thin double-layered epithelium and containing homogeneous secretion. Note stromal fibrosis and the calcific deposit. (B is from Ramzy I. Clinical cytopathology and aspiration biopsy. Norwalk, CT: Appleton-Lange, 1990).

Microscopic Features

The metaplastic cells are large, polygonal, with well-defined cell borders, and they form a single flat layer or papillary folds. The cytoplasm is abundant and has a large number of brightly eosinophilic refractile granules that represent mitochondria by electron microscopy. Many cells

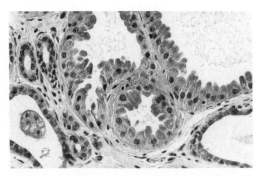

Figure 6.6. Apocrine metaplasia. Three ducts in the center are lined by large cells with granular cytoplasm that stains with eosin. The cytoplasm protrudes into the lumen, and the nuclei are slightly larger than those of the surrounding ducts. Note cystic dilatation of the metaplastic ducts. (From Ramzy I. Clinical cytopathology and aspiration biopsy. Norwalk, CT: Appleton-Lange, 1990.)

have a dome-like cytoplasmic protrusion toward the lumen, referred to as apocrine, or apical, bleb (Fig. 6.6). The nuclei are slightly oval or round, equally spaced, and although they may be large, their chromatin is uniform. Many nuclei contain single nucleoli. Occasionally, papillary infoldings may be seen in metaplastic foci. The presence of metaplasia is usually an assuring sign of the benign nature of a particular lesion, but malignant tumors of apocrine differentiation are known to occur (see Chapter 7).

Stromal Fibrosis and Inflammatory Cell Infiltrate

Diffuse fibrous tissue proliferation of the breast occurs in association with the reduction of the gland cell mass after menopause. Unlike this normal manifestation of aging, many patients develop fibrosis at a much younger age. This re-

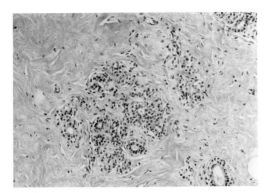

Figure 6.7. Fibrosis. Breast tissue in a postmenopausal patient showing stromal fibrosis, small ducts, and a lymphocytic infiltrate in the stroma.

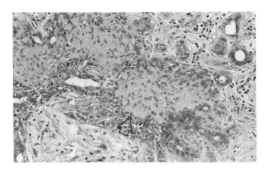

Figure 6.8. Myoepithelial hyperplasia. The stroma around the ducts contains nodules of proliferating myoepithelial cells (*arrow*), with small uniform nuclei and abundant pale eosinophilic cytoplasm.

sults in the formation of ill-defined areas of stromal fibrosis. In advanced disease, the fibrous tissue may produce distinct nodules that can be palpated within the softer breast tissue. These areas may be clinically and mammographically suspected of being a desmoplastic reaction to an infiltrative carcinoma, particularly when they are accompanied by calcification.

Microscopic Features

Fibrosis usually surrounds the breast acini and ducts. The loose connective tissue around the small ducts and acini within the lobules is gradually replaced by a more dense and solid mature collagenous fibrous tissue (Fig. 6.7). The collagen stains brightly eosinophilic and may eventually become hyalinized. Calcific deposits may be seen among areas of fibrosis.

An inflammatory cell infiltrate is often seen in association with stromal fibrosis and epithelial hyperplasia. Lymphocytes and histiocytes

predominate this infiltrate, with an occasional plasma cell or neutrophil. This infiltrate is not a reflection of infection, and the use of the term chronic cystic mastitis for this condition should be discouraged.

Epithelial Hyperplasia (Adenosis, Epitheliosis)

This term refers to benign hyperplastic proliferation of the epithelium of the terminal duct/lobule or larger ducts. There is some confusion in the use of these terms (8, 9). Adenosis denotes proliferation of the lobular elements, while epitheliosis refers to hyperplasia of ductal or lobular elements of the breast. Ductal hyperplasia and papillomatosis may develop with or without atypia. Sclerosing adenosis indicates proliferation of predominantly lobular elements. Other lesions that may be related include microglandular adenosis and myoepithelial hyperplasia.

Adenosis

This refers to enlargement of the lobules beyond the average range of 10 to 100 acini (10). The term is rarely used in the United States unless qualified, such as in the case of blunt adenosis or sclerosing adenosis. *Blunt duct adenosis* refers to enlargement of lobules, with change of the epithelium into columnar rather than cuboidal cells. The resulting two-layered structures have a blunt outline. The cells have hyperchromatic oval nuclei and show cytoplasmic protrusions into the lumen. The number of units within each lobule is not increased, and microcysts are often seen (9).

Secretory changes may occur in some foci, particularly in women who are receiving exogenous hormones. The cells become cuboidal with vacuolated cytoplasm, and the lumen is distended by the secretion. The latter stains positively for α-lactalbumin and casein (11).

Microglandular Adenosis

This is a recently recognized lesion characterized by proliferation of small acini, lined by a single layer of cuboidal cells (12, 13). No lobular pattern or myoepithelial cells are seen. The lesion may result in a mass, but unlike tubular carcinoma, there is no cellular atypia, cytoplasmic protrusion, or cellular bridging, and no in situ carcinoma in the surrounding tissues.

Hyperplasia of Myoepithelium

In some patients, particularly in menopause, the ductal epithelium becomes atrophic and is surrounded by several layers of hyper-

Table 6.2.   Atypical Hyperplasia and Intraductal (In Situ) Carcinoma

Atypical Hyperplasia	Intraductal Cribriform Carcinoma
Glandular spaces irregular, ill-defined	Punched-out, uniform round spaces
Necrosis and histiocytes in lumen rare	Necrosis present, with histiocytes
Hemorrhage, calcification rare	Common
Cells crowded with overlapping nuclei	Cells evenly spaced, no overlapping
Bridges have epithelium, myoepithelium with nuclei parallel to longitudinal axis	Only epithelium, no myoepithelium[a], nuclei lose polarity and lie across axis
Epithelial cell nuclei oval normochromic with rare nucleoli, rare mitosis	Nuclei round hyperchromatic, often with large nucleoli, mitosis frequent and abnormal
Apocrine metaplasia common	Less likely to be intimately mixed

[a]Except in the peripheral part.

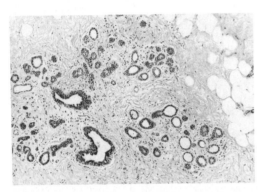

Figure 6.9.   Epithelial hyperplasia. In addition to stromal fibrosis, this breast shows cystic dilatation of the small terminal ducts in the lobules, forming microcysts.

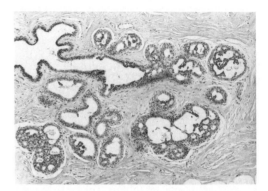

Figure 6.10.   Epithelial hyperplasia. The ducts are dilated and show proliferation of the epithelium. Note the cell bridges that cross the lumen.

plastic myoepithelial cells. These cells often radiate from the central ductal or acinar epithelium and have an eosinophilic cytoplasm that stains positively for myosin (Fig. 6.8). This finding may be part of sclerosing adenosis and appears to have little significance.

Intraductal Epithelial Hyperplasia (Without Atypia)

This condition, occasionally referred to as epitheliosis, is fairly common in postmenopausal women (14). The gross features are not specific, and the lesions are multifocal, with intricate mingling with fibrotic and cystic areas within the breast tissue.

Microscopic Features

The number of layers of epithelium increases, and the lumen outline becomes irregular. This is due to variation in the height of the epithelium and the presence of solid epithelial infoldings referred to as intraductal papillomatosis (Fig. 6.9). The lumen is distended by a mixture of epithelial and myoepi-

thelial cells. These cells form bridges that break the lumen into irregularly shaped spaces, unlike the uniform punched out spaces of cribriform intraductal carcinoma. The epithelial and myoepithelial cells are arranged along the longitudinal axes of the bridges (15). The nuclei of the epithelial cells are oval, irregularly spaced, and are not enlarged. They are cytologically bland, maintaining uniform distribution and the vesicular nature of the chromatin. Nucleoli and mitotic figures are rare. Myoepithelial cells have darker, smaller, more elongated nuclei, as compared with those of epithelial cells. A few lymphocytes may also be present. No necrosis is seen in benign epithelial hyperplasia, a feature that helps differentiate it from carcinoma (Table 6.2).

Intraductal "microscopic" papillomatosis is usually a part of epithelial hyperplasia (Fig. 6.10). The proliferating epithelial lining often folds within the lumen. The resulting papillary formations are usually small and, unlike true papillomas, they are almost always multiple, affect small ducts, and lack fibrovascular cores. Uniform nuclei and the presence of an outer myo-

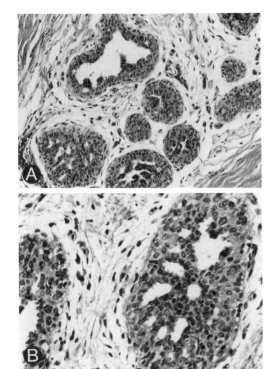

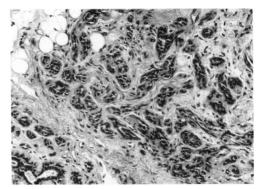

Figure 6.12. Sclerosing adenosis. The breast shows cords of epithelial cells surrounded by bands of dense fibrous tissue. The cords do not show a lumen, except in a rare focus, and the nuclei are not enlarged, irregular, or hyperchromatic. Note that the lobular pattern is partially preserved.

Figure 6.11. Atypical hyperplasia. **A,** The proliferation resulted in distension of the ducts by a mixed population of epithelial and myoepithelial cells. Note the bridges that divide the lumen into irregularly shaped spaces and the micropapillae. Contrast to the cribriform intraductal carcinoma illustrated in Chapter 7. **B,** Detail of two ducts to illustrate slight nuclear atypia. Such patients should be followed closely since they are at high risk for developing carcinoma.

epithelial cell layer supports the benign nature of these changes.

Atypical Epithelial Hyperplasia

Atypical ductal hyperplasias are lesions exhibiting borderline atypical cellular features that are not quite diagnostic of intraductal carcinoma. These lesions, however, are thought to be precancerous. In some studies, foci of intraductal carcinoma were reported in about half the cases (14).

Microscopic Features

In addition to histologic characteristics of hyperplasia, some features indicate atypia. These include dominance of the epithelial cell component over the myoepithelium, the presence of nuclear hyperchromasia and pleomorphism, a high nuclear-cytoplasmic ratio, and the presence of a few, but normal, mitotic

figures (Fig. 6.11). There is considerable overlap between these features and those of intraductal carcinoma, even on an ultrastructural level. Necrosis, however, is usually absent.

Sclerosing Adenosis

This is the outcome of epithelial and myoepithelial proliferation, accompanied by pronounced fibrosis. It is uncommon before 30 years of age but has been reported in 7 to 20% of breast biopsies. The lesions produce ill-defined masses of firm fibrous tissue that may mimic carcinoma grossly, including the presence of chalky streaks within the mass. Their consistency, however, is not as hard and cartilaginous as carcinoma, and most sclerotic lesions lack the yellowish-white areas of necrosis (Table 6.3). Occasionally, sclerosing adenosis produces a hard, central, dense fibrous core surrounded by softer lobulated areas.

Microscopic Features

Following an early cellular phase in which mitotic figures may be seen, bands of mature fibrous tissue surround the hyperplastic epithelium, compressing it into small distorted islands of ductal and acinar cells. The islands of distorted ducts and acini are surrounded by basement membrane material that can be demonstrated histochemically. In some areas, the epithelium is not identifiable as two layers, and differentiation from the "Indian file" arrangement of infiltrating carcinomas may be difficult, particularly in a frozen section. Perineural and vascular invasion has been reported in 2 to 3.9% of cases (16, 17). Careful examination usually reveals that the cell cord separates into two layers of epithelium-myo-

Table 6.3.   Sclerosing Adenosis and Carcinoma

Sclerosing Adenosis	Infiltrating Adenocarcinoma
Double layers when open	Single file or solid cord
Fibrocystic changes nearby	Fibrocystic changes not necessarily close
Lobular pattern partially preserved	Lobular pattern destroyed
No necrosis	Necrosis present
Apocrine metaplasia present	No apocrine metaplasia
Nuclei small, uniform, normochromic	Nuclei large with coarse chromatin, nucleoli
No intraductal carcinoma nearby	Foci of intraductal carcinoma nearby
No elastosis in adjacent stroma	Elastosis present

epithelium in some foci and that the nuclei are not enlarged, irregular, or hyperchromic (Fig. 6.12). Furthermore, the breast tissue retains its lobular pattern and may show apocrine metaplasia and unquestionably benign fibrous areas in the immediate vicinity. If, after careful study of a frozen section, there is doubt as to the nature of a lesion, the diagnosis of malignancy vs. benignancy should be deferred until permanent sections are prepared the next day.

A variant, referred to as *sclerosing papillary ductal proliferation* or radial scar, has been reported (18, 19). In this lesion, sclerotic hyperplastic ducts radiate from a central scar that is also rich in elastic tissue (20). Calcification may be prominent, but the cytologic features of malignancy are lacking.

Lobular Hyperplasia

Lobular hyperplasia, similar to lobular carcinoma, refers to a group of hyperplastic and neoplastic lesions characterized by certain morphologic and behavioral features. Although lobular hyperplasia and lobular carcinoma in situ (LCIS) are usually seen in the lobules, they are not limited to these structures and may extend to the interlobular ducts. Mixtures of lobular and ductal lesions may also be encountered and, in some cases, the differentiation may not be feasible.

Lobular hyperplasia is often multifocal or bilateral and has no characteristic gross features. Microscopically, there is partial filling of the acini by the hyperplastic cells. These cells do not occlude the lumen completely and, unlike sclerosing adenosis, the lobular architecture is not distorted (Fig. 6.13). The small round or cuboidal hyperplastic cells are not uniformly spaced, and they have scant cytoplasm. The uniform, round, or slightly ovoid nuclei are larger than those of normal cells but smaller than in ductal hyperplasia. They are crowded and overlap. The presence of a mixture of acinar, myoepithelial, and lymphocytic cells; the incomplete filling of the acini; the lack of distension of the lobules and terminal ducts, as well as the absence of active mitosis, differentiate lobular hy-

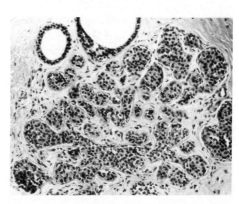

Figure 6.13.   Lobular hyperplasia. The lobules are partially filled by small cells with slightly enlarged nuclei and mixed with myoepithelial cells. Note preservation of lobular architecture and lack of mitosis.

perplasia from LCIS. However, atypical lobular hyperplasia is associated with an increased risk of developing carcinoma. The risk varies from 12 to 25%, with the higher figure associated with young age (below 45 years) and the presence of severe atypia (21, 22).

Juvenile (Virginal) Hypertrophy

The increase in the circulating estrogens at the time of menarche induces the development of the breast. Juvenile hypertrophy may be a manifestation of increased secretion of estrogenic hormones due to hypothalamic, hypophysial, adrenal, or ovarian dysfunction, such as the development of a granulosa cell tumor. It may also be the result of increased sensitivity of the tissues to normal levels of the hormone, and it may be associated with precocious puberty. Hypertrophy may be bilateral and is reflected histologically by ductal and stromal proliferation. The ducts are dilated and enlarged, with tufting of individual epithelial cells into the lumen. The stroma may be edematous or myxoid, or it may exhibit an increase of adipose tissue. However, the contribution

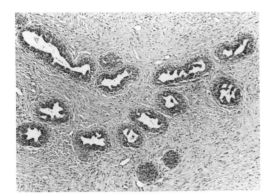

Figure 6.14. Juvenile hypertrophy. The proliferation is predominantly ductal and stromal, not acinar. There is tufting of individual cells within the ductal lumen.

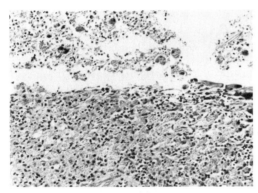

Figure 6.15. Galactocele. The epithelial lining has been destroyed, and the lumen of the distended duct contains cell debris, foam cells, and some chronic inflammatory cells. The periductal tissues are heavily infiltrated by chronic inflammatory cells, including histiocytes, lymphocytes, and plasma cells.

from terminal acinar epithelium is minimal (Fig. 6.14). In men, hypertrophy is referred to as gynecomastia and may result from excess estrogen such as is caused by inadequate conjugation of estrogen in cirrhosis. Discussion of this disorder, however, is beyond the scope of this book.

Galactocele

This is a cystic dilatation of one of the major ducts at the areola, often occurring as the result of obstruction during lactation (23). A few cases are associated with galactorrhea and the use of oral contraceptives. The contents are milky white and consist of a large number of lipid-rich foam cells and a few cuboidal ductal cells, in addition to granular eosinophilic secre-

Table 6.4. Benign Neoplasms of Breast

Duct papilloma	Juvenile fibroadenoma
Fibroadenoma	Granular cell myoblastoma
Cystosarcoma phyllodes[a]	Pleomorphic adenoma
Florid adenoma of nipple	Hemangioma
Tubular adenoma	Fibroma
Adenoma of medium ducts	Schwannoma
Lactating adenoma	Lipoma
Florid multiple papillomatosis	

[a]These tumors have a tendency to recur, and some behave aggressively as sarcomas.

tions and lipid. The cyst is originally lined by the double-layered epithelium of mammary ducts. However, the distension often causes the epithelium to become stretched or destroyed, and many galactoceles may be lined by nothing more than foam cells (Fig. 6.15). Secondary infection is accompanied by an inflammatory exudate in the lumen and in the surrounding tissues.

BENIGN NEOPLASMS

Benign neoplasms of the breast may be epithelial or stromal. Papillomas of the mammary ducts are not as common as fibroadenomas. Other benign neoplasms of the breast are rare and include florid, tubular, large duct, apocrine, and pleomorphic adenomas; granular cell tumors; and other soft neoplasms (Table 6.4). Although cystosarcoma phyllodes is a neoplasm with a variably aggressive behavior, it will be considered with the benign tumors.

Duct Papilloma

Intraductal papillomas are uncommon, but an incidence as high as 20% has been reported in women over 70 years old (14). Most of these, however, are asymptomatic, and in surgical specimens, papillomas are detected in less than 0.4% of cases (24–26). The clinically manifest tumors usually affect middle-aged women. They present with a bloody or straw-colored nipple discharge in about 75% of cases, allowing cytologic detection of the neoplasm in smears prepared from the fluid. Contrast medium mammography may reveal the lesion, and a dye is often injected at the time of surgery to help localize the mass. The solitary tumors are benign and have only a minimal malignant potential, unlike multiple papillomas (25, 26).

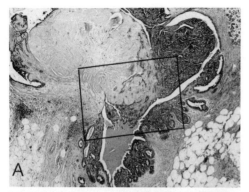

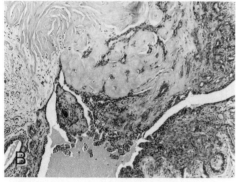

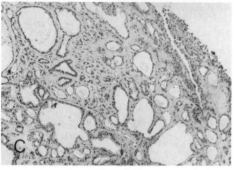

Figure 6.16. Ductal papilloma. **A**, A low-power view of a papilloma distending the lumen of a duct within the fibroadipose breast tissue. **B**, At higher magnification, the tumor shows fibrous as well as densely cellular areas. Note secretion in the lumen that caused a nipple discharge in this patient. **C**, A papilloma with glandular spaces within the core of the papillary fronds.

Gross Features

Papillomas do not produce any palpable swelling except in a few cases, where an ill-defined subareolar mass may be palpated. In most cases, the neoplasm is less than 0.5 cm across. It appears as a friable, soft, yellowish-pink polypoid lesion that protrudes into the lumen of a major duct. Cystic dilatation of the duct may occur, and the tumor is then referred to as cystadenoma or intracystic papilloma.

Microscopic Features

Benign papillary neoplasms form complex papillary fronds that consist of fibrovascular connective tissue cores, covered by epithelial cells. These epithelial cells possess uniform round or oval nuclei that are bland, normochromic, and have a uniformly distributed chromatin. Their polarity is maintained, being oriented perpendicularly to the basement membrane (Fig. 6.16). The cytoplasm is moderate to scant, and apical protrusions as well as apocrine metaplasia are fairly common. A layer of myoepithelial cells separates the surface epithelial cells from a well-defined basement membrane. The few mitotic figures seen are normal.

There is some overlap between the features of duct papillomas and epithelial proliferation associated with fibrocystic changes. However, the presence of complex branching of the epithelium and the large size of the involved duct favor the diagnosis of papilloma, particularly when a single lesion is encountered. Differentiation from papillary carcinoma may be difficult, particularly at frozen sections, since necrosis and hemorrhage may occur in papillomas. Fibrosis of the peripheral zone follows, entrapping some cells that may be misinterpreted as infiltrating the duct wall. However, lack of nuclear hyperchromasia or significant atypia and the presence of myoepithelial cells support the benignancy of the lesion (Table 6.5).

Fibroadenoma

Fibroadenomas are the most common benign breast neoplasms, and it is estimated that 10 to 25% of women have one or more of these tumors (7). The neoplasms are encountered in all age groups, but particularly in young adults, and are thought to be of lobular origin. They are estrogen-dependent neoplasms that are often associated with menstrual irregularities and can enlarge rapidly during pregnancy. After menopause, the tumors often regress and become hyalinized. A juvenile subtype affects adolescents and is characterized by rapid growth.

Gross Features

Fibroadenomas are freely mobile neoplasms, with a rubbery-firm consistency. They are well defined, lobulated, and surrounded by a fibrous capsule and compressed breast tissue (Fig. 6.17). The pink or tan white cut surface

Table 6.5. Papilloma and In Situ Papillary Carcinoma

Papilloma	Papillary Carcinoma
Complex branching and gland pattern with fibrovascular stalk	Cribriform, with thin stalks that may be lacking in some solid areas
Two cell types, epithelial and myoepithelial, with epithelium forming a single layer	Only epithelial cells, often in multiple layers with loss of polarity
Epithelial nuclei are small normochromic with a rare, and normal, mitosis	Nuclei are large hyperchromatic, with frequent, and maybe abnormal, mitosis
Peripheral fibrosis entraps outer cells	True invasion of periductal tissues
Apocrine change is common	Apocorine change is rare

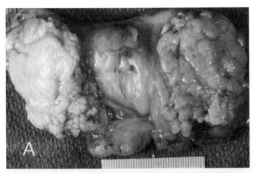

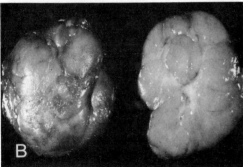

Figure 6.17. Fibroadenoma. **A**, The tumor is well-defined from the surrounding breast tissue, and the cut surface shows clefts. **B**, Lactating fibroadenoma. Note well-defined capsule. (Courtesy of Dr. Mary R. Schwartz, Baylor College of Medicine, Houston, Texas.)

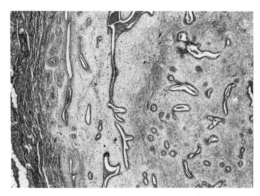

Figure 6.18. Fibroadenoma. Proliferation of ducts and stroma produces this pericanalicular pattern. The stroma in the vicinity of the glands is loose and pale, while around lobules of neoplastic tissue, a denser, darker staining collagenous stroma is evident.

bulges over the capsule, and fine linear slits and fibrous trabeculae may be visible. Fibroadenomas vary in size, with the majority being 1 to 3 cm in diameter, and multiple neoplasms are seen in about 20% of cases. Microscopic lesions, often seen in association with epithelial hyperplasia, probably represent a fibroadenomatoid pattern of hyperplastic lesions rather than true neoplasia. "Giant" fibroadenomas are more common in adolescents, particularly blacks around 10 to 20 years old. These tumors tend to grow rapidly and are often 10 or 12 cm in diameter (27). The large size of some tumors

is not an indication of malignancy, and local excision with nipple preservation is adequate and allows subsequent normal development of the breast.

Microscopic Features

Fibroadenomas have two major components: epithelial and stromal. The proliferation of these two components results in either a pericanalicular or an intracanalicular pattern. This classification, however, has no prognostic significance, and although these two patterns are morphologically distinct, most tumors show a mixture of both types.

In the *pericanalicular type*, the neoplastic stroma surrounds epithelium-lined tubules. The epithelium consists of two layers, an inner cuboidal and an outer myoepithelial. The epithelial cells are uniform and equally spaced. Some cells have large nuclei with occasional small round nucleoli, but mitotic figures are rare. The glands are surrounded by a zone of concentrically arranged loose edematous stroma, while dense collagenous

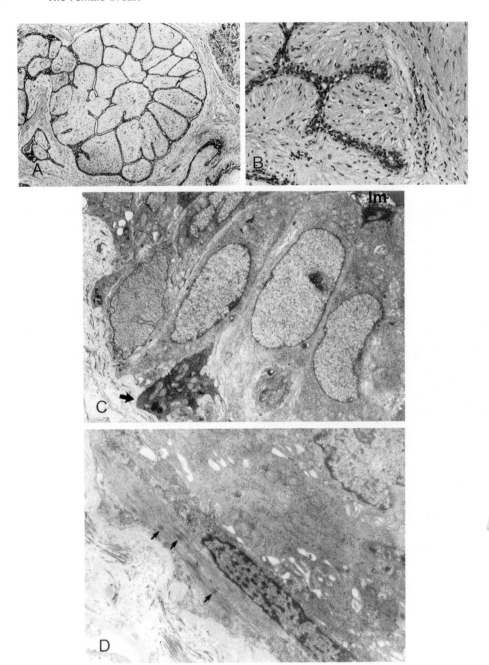

Figure 6.19. Fibroadenoma. **A**, An intracanalicular pattern is produced by the proliferation of stroma within stretched out ducts. **B**, Higher magnification showing the double-layered structure of the compressed epithelium at areas where it separates to form a lumen. **C**, Electron micrograph showing an orderly architecture of the epithelial cells around a lumen (*Lm*). A myoepithelial cell (*arrow*) is seen at the base of the epithelium. **D**, Smooth muscle features of a myoepithelial cell include collections of thin filaments with focal densities (*arrows*) arranged parallel to the longitudinal axis of the cell. (From Ramzy I. Clinical cytopathology and aspiration biopsy. Norwalk, CT: Appleton-Lange, 1990.)

stroma forms broad bands around clusters of glands and loose stroma (Fig. 6.18). Elastic tissue is usually lacking in the stroma of these neoplasms, but smooth muscle fibers may be seen, particularly in lesions close to the nipple.

In the *intracanalicular type*, stromal proliferation stretches the epithelium in various directions, forming distorted slit-like structures that appear to be invaginated by the stroma (Fig. 6.19). The double-layered epithelium is more difficult to demonstrate than in the pericanalicular type, since the stretching results in attenuation of the epithelium and fusion of the two layers on each side of the gland.

Secretory changes may be observed in some fibroadenomas with or without pregnancy and lactation (28). Under these circumstances, infarcts may also develop, and malignancy may be clinically suspected. Fibroadenomas often become hyalinized or show areas of calcification, particularly after menopause. Squamous, myxomatous, osseous, and cartilaginous metaplasias have been reported in fibroadenomas. In exceptionally rare conditions, an in situ adenocarcinoma may develop within a fibroadenoma (29, 30).

Cystosarcoma Phyllodes

These uncommon tumors of mammary stroma and ducts are responsible for about 1% of fibroepithelial breast tumors. They affect patients between the fourth and ninth decades of their life. Although they have a tendency to recur, a manifestation of the aggressive nature or incomplete excision of the tumor, lymph node, and distant metastases are rare.

Gross Features

Cystosarcoma phyllodes present as well-defined, rapidly growing swellings. They are generally large, averaging about 5 to 8 cm in diameter, with some much larger ones reported (31, 32). The large neoplasms may ulcerate through the attenuated skin. Cystosarcomas are lobulated and fleshy, with firm nodularity. On cut section, the neoplasm has a leaf-like appearance because of the presence of linear slits. Gray nodules of firm tissue are separated by white fibrous trabeculae. In addition, areas of myxoid, gelatinous, or cartilaginous consistency may be present.

Microscopic Features

Cystosarcoma phyllodes may be histologically benign, or it may be malignant. This separation, however, is not uniformly accepted since borderline and mixed types are encountered. In addition, the recurrence rate has been reported in some series as 8% for tumors classified as malignant, and 18% for those initially classified as benign, possibly a reflection of less extensive resection in the latter case (33). Because of these difficulties in separating the

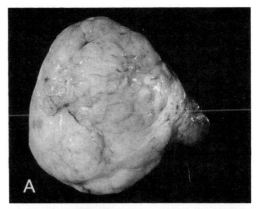
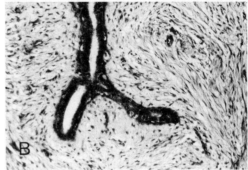

Figure 6.20. Cystosarcoma phyllodes. **A**, A large fleshy lobulated gray tumor that was growing rapidly. (Courtesy of Dr. Mary R. Schwartz, Baylor College of Medicine, Houston, Texas.) **B**, A cellular stroma with slight nuclear pleomorphism. The ductal epithelial component is similar to that seen in intracanalicular fibroadenoma in this "benign" form of cystosarcoma.

members of this spectrum, both types should be considered as potentially aggressive neoplasms.

Benign cystosarcoma phyllodes represents a giant fibroadenoma that is predominantly of the intracanalicular variety. The stroma, however, is more prominent, cellular, and dense, and mitotic figures may be seen. Myxoid, cartilaginous, and other forms of mesenchymal metaplastic changes may be present. Leaf-like papillary processes of epithelium and stroma invaginate the ducts, stretching the ducts to form epithelial spaces. These slits are lined by the usual double layer of uniform ductal and myoepithelial cells (Fig. 6.20). Squamous metaplasia is common, but cysts and apocrine metaplasia are rare.

Malignant cystosarcoma phyllodes is a rare, highly cellular true sarcoma, with nuclear pleomorphism and hyperchromasia of the stromal cells. The cells are arranged in a disorderly fashion, and abundant mitotic figures as well

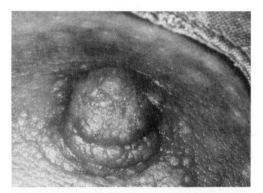

Figure 6.21. Florid nipple adenoma. Papillary proliferation within a large lactiferous duct in the areola. This tumor has resulted in ulceration of the epidermis. (Courtesy of Dr. Don A. Gard, Baylor College of Medicine, Houston.)

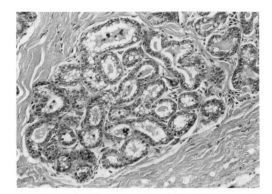

Figure 6.22. Lactating adenoma. Note uniformity of the glands and the secretory activity of the epithelium.

as necrosis and hemorrhage are seen. Foci that morphologically resemble myxoid liposarcoma or fibrosarcoma may be present. The glands are widely separated by broad bundles of stroma that may dominate the neoplasm. Carcinomas, usually of the lobular type, rarely develop within a cystosarcoma (34).

Recurrence occurred in 30% of patients with cystosarcoma studied by Norris and Taylor (31). Although no solid criteria for benign behavior were observed, those associated with less likelihood for recurrence included: size less than 4 cm; mitotic figures below 3 per 10 high-power fields; a pushing margin; and the lack of nuclear pleomorphism. Distant metastases usually involve the lungs, bones, and pleura and may consist of the sarcomatous elements only (35).

Other Benign Tumors

Florid Adenoma of Nipple

This neoplasm, also referred to as subareolar duct papillomatosis, appears as a nodule in the areola that frequently ulcerates and, as a result, may be confused with Paget's disease. The 1- to 2-cm single, well-defined but not encapsulated nodule may be associated with crust formation and a serosanguinous nipple discharge. Histologically, the lesion is similar to syringocystadenoma papilliferum of the skin. It consists of ducts of various sizes, with intraductal papillary proliferation of uniform epithelial cells (Fig. 6.21). A layer of myoepithelial cells is often seen in some areas of the lesion. Solid nests of epithelial cells may be present within the ducts. Fibrosis may result in areas similar to those in sclerosing adenosis. Mitotic figures are sparse, and necrosis is not

seen except in association with surface ulceration and inflammation.

Tubular Adenomas

These uncommon neoplasms are of lobular origin. They differ from fibroadenomas in that their scant stroma is not neoplastic but is just enough to support the neoplastic epithelium. The small crowded glands are lined by a layer of cuboidal epithelium surrounded by myoepithelium.

Adenoma of Medium Ducts

This entity has been described by Azzopardi and Salm in 1984 (36). In these, epithelial and myoepithelial cells distend the duct lumen, and the lesion may be surrounded by a fibrotic wall or may show a central radiating fibrous core. Apocrine metaplastic changes are common in these lesions.

Lactating Adenomas and Lactating Fibroadenomas

Some adenomas and fibroadenomas manifest pronounced secretory activity (Fig. 6.22). Such activity may be associated with pregnancy or lactation but may occur independent of these conditions. Lactating tumors often show frequent mitotic figures and necrosis.

Granular Cell Tumors

These are benign neoplasms, probably of Schwann cell origin. They present as a hard well-defined or poorly defined mass that may resemble carcinoma. The epithelium-like polygonal cells have abundant granular cytoplasm and central small uniform nuclei that lack the usual nuclear criteria of malignancy. The overlying skin often shows pseudoepitheliomatous hyperplasia.

Florid (Multiple) Papillomatosis

Unlike solitary papillomas, this condition involves the terminal ducts and tends to affect younger patients. It usually presents as a mass with no nipple discharge. It is much less common than solitary lesions and is associated with carcinoma in about 25% of cases, hence its clinical significance (37). They tend to recur in about half the cases, and carcinoma has been reported to develop in 4 to 10 years following the detection of these lesions (26). Over 100 papillomas may be encountered in the same patient, and in 25% of cases, both breasts are involved. Microscopically, the lesions are similar to solitary papillomas. However, areas of atypia with epithelial stratification and nuclear hyperchromasia are seen more frequently. Transitional foci to intraductal carcinoma may also be encountered (38, 39).

Juvenile Papillomatosis (Fibroadenoma)

This lesion affects mostly patients in their 20s. The lesion is accompanied with extensive intraductal papillomatosis and cyst formation, resulting in a "Swiss cheese" appearance. It presents as a mass that resembles a fibroadenoma and is bilateral. The presence of apocrine metaplasia, the extent of the cyst formation, and the infrequent mitotic figures support a benign diagnosis, even when necrosis is present. A family history of breast carcinoma has been reported in 28% of the cases, and it appears that the patients themselves may be at high risk of developing carcinoma (40).

Pleomorphic Adenoma

These are rarely encountered in the breast. They have a cartilaginous consistency that leads to suspicion of malignancy. However, they are well-defined and have a characteristic histologic appearance. Other tumors of skin and soft tissues, such as lipomas, angiomas, leiomyomas, neurofibromas, and schwannomas may also be encountered.

CYTOLOGY OF BENIGN BREAST DISEASE

Aspiration biopsy cytology can play a role in the diagnosis of benign breast disease (41–44). A brief outline of the cytologic features of the common lesions follows, but for a more detailed discussion, the reader is referred to cytopathology texts (45).

Solid lesions of the breast can be aspirated using thin (No. 23-gauge) needles. Large cysts

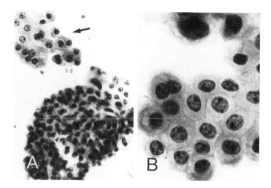

Figure 6.23. Aspirate from breast mass. The patient had fibrocystic and hyperplastic changes. **A,** Note cohesive sheet of ductal cells with small amounts of cytoplasm, as compared to the abundant cytoplasm of the apocrine cells at arrow. **B,** A higher magnification of a sheet of apocrine metaplastic cells with well-defined cell borders and abundant granular cytoplasm.

may be associated with enough pain to necessitate aspiration to relieve tension and to help to reassure a patient if open biopsy is not contemplated. Examination of straw-colored or clear fluids aspirated from all cysts may not be cost-effective in terms of cancer detection. However, hemorrhagic cyst fluids should always be submitted to the laboratory, in view of the possibility of malignancy. Carcinoma was detected in 1 to 1.7% of aspirated cysts; the fluid in some of these was straw-colored, and the mass disappeared following the procedure (46).

Lesions with prominent hyperplasia and papillomatosis produce cellular aspirates, while fibrotic lesions, such as sclerosing adenosis, result in scant cellular specimens. The aspirate may contain ductal, apocrine, and foam cells in addition to stromal and inflammatory cells. Ductal epithelial cells appear in small clusters or sheets (Fig. 6.23). They are cuboidal, uniformly spaced, and have small nuclei, with finely granular chromatin. Apocrine cells are usually in sheets, and their cytoplasm is well-defined and coarsely granular. The nuclei are large, with prominent single central nucleoli but lack the coarsely granular chromatin of malignant cells. Foam cells, probably of epithelial origin, and histiocytes are frequently observed in cyst fluids (Fig. 6.24). Myoepithelial cells appear as dark small round, lymphocyte-like, or spindly naked nuclei.

Some aspirates of fibroadenomas are scanty cellular, while others show abundant epithelial and stromal cells (Fig. 6.25). The epithelium forms broad sheets of cohesive, uniform, and equally spaced ductal cells. Branching epithelial formations that resemble "antler horns"

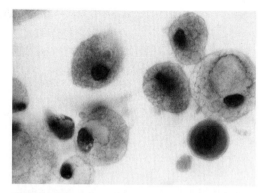

Figure 6.24. Foam cells. These cells were seen in a nipple discharge from a pregnant patient.

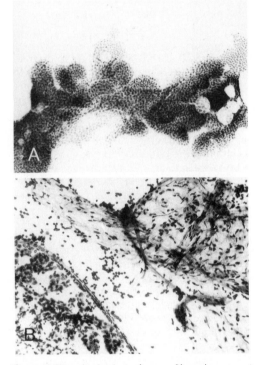

Figure 6.25. **A**, Aspirate from a fibroadenoma. A sheet of uniform epithelial cells in a "deer antler" shape, characteristic of intracanalicular growth pattern. **B**, A mixture of spindled fibrous stromal cells and epithelial cells, aspirated from a breast with fibrocystic changes. (From Ramzy I. Clinical cytopathology and aspiration biopsy. Norwalk, CT: Appleton-Lange, 1990.)

may be seen. Stromal cells are arranged randomly or in fascicles, and mitotic figures are rare. The cytologic features of fibroadenomas may overlap with those of fibrocystic changes.

Papillomas often present with a nipple discharge, allowing detection by cytologic examination of the fluid. Needle aspiration may also be feasible in the rare occasion where a definite mass is palpable. Papillary fronds as well as isolated ductal cells with uniform round or oval nuclei may be seen. The complex branching of the epithelium and the observation of abundant foam cells and elongated ductal cells favor the diagnosis of papilloma over fibrocystic changes. Differentiation from papillary carcinoma may be difficult cytologically as well as histologically.

Although a positive cytologic diagnosis of cancer is a reliable indicator of the presence of malignancy, there are limitations to a negative diagnosis. Rendering such negative diagnosis can only confirm the clinical impression of the benign nature of a lesion. If the aspiration biopsy is negative and malignancy is clinically suspected, an open biopsy should be performed without hesitation.

REFERENCES

1. Davies JD. Hyperelastosis, obliteration and fibrous plaques in major ducts of the human breast. J Pathol 1973;110:13–26.
2. Adair FE, Munzer JT. Fat necrosis of the female breast. Report of one hundred ten cases. Am J Surg 1947;74:117–128.
3. Berkowitz GS, Kelsey JL, Livolsi VA, et al. Exogenous hormone use and fibrocystic breast disease by histopathologic component. Int J Cancer 1984;34:443–449.
4. Walsh PV, McDicken IW, Bulbrook RD, et al. Serum oestradiol-17 and prolactin concentrations during the luteal phase in women with benign breast disease. Eur J Cancer Clin Oncol 1984;20:1345–1351.
5. Li Volsi VA, Stadel B, Kelsey JL, et al. Fibrocystic breast disease in oral contraceptive-users: histopathological evaluation of epithelial atypia. N Engl J Med 1987;299:381–385.
6. Consensus meeting: is fibrocystic disease of the breast precancerous? Arch Pathol Lab Med 1986;110:171–173.
7. Frantz VK, Pickren JW, Melcher GW, et al. Incidence of chronic disease in so-called "normal breasts"; a study based on 225 post mortem examinations. Cancer 1951;4:762–783.
8. Azzopardi JG. Problems in breast pathology. In: Bennington JL, ed. Major problems in pathology, vol 11. Philadelphia: Saunders, 1979.
9. Sloane JP. Biopsy pathology of the breast. New York: John Wiley & Sons, 1985.
10. Bonser GM, Dossett JA, Jull JW. Human and experimental breast cancer. London: Pitman Medical Publications, 1961.
11. Earl HM. Markers of human breast differentiation and breast carcinomas and characterization of monoclonal antibodies to human casein [Dissertation]. London University, 1985. (Quoted by Sloane, ref 9.)

12. Clement PB, Azzopardi JG. Microglandular adenosis of the breast: a lesion simulating tubular carcinoma. Histopathology 1983;7:169–180.

13. Rosen PP. Microglandular adenosis: a benign lesion simulating invasive mammary carcinoma. Am J Surg Pathol 1983;7:137–144.

14. Kramer WM, Rush BF. Mammary duct proliferation in the elderly: a histopathologic study. Cancer 1973;31:130–137.

15. Ahmed A. Ultrastructural aspects of human breast lesions. Pathol Annu 1980;15:411–443.

16. Davies JD. Neural invasion in benign mammary dysplasia. J Pathol 1973;109:225–231.

17. Taylor HB, Norris HJ. Epithelial invasion of nerves in benign diseases of the breast. Cancer 1967;20:2245–2249.

18. Fenoglio C, Lattes R. Sclerosing papillary proliferations in the breast. Cancer 1974;33:691–700.

19. Nielsen M, Jensen J, Andersen JA. An autopsy study of radial scar in the female breast. Histopathology 1985;9:287-295.

20. Tremblay G, Buell RH, Seemayer TA. Elastosis in benign sclerosing ductal proliferation of the female breast. Am J Surg Pathol 1977;1:155–159.

21. Page DL, Vander Zwagg R, Rogers LW, et al. Relation between component parts of fibrocystic disease complex and breast cancer. J Natl Cancer Inst 1978;61:1055–1063.

22. Toker C. Small cell dysplasia and in situ carcinoma of the mammary ducts and lobules. J Pathol 1974;114:47–52.

23. Winker JM. Galactocele of the breast. Am J Surg 1964;108:357–360.

24. Sandison AT. A study of surgically removed specimens of breast, with special reference to sclerosing adenosis. J Clin Pathol 1958;11:101–109.

25. Haagensen CD. Diseases of the breast, 2nd ed. Philadelphia: Saunders, 1971.

26. Murad TM, Contesso G, Mouriesse H. Papillary tumors of large lactiferous ducts. Cancer 1981;48:122–133.

27. Stromberg BV, Golladay ES. Cystosarcoma phyllodes in the adolescent female. J Pediatr Surg 1978;13:423–425.

28. Bailey AJ, Sloane JP, Trickey BS, et al. An immunocytochemical study of lactalbumin in human breast tissue. J Pathol 1982;137:13–23.

29. Buzanowski-Konakry K, Harrison EG Jr, Payne WS. Lobular carcinoma arising in fibroadenoma of the breast. Cancer 1975;35:450–456.

30. Fondo EY, Rosen PP, Fracchia AA, et al. The problem of carcinoma developing in a fibroadenoma: recent experience at Memorial Hospital. Cancer 1979;43:563–567.

31. Norris HJ, Taylor HB. Relationship of histologic features to behavior of cystosarcoma phyllodes: analysis of ninety-four cases. Cancer 1967;20:2090–2099.

32. Hart WR, Bauer RC, Oberman HA. Cystosarcoma phyllodes. A clinicopathologic study of 26 hypercellular periductal stromal tumors of the breast. Am J Clin Pathol 1978;70:211–216.

33. Hajdu SI, Espinosa MH, Robbins GF. Recurrent cystosarcoma phyllodes: a clinicopathologic study of 32 cases. Cancer 1976;38:1402–1406.

34. Rosen PP, Urban JA. Coexistent mammary carcinoma and cystosarcoma phyllodes. Breast 1975;1:9–15.

35. Lindquist KD, van Heerden JA, Weiland LH, et al. Recurrent and metastatic cystosarcoma phyllodes. Am J Surg 1982;144:341–343.

36. Azzopardi JG, Salm R. Ductal adenoma of the breast: a lesion which can mimic carcinoma. J Pathol 1984;144:15–23.

37. Murad TM, Pritchett P. Malignant and benign papillary lesions of the breast. Hum Pathol 1977;8:379–390.

38. Ohuchi N, Abe R, Kasai M. Possible cancerous change of intraductal papillomas of the breast: a 3-D reconstruction study of 25 cases. Cancer 1984;54:605–611.

39. Papotti M, Gugliotta P, Ghiringhello B, et al. Association of breast carcinoma and multiple intraductal papillomas: an histological and immunohistochemical investigation. Histopathology 1984;8:963–975.

40. Rosen PP, Holmes G, Lesser ML, et al. Juvenile papillomatosis and breast carcinoma. Cancer 1985;55:1345–1352.

41. Abele JS, Miller TR, Goodson WH III, et al. Fine-needle aspiration of palpable breast masses. A program for staged implementation. Arch Surg 1983;118:859–963.

42. Frable WJ. Needle aspiration of the breast. Cancer 1984;53:671–676.

43. Kreuzer G. Aspiration biopsy cytology in proliferating benign mammary dysplasia. Acta Cytol 1978;22:128–132.

44. Kline TS, Joshi LP, Neal HS. Fine-needle aspiration of the breast: diagnoses and pitfalls. A review of 3545 cases. Cancer 1979;44:286–292.

45. Ramzy I: Clinical cytopathology and aspiration biopsy. Fundamental principles and practice, chapter 22. Norwalk, CT, Appleton-Lange, 1990.

46. McSwain GR, Valicenti JF, O'Brien PH. Cytologic evaluation of breast cysts. Surg Gynecol Obstet 1978;146:921–925.

7

Pathology of Malignant Neoplasms

Ibrahim Ramzy

Carcinoma of the breast is responsible for 27% of all cancers occurring in women, with over 136,000 new cases of invasive disease and at least 5000 additional cases of in situ carcinoma diagnosed every year in the United States. The disease remains the leading cause of cancer mortality in females in all ages combined, accounting for 18% of cancer deaths, and was only recently surpassed by lung cancer in some states (1). This chapter deals with the gross and microscopic features of breast carcinomas and sarcomas and the morphologic parameters that may predict the outcome of these malignancies. It also seems appropriate to discuss the role and limitations of cytologic diagnosis of malignant tumors of the breasts by examination of nipple secretions and aspirates of solid lesions.

CLASSIFICATION

Most breast malignancies are primary epithelial carcinomas, with only a small number of sarcomas and metastatic tumors reported. Although the terminal ductules are probably the source of almost all cancers, neoplasms are traditionally classified into ductal and lobular carcinomas (2–4). This designation is based on morphologic, clinical, and prognostic characteristics rather than on the exact site of origin. Some lesions, such as papillary carcinoma, clearly originate within the ducts, while the early stages of other "ductal" tumors have a lobular configuration. Furthermore, a considerable degree of overlap of histologic and cytologic features exists between ductal and lobular neoplasms, and about half the cases have features of both types. Each of these entities can be an in situ or an infiltrative carcinoma, and several clinicopathologic variants of ductal carcinoma have been recognized (Table 7.1).

DUCTAL ADENOCARCINOMA

This is the most common type of breast carcinoma. In situ carcinomas rarely manifest any symptoms, and by the time patients seek medical advice, the tumor is usually in the infiltrative stage. About 40% of the cases show evidence of spread to the regional nodes at the time of diagnosis, and distant metastases are demonstrated in 8% of cases. In addition, many neoplasms are multicentric, and areas of in situ carcinoma are often observed in association with invasive tumors. The disease is slightly more common in the left breast, and in 50% of cases, the tumor is located in the upper outer quadrant. The central part of the breast is involved in about 20% of cases, while each of the remaining quadrants is affected in 10% of cases.

Ductal Adenocarcinoma In Situ

In situ or intraductal carcinomas (DCIS) are uncommon, with foci detected in 1 to 4% of breasts after thorough examination at autopsy (5). Most cases are discovered incidentally during mammography or other imaging techniques, with the exception of intraductal papillary carcinomas, which may present with a bloody nipple discharge. Some lesions are surrounded by fibrosis or are large enough to be palpated. About one-third of the patients have more than one focus of in situ carcinoma, but bilaterality is rare (6). By definition, the basement membrane zone surrounding the duct remains intact. However, breaks through the basal lamina can be demonstrated ultrastructurally, and extensive study reveals microinvasion in 20% of mastectomy specimens following biopsy diagnosis of in situ carcinoma. This is particularly true in tumors larger than 2.5

Table 7.1.   Malignant Tumors of the Breast: Classification and Incidence[a]

Ductal Adenocarcinoma		Other Rare Variants of Carcinoma	
In situ ductal carcinoma,	5	Carcinoid tumor	
includes intracystic & Paget's		Secretory (juvenile) carcinoma	
Infiltrative duct carcinoma		Squamous cell carcinoma	
NOS, with desmoplasia	72	Adenoid cystic carcinoma	
Medullary carcinoma	3	Lipid-rich carcinoma	
Mucinous carcinoma	2	Carcinoma with osseous or chondromatous	
Papillary carcinoma	1	metaplasia	
Inflammatory carcinoma[b]	2–4	Spindle cell (pseudosarcomatous)	
Paget's disease	2		
Apocrine duct carcinoma		**Sarcoma and Carcinosarcoma**	
Tubular carcinoma	2	Cystosarcoma phyllodes, malignant	
		Angiosarcoma	
Lobular Adenocarcinoma		Leiomyosarcoma	
Lobular carcinoma in situ	3	Neurosarcoma	
Infiltrating lobular carcinoma	10–15	Malignant lymphoma	
Signet-ring cell variant		Carcinosarcoma	
		Mixed tumors	

[a]Incidence given as percent of all malignant breast tumors. As a group, ductal carcinomas are responsible for 75 to 80%, lobular carcinomas for 10 to 20% and sarcomas for 0.5 to 1% of all breast malignancies.
[b]Inflammatory carcinoma is a specific clinical but not a histologic type.

cm. Large tumors are also responsible for the 1 to 2% of cases that show metastasis (7). It has been estimated that half the patients with post-surgical residual in situ carcinomas will develop infiltrative carcinoma in the ipsilateral breast within 10 years (6). It is of interest to note that ultrastructural evidence of basal lamina invasion by neoplastic cells has been demonstrated in many cases of carcinoma classified as intraductal by light microscopy (8, 9).

Several morphologic patterns of in situ ductal carcinomas are recognized. These include the solid, comedo, cribriform, papillary, and mixed types. Some of these have a characteristic gross appearance, while most have no specific features on examination of the breast. Since ductal carcinoma may occur within the lumen of a cyst, the presence of a cyst should not exclude the possibility of malignancy or negate the need for careful sampling of the suspected areas.

Solid Intraductal Carcinoma

Breasts harboring foci of intraductal carcinoma may exhibit areas of induration. Some neoplasms are associated with fibrosis, cysts, and hyperplastic areas. *Microscopically,* the ducts are distended by a solid core of neoplastic cells. These cells, which are larger than those of normal ducts, are not mixed with myoepithelial cells. They possess large pleomorphic nuclei, with thick nuclear membranes and coarsely granular chromatin, and many have large nucleoli (Fig. 7.1). Focal individual cell necrosis may be seen, and mitotic figures are often present. Stromal reaction around the involved duct, in the form of lymphocytic infiltrate or fibrosis, is minimal, and no evidence of elastosis is seen.

Comedocarcinoma

Comedocarcinoma should be suspected when, in addition to the presence of slight induration of the resected breast tissue, tiny creamy paste-like necrotic material can be expressed from the cut surface. In this type, the ducts are distended by neoplastic cells similar to those of the solid-type tumor. However, the neoplastic cell mass shows central necrosis, with eosinophilic granular or homogeneous material replacing the cells in the center (Fig. 7.2). This material consists of cytoplasmic and nuclear debris and may show focal calcification.

Cribriform Carcinoma

In cribriform carcinoma, the neoplastic cell masses that fill the distended ducts develop multiple holes, giving the cell mass a cribriform, or sieve-like, pattern. Unlike the irregular spaces observed in atypical ductal epithelial hyperplasia, the spaces in carcinoma are usually round, well-defined, and uniform in appearance (Figs. 7.3 and 7.4). The neoplastic cells are evenly spaced and show nuclear enlargement, hyperchromasia, and pleomorphism, with coarsely granular and irregularly distributed chromatin. Nucleoli are prominent, and mitotic figures are often seen. Although cytologic atypia may be minimal in cribriform carcinomas, the malignant cells within the

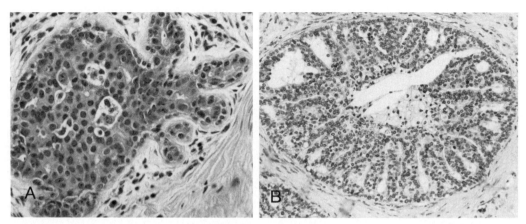

Figure 7.1. Intraductal carcinoma. **A**, Solid type showing distended duct in the terminal lobular unit. The presence of early necrosis within the tumor cell mass is a feature of malignancy. **B**, Intraductal carcinoma, showing a "roman column" pattern.

ducts do not overlap and are not mixed with myoepithelial cells. Table 6.2 (Chapter 6) lists some helpful features for differentiation of this type of carcinoma from atypical hyperplasia.

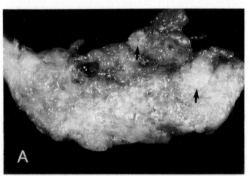

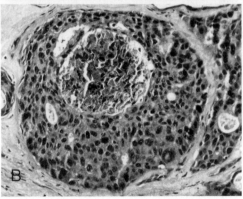

Figure 7.2. Intraductal carcinoma, comedo type. **A**, Resected specimen with solid ducts with central necrosis at *arrow* (Courtesy of Dr. Mary Schwartz, Baylor College of Medicine, Houston, Texas). **B**, Distended duct with necrotic tumor cells in center.

Intraductal Papillary Carcinoma

These tumors differ from the other types of intraductal carcinoma in that they may present early with a bloody nipple discharge, particularly when they involve a large duct. The neoplasm may be visualized as small papillary growth within the lumen of a large duct. It may result in obstruction, causing retention of secretions or of altered blood and distention of the distal part of the affected duct (Fig. 7.5). Microscopically, the papillary fronds consist of a delicate central core of vascular stroma surrounded by several layers of epithelial cells (10, 11). The fronds share a community border and often show complex branching. When these

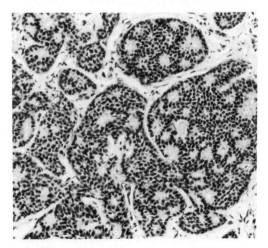

Figure 7.3. Intraductal carcinoma, cribriform type. Note the well-defined round or oval spaces in the cribriform area.

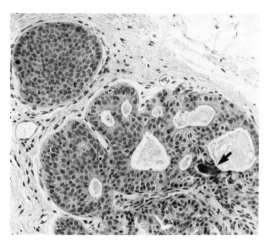

Figure 7.4. Intraductal carcinoma, mixed cribriform and solid patterns. Calcium deposits are evident (*arrow*).

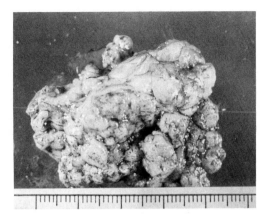

Figure 7.5. Intraductal carcinoma, papillary type. This 3.5-cm papillary tumor was distending the lumen of one of the large lactiferous ducts.

branches fuse together, they result in the formation of solid cell bridges where the stroma is scant or is completely lacking. The thickness of the epithelium and number of cell layers is variable, but myoepithelial cells are not part of the neoplasm, and apocrine metaplasia is rare. The epithelial cells have large hyperchromatic nuclei with prominent irregular nucleoli and coarse chromatin. The stroma may be fibrotic. Blood, inflammatory cells, and evidence of necrosis may be present, but the basement membrane zone is intact. Calcific deposits may be seen within the duct lumen, and lamellated psammoma bodies are occasionally encountered. The main features that differentiate papillary carcinomas from papillomas were summarized in Table 6.5 (Chapter 6).

Other Types of Intraductal Carcinoma

A multicystic variety of intraductal carcinoma has been reported by Rosen and Scott (12). The cysts are distended by an eosinophilic material, and the lining epithelium may be deceptively bland. In such cases, the diagnosis of carcinoma should not be made unless definite areas of malignancy are demonstrated.

Infiltrative Ductal Adenocarcinoma

Invasion of the stroma by neoplastic cells results in several morphologic variants of breast carcinoma. Some of these variants have distinctive clinical manifestations with prognostic implications. More than one type can be present in the same breast, and differentiation between these variants is not always feasible, particularly in frozen sections. The variants include

duct carcinoma with desmoplastic reaction, medullary carcinoma, mucinous carcinoma, papillary carcinoma, inflammatory carcinoma, Paget's disease, apocrine carcinoma, tubular carcinoma, and some rare types.

Infiltrative Ductal Carcinoma, Nonspecified or Desmoplastic

This type of ductal carcinoma accounts for most breast cancers that present at an infiltrative stage. It affects women in their 4th to 7th decades of life and is characterized by an extensive desmoplastic reaction of the stroma that is associated with the development of a hard, usually painless mass.

Gross Features

A poorly defined area of induration can usually be palpated within the softer breast tissue. At the time of open biopsy, most neoplasms are 1 to 3 cm in diameter. Tumors are rarely encountered when they are still of microscopic size, although mammography and self-examination help to bring some of these early lesions into light. Other tumors reach a size of 10 or 15 cm, often because of patient denial or lack of knowledge, before the patient seeks medical advice. The mass has a hard consistency and offers a cartilaginous gritty resistance while cutting the specimen. The cut surface is depressed due to retraction of the fibrous tissue. It is grayish-white with tiny foci of yellow streaks of elastic tissue radiating from the center with areas of necrosis as well as calcific deposits. The outer margin of the mass is irregular, with tapering processes that extend into the surrounding adipose tissue (Fig. 7.6).

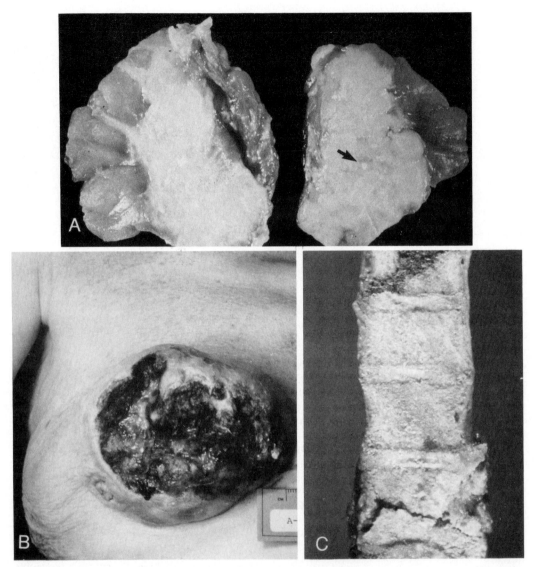

Figure 7.6. Infiltrating ductal carcinoma. **A,** Note the irregular infiltrating contour of the lesion and the creamy areas of necrosis (*arrow*) and the retracted cut surface. **B,** A late case with extensive skin ulceration. **C,** Vertebral metastases at autopsy, with both osteoblastic and osteolytic deposits and pathologic fracture.

The fibrous bands cause retraction of the nipple and wrinkling of the thick overlying skin to produce a characteristic "peau d'orange" appearance. The neoplasm may also be fixed to the underlying soft tissues or to the skin. Although necrosis is often present, areas of hemorrhage are uncommon. Ulceration of the nipple or other parts of the skin is uncommon, except in advanced cases.

Microscopic Features

The epithelial cells are arranged in cords, trabeculae, or as small clusters. The cells often form long one- or two-cell-thick cords, referred to as an "Indian file" pattern; such a pattern, however, is also characteristic of lobular carcinomas. Ductal carcinoma cells often form small nests of a few cells each, as well as larger groups (Fig. 7.7). The nuclei of the malignant cells are large, often three or four times the size of a red blood cell, and are pleomorphic. The nuclear contours are irregular; the nuclear membranes are thick; and the chromatin is coarsely clumped. Nucleoli are prominent; nuclear and cytoplasmic molding is evident; and mitotic figures are often encountered. The ma-

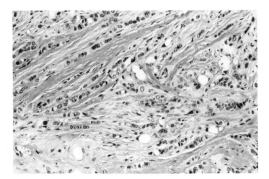

Figure 7.7. Infiltrating ductal carcinoma, desmoplastic reaction. Large tumor cells infiltrate in small groups. Note the large nuclei, compared with lymphocytes or RBCs, and the stromal fibrosis.

lignant cells have an abundance of organelles, and some show intracellular lumina, with intraluminal microvilli and electron-dense mucinous material (Fig. 7.8). Cilia may be rarely seen.

The neoplastic epithelial cells are surrounded by basal laminae and an abundant dense collagenous stroma (Fig. 7.9). This collagen, unlike that of benign breast tissue, consists of large amounts of type V fibrillary variety (13). The stroma is also rich in elastic tissue, which is diffusely arranged but is also concentrated around ducts and vessels (14). Foci of hydroxyapatite calcification, including lamellated psammoma bodies, are common. Calcific deposits may also be seen among groups of epithelial cells. Myoepithelial cells are present within the stroma, as demonstrated by actin and myosin stains, but they do not form an integral part of the proliferating neoplastic cells. Lymphocytes are not abundant in the desmoplastic type. Most of these are a mixture of T-inducer and T-suppressor, unlike those in the normal breast, which are predominantly suppressor (15). Necrosis is often associated with a chronic inflammatory or foreign body granulomatous reaction, and in some cases, fat necrosis is encountered near carcinomatous foci.

Although most carcinomas possess large pleomorphic nuclei, the neoplastic cells in some tumors may have intermediate or small nuclei. Carcinomas consisting of medium-sized cells have deceptively bland nuclei. These nuclei, however, are still more than double the size of those of adjacent normal ductal cells. Tumors of the small cell type, which account for 25% of cases of breast carcinomas, may be difficult to differentiate from sclerosing adenosis. Table 6.3 (Chapter 6) lists some of the differentiating features. Necrosis and the lack

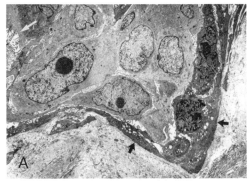

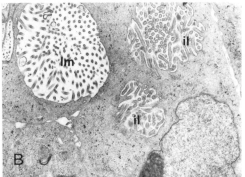

Figure 7.8. Ultrastructure of ductal carcinoma. **A,** An intraductal component showing preservation of myoepithelial cells (*short arrow*) and prominence of the nucleoli of the neoplastic cells. *Long arrow* points to an intercellular lumen lined by microvilli. **B,** Malignant ductal cells with multiple intracytoplasmic lumens (*il*) lined by microvilli and an intercellular lumen (*lm*). (Electron micrographs courtesy of Dr. Janine K. Mawad, Baylor College of Medicine, Houston, Texas.)

of myoepithelial cells are important indications of malignancy in such neoplasms of cytologically bland cells. Table 7.2 summarizes the features of ductal carcinoma.

Medullary Carcinoma

This neoplasm is responsible for about 5% of breast carcinomas. Medullary carcinomas usually present as large tumors that are well-circumscribed but not encapsulated. They have a softer consistency than desmoplastic tumors. Their cut surface has a homogeneous encephaloid appearance, is grayish pink or tan, and because of the lack of fibrosis, it does not retract from the surface (Fig. 7.10). Hemorrhage and necrosis are often seen, but the skin overlying the bulky deep-seated tumors is not involved and rarely ulcerates.

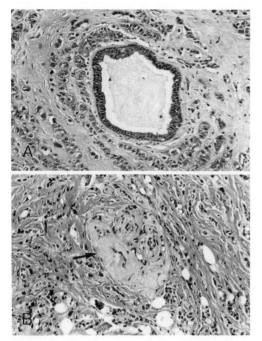

Figure 7.9. Infiltrating ductal carcinoma with desmoplasia **A**, Concentric cords of tumor cells and fibrosis surrounding a benign but distended duct. Note the myoepithelial layer and the small size of the normal duct nuclei, compared to that of the cancer cells. **B**, Stromal elastosis is evident as a pale area at *arrow*.

Microscopic Features

Most of the neoplastic cells of medullary carcinomas are arranged in large nodules of several hundred cells each in a syncytial pattern. In other areas, the cells form interconnecting cords. The individual cells are large, pleomorphic, and have large, pleomorphic, vesicular nuclei, with nuclear membrane folds

Table 7.2.   Features of Ductal Adenocarcinoma

Hard irregular mass, with retraction from skin
  surface
Gritty cartilaginous resistance on cutting
Grayish-white with yellow streaks of elastosis
Cords, trabeculae, and small nests of tumor cells
Large hyperchromatic nuclei, disorderly oriented,
  some eccentric
Large irregular and multiple nucleoli
Frequent mitotic figures seen; some are abnormal
Some tumors consist of cells with small bland
  nuclei
Fibrosis and elastosis of stroma
Necrosis, calcification and, occasionally, fat
  necrosis

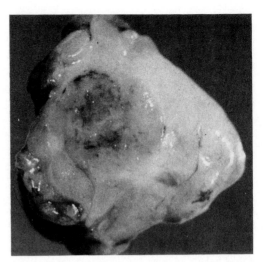

Figure 7.10. Medullary carcinoma, showing a large homogeneous mass with a grayish-pink cut surface that did not retract.

and prominent nucleoli. The cytoplasm is usually abundant and basophilic, and mitotic figures are frequent (Fig. 7.11). Deposition of basal lamina and the proliferation of myoepithelial cells are not features of this tumor (16). The nodules and cords are separated by thin connective tissue trabeculae in which variable numbers of lymphocytes, macrophages, and plasma cells are seen. Most lymphocytes are T cells, and their presence may be correlated with better long-term survival. Necrosis and hemorrhage are often seen in the background, but calcification is uncommon. The epithelial cells of typical medullary carcinoma do not form glands, but focal squamous metaplasia is not uncommon. Differentiation from malignant lymphoma may be difficult at times, but immunohistochemical studies can be helpful.

Tumors showing the typical pattern described above account for less than 5% of breast cancers (17). They have a better prognosis than nonmedullary ductal carcinomas, although they have the same tendency to spread to lymph nodes (18). The 10-year survival rate is about 85%, particularly for patients with small tumors (Table 7.3). Atypical varieties of medullary carcinoma are not uncommon and have a less favorable prognosis. The atypical features include extensive marginal infiltration, few lymphocytes, desmoplastic reaction, less than 75% syncytial growth pattern, or displaying tubular pattern. Such tumors may be classified as infiltrating duct carcinoma with medullary features, and their 10-year survival rate has been reported at 64% (19).

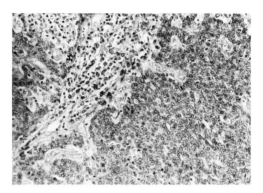

Figure 7.11. Medullary carcinoma. The neoplastic cells are large and are arranged in large sheets and nests. The stroma is not desmoplastic, and it is infiltrated by lymphocytes. (From Ramzy I. Clinical cytopathology and aspiration biopsy. Norwalk, CT: Appleton-Lange, 1990.)

Mucinous Carcinoma

Many breast carcinomas show evidence of focal mucin production. However, in mucinous tumors, also referred to as colloid carcinomas, mucin is produced in large quantities, resulting in bulky neoplasms that often reach 10 cm or more in diameter. This type of tumor accounts for 2 to 5% of breast carcinomas. The neoplasms are well-circumscribed, nonencapsulated, and are usually firm with multiple lobules or spaces distended with mucin. These have a characteristic gelatinous bluish or grayish-pink cut surface with a translucent glistening appearance (Fig. 7.12).

Microscopic Appearance

Nests, cell balls, and isolated cancer cells are seen, surrounded by pools and streaks of extracellular mucin. The cells have pleomorphic nuclei, and only a few of these are pushed to the side by intracellular mucin, producing a signet-ring appearance. Pale eosinophilic or basophilic mucinous pools may replace most of the neoplastic cells. These pools are separated by bands of collagenous fibrous tissue (Fig.

Table 7.3. Features of Medullary Carcinoma

Large but circumscribed deep lesion
Soft-to-firm consistency
No fibrosis or skin retraction
Large cells in a syncytial growth pattern
Moderate or marked nuclear pleomorphism
Mononuclear lymphocytic-plasmacytic infiltrate
Gland formation and calcification uncommon
Typical cases have an 85% 10-year survival rate

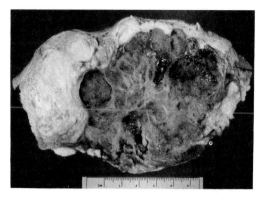

Figure 7.12. Mucinous carcinoma. Note the trabeculae separating pools of mucin, resulting in the glistening cut surface of this large tumor.

7.13). This mucinous material, as well as the intracellular material, stains positively with mucicarmine, periodic acid-Schiff (PAS) and other stains for mucin. The stroma does not show lymphocytic infiltrate or elastosis, and necrosis is not a feature of this tumor. Ultrastructurally, the epithelial cells are rich in dilated rough endoplasmic reticulum and possess a well-developed Golgi apparatus (20). Mucin is seen within membrane-bound structures (Fig. 7.14).

Pure mucinous tumors in which the mucoid pattern forms the bulk of the mass has a relatively favorable prognosis and less tendency to spread to lymph nodes than desmoplastic tumors. If a nonmucinous component is encountered, the tumors are classified as mixed mucinous, and these do not share the same favorable outcome as pure tumors. The classification of mucinous tumors into type A, where ≥75% of their bulk consists of extracellular mucin, and type B with <50% as extracellular mu-

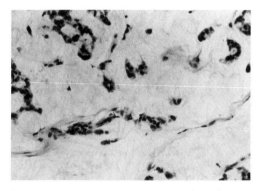

Figure 7.13. Mucinous carcinoma. Lakes of mucin surround the neoplastic cells, some of which have a signet-ring appearance, when seen at higher magnification.

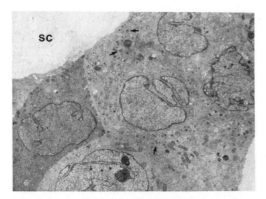

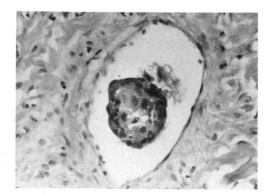

Figure 7.14. Mucinous carcinoma. Electron micrograph showing nuclear irregularity, large number of mucin granules (*arrows*), and the extracellular finely granular material (*SC*) consisting of secreted mucopolysaccharides. (Electron micrographs courtesy of Dr. Janine K. Mawad, Baylor College of Medicine, Houston, Texas.)

Figure 7.15. Inflammatory carcinoma. Tumor cells distend a dermal lymphatic.

cin, is not widely used. In type B, many sheets of neoplastic cells containing dense core granules are present. Carcinomas consisting entirely of single signet-ring cells are considered to be of lobular origin and have a less favorable prognosis than pure mucinous carcinoma.

Papillary Carcinoma

Infiltrative papillary carcinoma is responsible for less than 1% of breast cancers. Unlike desmoplastic neoplasms, papillary lesions may present with serous or bloody nipple discharge. A large duct in the subareola is often involved, and obstruction by a large tumor, cyst formation, and hemorrhage are common. The gross characteristics are similar to those of intraductal papillary carcinomas, and differentiation is not always feasible (10). However, the presence of areas of induration in the surrounding stroma strongly suggests an infiltrative growth.

Microscopic Features

The papillae are complex, with multiple layers of epithelial cells showing cytologic and histologic features of malignancy, as in intraductal papillary carcinoma. In addition, the neoplastic cells infiltrate the surrounding stroma, often losing their papillary configuration, and inducing fibrosis and lymphocytic infiltrate. Lymph node metastases are late but may manifest papillary formation.

Inflammatory Carcinoma

A rare clinical subtype of infiltrative ductal carcinoma, inflammatory carcinoma, is encountered mostly in young patients, often during the postpartum period or during pregnancy. However, the tumor may also be seen in older patients and nonpregnant patients. The neoplasm grows rapidly and is characterized by marked swelling, tenderness, and redness of the affected breast, similar to the manifestations of acute mastitis. The skin is red and diffusely thickened.

Microscopic Features

The neoplasm shows one of the various types of infiltrative ductal carcinoma described above. The histologic hallmark of inflammatory carcinoma, however, is the presence of nests of neoplastic cells within the lumina of small lymphatics and blood vessels in the superficial dermis (Fig. 7.15). This causes obstruction and dilatation of these channels and the characteristic clinical presentation. Aspiration of subcutaneous tissues or sampling by a core biopsy determines the neoplastic nature of the mass and rules out acute mastitis. The prognosis is grave, and less than 5% of the patients survive for 5 years (21).

Paget's Disease

This type of carcinoma is responsible for 2% of cases of breast cancer (22, 23). The adenocarcinoma affects menopausal or perimenopausal patients and involves the nipple, areola and, rarely, the vulva. A pruritic red and eczematoid skin lesion develops and is often associated with bleeding and covered by a crust (Fig. 7.16). The skin lesions are almost always associated with infiltrating or intraductal carcinoma of the deep parts of the breast. The deeply

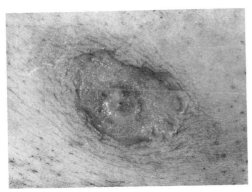

Figure 7.16. Paget's disease. Ulceration and excoriation of the nipple and areola in a 59-year-old patient. (Courtesy of Dr. Mary R. Schwartz, Baylor College of Medicine, Houston, Texas.)

seated masses are indistinguishable from carcinomas with fibrosis which were previously described. It has been suggested that Paget's disease starts at the dermoepidermal junction, from multipotent cells that can differentiate into glandular as well as squamous cells. The presence of desmosomes and melanosomes supports a squamous cell origin. Unlike squamous cells, however, Paget's cells are strongly positive for mucin and epithelial membrane antigen. This suggests that they are glandular, of breast duct origin, rapidly spreading to the skin surface as well as to the deeper parts of the breast.

Microscopic Features

In addition to the intraductal or infiltrating ductal carcinoma present in the deep breast tissues, the skin of the nipple and areola is infiltrated by large neoplastic cells, referred to as Paget's cells. These cells have abundant clear or vacuolated cytoplasm that stains positively for mucin. They have large irregular nuclei with prominent nucleoli. The cells form clusters within the epidermis or infiltrate the superficial layers of the epidermis as isolated cells. The surrounding squamous cells are normal in appearance, with no evidence of nuclear enlargement or pleomorphism (Fig. 7.17). The characteristic cells may also be seen in touch smears, prepared by gently scraping the skin surface, after moistening the lesion with saline for few minutes to soften the crust. Although Paget's cells may contain melanin granules, primary melanomas are exceptionally rare in the nipple.

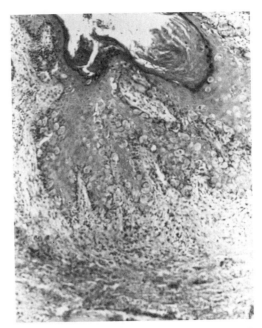

Figure 7.17. Paget's disease. Large cells with pale mucinous cytoplasm and pleomorphic nuclei are seen infiltrating the epidermis.

Apocrine Duct Carcinoma

Carcinomas with apocrine differentiation are rare and have no gross features that differentiate them from other ductal carcinomas. Microscopically, however, these tumors consist of characteristic large cells, with clear or eosinophilic granular or homogeneous cytoplasm and large hyperchromatic nuclei with coarse chromatin. Unlike benign apocrine cells, the malignant cells form solid nests or small glandular spaces that infiltrate the stroma in small groups (Fig. 7.18). Large cystic spaces are rarely encountered, as in benign metaplastic lesions.

Tubular Carcinoma

Tubular carcinomas are responsible for about 5% of breast cancers, with higher figures reported in series detected by mammography. The neoplasms are characterized by the formation of tubular structures that infiltrate the mammary stroma (24, 25). They present as a hard, stellate-shaped mass in the breast, and most neoplasms are less than 1 cm in diameter.

Microscopic Features

The epithelial cells form small well-defined tubules that are lined by a single layer of relatively uniform cells of slightly larger size than normal ductal cells. The cytoplasm often shows

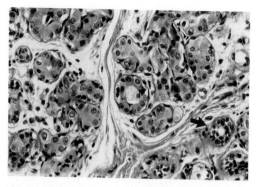

Figure 7.18. Apocrine carcinoma. The cells are large and have a dense eosinophilic (dark) cytoplasm. Compare the size of the neoplastic nuclei with that of normal lobule at *arrow*.

apical protrusions toward the lumen, and the nuclei usually possess prominent nucleoli. The stroma shows hyalinized fibrosis and peritubular and perivascular elastosis. Calcification may be present, but lymphocytic infiltrate is minimal, and the proliferation of myoepithelial cells is not evident. Necrosis, mitotic figures, and hemorrhage are not features of this type of carcinoma. Unlike sclerosing adenosis, the tubules in carcinoma are dilated, disorganized, and widely separated from each other by stroma (Fig. 7.19). Basement membrane and myoepithelial antigens cannot be demonstrated by immunocytochemistry in tubular carcinomas.

In addition to the pure tubular carcinoma described above, the tumors may be sclerotic or may be mixed with other carcinomas. Tubular carcinomas are often bilateral and multicentric and may contain mucin, ·features that are shared with lobular carcinoma. Foci of in situ or infiltrating lobular carcinoma are often pres-

ent in tubular carcinoma, and the term tubulolobular carcinoma has been suggested for such cases (26). A desmoplastic ductal carcinoma component is encountered in more than half the cases. The prognosis of this mixed desmoplastic and tubular variety is worse than that of pure tubular tumors that have a favorable outcome, with nodal metastases reported in 19% and 6% of cases, respectively (27).

LOBULAR ADENOCARCINOMA

About 10 to 20% of cases of breast cancer are classified as lobular carcinomas, and half of the cases are in situ (LCIS), while the other half present in an infiltrative phase (ILC). Lobular tumors are characterized by primary involvement of the lobules, although they may also extend into the large ducts or be associated with ductal carcinoma. Lobular carcinomas involve the upper-outer quadrant of the breast in most cases, are often multifocal, and when the contralateral breast is sampled, about one-third show foci of carcinoma (28). Long follow-up studies showed that about 30% of the patients with in situ lobular carcinoma develop infiltrative carcinoma after an average 16-year interval (29). The invasive tumors occur in the ipsilateral or contralateral breasts with almost equal frequency, and the majority are *ductal*.

Lobular Carcinoma In Situ (LCIS)

Lobular carcinomas are difficult to detect clinically or radiologically during the in situ stage, since they involve small terminal lobules and are almost never palpable. Most cases are diagnosed incidentally during mammography for routine screening or for fibrocystic lesions, and the majority occur during the reproductive years.

Microsopic Features

The lobules are distended and filled by neoplastic epithelial cells. The majority of these neoplastic cells are uniform and small (type A), but they are larger than those of the surrounding normal lobules and may contain a rare micronucleolus. The cytoplasm is scant and clear, and some cells have a signet-ring appearance. The cytoplasmic vacuoles of these signet-ring cells are mucicarmine-positive and occasionally show a central dense body (Fig. 7.20). The small type A cells are intermingled, within the same acinus, with larger but less common "type B" cells. The latter type have large hyperchromatic pleomorphic nuclei with prominent nucleoli (29). The involved lobular acini often surround a normal-appearing in-

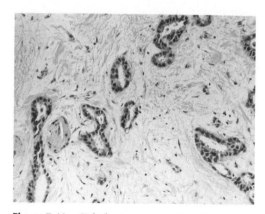

Figure 7.19. Tubular carcinoma. The disorganized glands are widely separated by fibrous stroma and are usually lined by a single layer of neoplastic cells.

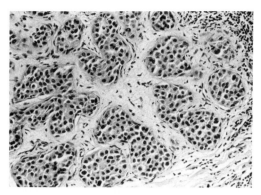

Figure 7.20. Lobular carcinoma in situ. The lobules are distended by rather uniform cells, leaving minimal or no lumen. Compare cell size with lymphocytes in *upper-right corner*.

tralobular duct, lined by small ductal epithelial cells and myoepithelium. Occasionally, the tumor cells spread under the ductal epithelium in a pagetoid fashion, lifting it up towards the lumen or replacing the small ductal cells with the larger LCIS cells. Table 7.4 lists the features of lobular carcinoma.

In situ lobular carcinoma should be differentiated from lobular hyperplasia (Table 7.5). Unlike hyperplasia, the acini in LCIS are filled with cells, leaving no residual lumen. Myoepithelial cells and lymphocytes do not constitute a part of the proliferating cell mass. LCIS should be differentiated from ductal carcinoma in situ involving the terminal ducts and lobules. Ductal tumors show necrosis, nuclear pleomorphism, and mitotic activity, features that are usually lacking in LCIS.

Infiltrating Lobular Carcinoma (ILC)

The infiltrative stage of lobular carcinoma is more difficult to define than LCIS. It has been estimated that 2 to 14% of infiltrative breast carcinomas are of lobular type, and the tumor appears to be more common in blacks than in caucasians (30).

Table 7.4. Features of Lobular Adenocarcinoma

Incidental finding or may present as a soft or firm mass
Lobules distended with small and some large cells
Small cells have central nucleoli, while the large cells have large pleomorphic nuclei with irregular nuclear membranes
Intracytoplasmic vacuoles and signet-ring cells
Sclerotic stroma

Gross Characteristics

Infiltrating lobular carcinoma (ILC) may be indistinguishable from infiltrating ductal carcinoma. Although they may produce multiple or single nodules, these tumors have more of a tendency to be multifocal, as compared with ductal carcinomas. Nodules of infiltrative lobular carcinoma are frequently palpable, although some are difficult to localize, and occasionally no masses are encountered.

Microscopic Features

The breast stroma is infiltrated by small uniform neoplastic cells that are often arranged in a single "Indian file" pattern, with bands of fibrous tissue in between. The neoplastic cells frequently form concentric layers around normal ducts, giving a "target-like or bull's eye" appearance. Other cells may be arranged in short chains, tubules, or as broad sheets of poorly cohesive cells that can be mistaken for lymphomas. The cells have relatively large dark nuclei that are piled up and have prominent nucleoli (Fig. 7.21). The neoplastic cells have abundant rough endoplasmic reticulum (RER) and a prominent Golgi apparatus. Stromal necrosis is not a prominent feature of infiltrating lobular carcinoma, but foci of LCIS are frequently encountered (31).

Signet-ring cell carcinoma is considered by many authors as a variant of ILC in which the predominant neoplastic cells have vacuoles that push the nuclei to the side (32). The vacuoles are weakly positive for mucicarmine and PAS, and occasionally a condensed intravacuolar inclusion may be seen (Figs. 7.22 and 7.23). The presence of estrogen receptors in the neoplastic cells supports a mammary derivation. The signet-ring cell pattern is associated with poor prognosis.

The differentiation between medullary and infiltrating lobular carcinomas may be difficult. Lobular carcinoma cells, however, tend to be smaller, with round or oval eccentric nuclei that frequently have a flat surface on one side. Cases showing a mixture of large cells with a desmoplastic ductal carcinoma pattern and smaller cells with lobular pattern are found frequently. Since survival studies indicate a prognosis similar to that with ductal carcinoma, such cases are usually classified as ductal carcinomas with "lobular pattern."

OTHER CARCINOMAS

Breast carcinomas cells reaching the skin may have melanin in their cytoplasm and should be differentiated from malignant melanoma. Some tumors, probably lobular in ori-

Table 7.5. Lobular Hyperplasia and Lobular Adenocarcinoma

Lobular Hyperplasia	Lobular Adenocarcinoma
Incomplete filling, residual lumen	Complete filling, no residual lumen
Mixed epithelial and myoepithelial cells	Epithelial cells not mixed with myoepithelium
Cells crowded	Monotonous cells with less overlapping
Mitosis rare	Mitosis present

gin, consist of histiocyte-like neoplastic cells, while others are formed of spindled epithelial cells (33). A variety of mesenchymal changes may also be seen in some carcinomas. These include myxoid, osseous, cartilaginous, or spindle cell metaplasias, and the presence of these elements may give the impression of a mixed tumor. Chondroosseous metaplasia has been linked with poor prognosis. Osteoclast-like giant cells are encountered in exceptional cases. Mucoepidermoid carcinoma, carcinoids, and a glycogen-rich clear cell carcinoma have also been reported. Some of the rare forms of carcinoma deserve further consideration below.

Squamous Carcinoma

True squamous cell cancers, including an acantholytic variant, have been reported (34, 35). However, most squamous elements encountered in breast tumors are the result of metaplasia in adenocarcinomas (Fig. 7.24). Metaplastic tumors behave similarly to the common types of breast cancer and should not be confused with primary squamous carcinoma of the breast or with metastatic squamous carcinoma elsewhere.

Adenoid Cystic Carcinoma

This forms a firm, small, nodular lesion, usually under the areola. It has the same histologic features as adenoid cystic tumors seen in other organs, with true and pseudoglandular formations. The true glands contain muci-carmine-positive material in their lumina, while the pseudoglands contain basal laminar material as demonstrated by PAS and electron microscopy. The tumor progresses slowly, and the prognosis is better than that for infiltrating ductal carcinoma and that of adenoid cystic tumors at other sites (36, 37).

Secretory (Juvenile) Carcinoma

This tumor tends to affect children and adolescents. Its cells are uniform, bland, and have cytoplasmic vacuoles that are rich in acid mucopolysaccharides. The neoplasm has an excellent prognosis (38).

Lipid-Rich Carcinoma

These are rare tumors that have a softer consistency than desmoplastic neoplasms and consist of cells with clear lipid-rich cytoplasm (39). The tumors metastasize to lymph nodes, giving the appearance of reticuloendotheliosis and occult metastases, unlike other breast tumors, which involve the orbit rather than the globe (40).

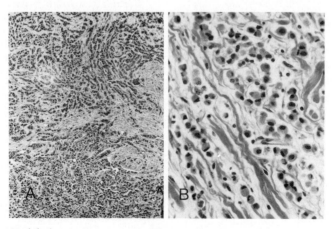

Figure 7.21.   Infiltrative lobular carcinoma. **A,** Neoplastic cells infiltrating the breast tissue in an "Indian file" pattern. **B,** Higher magnification of the small nests and cords of tumor cells.

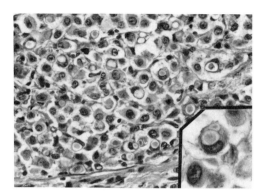

Figure 7.22. Signet-ring cell carcinoma. The nuclei of many cells are pushed aside by a large single cytoplasmic vacuole. Note the dense core of secretory material in the center of vacuoles (*insert*). (From Ramzy I. Clinical cytopathology and aspiration biopsy. Norwalk, CT: Appleton-Lange, 1990.)

Metastatic Carcinoma

Most metastases to the breast originate in the contralateral breast, and may be considered as second primary. Melanomas, gastrointestinal, and ovarian carcinomas may also metastasize to the breast. The recognition of these as metastatic is essential to avoid unnecessary mastectomy.

BREAST SARCOMAS

Sarcomas constitute about 0.5 to 1% of breast neoplasms and usually affect postmenopausal patients. The most common variety is

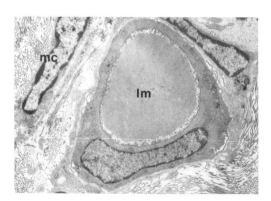

Figure 7.23. Infiltrative lobular carcinoma. A signet-ring cell with a central lumen (*lm*) that is lined by microvilli and is distended with secretion, displacing the nucleus peripherally. Reactive mesenchymal cells (*mc*) and collagenous stroma surround the neoplastic epithelial cell. (Electron micrograph courtesy of Dr. Janine K. Mawad, Baylor College of Medicine, Houston, Texas.)

malignant cystosarcoma phyllodes, which has been previously considered (Chapter 6). Angiosarcomas are sometimes seen in the breast, while malignant lymphomas, stromal sarcoma, liposarcoma, myosarcoma, and other sarcomas are extremely rare (Table 7.1). Care should be exercised to avoid interpreting atypical fibrous proliferation in benign conditions as indicative of sarcoma. Metaplastic mesenchymal elements, particularly cartilage and bone, occur in carcinomas, but they are morphologically bland. True mixed tumors exist, and they exhibit pleomorphic malignant morphologic features in their mesenchymal and epithelial elements (41).

Lymphangiosarcoma

These sarcomas develop at the site of the massive lymphedema occasionally following mastectomy (42). They present as ecchymotic nodules, often as late as 5 to 25 years after mastectomy. Histologically, the neoplasm consists of pleomorphic plump endothelial cells, lining vascular channels, and arranged in solid nests. The prognosis is poor.

Lymphoma and Leukemia

Primary involvement of the breast with lymphoma is rare, and most cases occur as a part of systemic involvement by the disease. Hodgkin's and non-Hodgkin's lymphomas have been reported (Fig. 7.25), as well as leukemia and myeloma (43). Pseudolymphomas, with formation of follicle and germinal centers, may also be encountered in the breast.

PATHOLOGIC FACTORS OF PROGNOSTIC SIGNIFICANCE

The main morphologic indicators of prognostic significance in breast carcinoma can be considered in two groups: those related to the primary tumor mass and those reflecting the spread of the neoplastic cells to the skin, lymph nodes, and surrounding tissues as well as to distant organs (Table 7.6).

The Primary Tumor

Tumor Type

As expected, intraductal and in situ lobular tumors have a better prognosis than infiltrative counterparts. Among the latter, medullary, tubular, Paget's, adenoid cystic, and mucinous carcinomas tend to have a better outcome than desmoplastic tumors. Inflammatory and lipid-rich tumors have the worst prognosis.

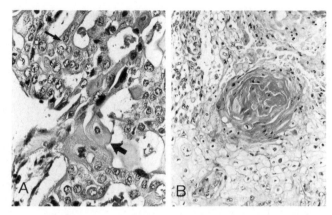

Figure 7.24.   Metaplastic carcinoma. **A**, The tumor shows columnar cells and gland formation (*thin arrow*), while in other areas (*thick arrow*), the cells have an abundant cytoplasm with keratinization associated with nuclear pyknosis, evidence of squamous differentiation. **B**, The lymph node metastases were almost entirely of squamous type.

Tumor Size

The doubling time for breast carcinoma varies from 30 to 209 days. However, neoplasms with greatest diameters of 3 cm or more usually have a poorer prognosis than tumors that are 2 cm or less in diameter (44, 45).

Tumor Grade

This can be assessed by evaluation of nuclear pleomorphism, formation of tubules, and the number of mitotic figures. Nuclei can be

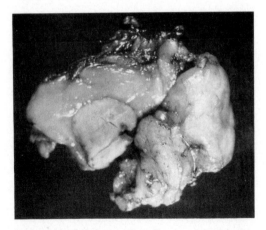

Figure 7.25.   Malignant lymphoma, primary breast involvement. The neoplasm forms a well-defined homogeneous mass that stands out from the surrounding breast tissue. Microscopically, this proved to be a non-Hodgkin's lymphoma, large-cell lymphocytic type.

classified into three grades, corresponding to minimal, moderate, and marked pleomorphism. The degree of differentiation, as manifested by tubule formation, can be also classified into three grades (Table 7.7).

Receptor and Other Assays

The standard estrogen receptor assay requires about 0.5 g of fresh tumor tissue obtained soon after the biopsy is submitted for frozen section and preserved by freezing. Histologic and cytologic material can also be immunostained for estrogen receptors and for *neu* oncogene (Fig. 7.26), and successful quantitative evaluation has been reported by some workers (46). Other immunohistochemical stains may play a role in the diagnosis but have no prognostic value. Nearly all breast carcinomas are positive for epithelial membrane antigen (EMA) and cytokeratin, while staining for carcinoembryonic antigen (CEA) is less consistent. Actin and myosin are rarely positive, and they indicate the presence of myoepithelial cells in the stroma, but not as part of the neoplastic epithelial cells. Type IV collagen and laminin, the basement membrane components that are seen around benign and normal breast epithelial cells, are rarely seen around carcinoma cells (13).

Spread of Breast Carcinoma

Breast cancer cells may spread by direct extension, as well as through lymphatics and/or blood vessels. The vascular supply and lym-

Table 7.6. Staging of Breast Cancer[a]

Stage	T[b]	N[c]	M[d]
I	1, 2	0	0
II	1, 2	1	0
III	1, 2	2	0
	3	0,1,2	0
IV	1,2,3	0,1,2	1

[a]Modified from the American and International Classifications.
[b]T—Primary tumor
  T1 <2 cm in greatest diameter, no skin involvement
  T2 >2 cm in greatest diameter or with skin involvement or nipple retraction
  T3 Any size with skin infiltration, ulceration, edema, pectoral muscle, or chest wall infiltration
[c]N—Regional lymph nodes
  N0 Axillary not palpable
  N1 Axillary palpable but movable
  N2 Axillary palpable and fixed (to other nodes or structures), or infraclavicular
[d]M—Distant metastases
  M0 No evidence
  M1 Clinical or radiologic evidence

phatic drainage of the breast is discussed in detail in Chapter 1.

Local Spread and Recurrence

The neoplastic cells infiltrate the fibroadipose tissues, extending to the skin as well as to the deep fascia and muscle. The tumor spreads along lactiferous ducts, and the nipple is involved in about 5 to 10% of cases. Such infiltration is associated with a decrease in the 5-year survival rate. Breast carcinomas are notorious for their tendency to recur up to 10 or 20 years after treatment. The local recurrence may involve the mastectomy site, or it may appear in

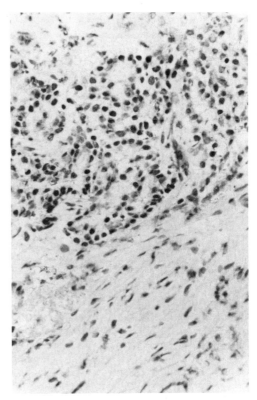

Figure 7.26. Estrogen receptors demonstrated in the nuclei of breast carcinoma cells that stained dark brown by immunoperoxidase technique. (Case courtesy of Lynn Dressler, MS, Albuquerque, New Mexico.)

other parts of the skin and soft tissues, including the contralateral breast (see below).

Lymph Node Metastases

These typically play an important role in determining the outcome for the patient. The ab-

Table 7.7. Tumor Grading System for Breast Carcinoma

Histologic Factors	Number of Points Awarded		
	Slight	Moderate	Marked
Loss of tubular arrangements of cells	1	2	3
Variation in nuclear size, shape and staining[b,c]	1	2	3
Frequency of hyperchromatic nuclei and mitoses	1	2	3
Total points:			
3–5: low malignancy (grade I)			
6,7: intermediate malignancy (grade II)			
8,9: high malignancy (grade III)			

[a]Modified from Bloom HJG, Richardson WW. Histologic grading and prognosis in breast cancer. A study of 1409 cases, of which 359 have been followed for 15 years. Br J Cancer 1957; 11:359–377.
[b]Prominent or multiple nucleoli raise the score to 3.
[c]This system of nuclear grading differs from that suggested by Black and his colleagues, in which the nuclei are graded from 0 to IV, with 0 being the *least* differentiated and IV being the best differentiated nuclei (64).

solute number, rather than the ratio of involved nodes, seems to have a good correlation with prognosis. Patients who have four or more nodes appear to do poorly (47–49). The axillary nodes are involved in over 75% of all cases showing systemic spread of the neoplasm. The internal mammary nodes are involved in about 8% of extended radical mastectomy specimens, particularly in those tumors located in the upper medial quadrant. There is also some evidence to suggest that infiltration of the perinodal adipose tissue is associated with worsening prognosis.

Hematogenous Spread

This method of spread, seen in about 5% of cases, correlates with unfavorable outcome. Evidence of vascular invasion may be seen in the breast tissue around the tumor. An attempt should be made to identify a rim of endothelial cells or some red blood cells around the nest of tumor cells, since shrinkage during preparation may cause false interpretation of invasion of lymphatics or blood vessels (50). In some cases, it may be necessary to stain for factor VIII to outline the endothelium. The presence of a nest at a distance from the main tumor, particularly if the contour of this nest does not conform to the outline of the tubular space, is further support of true vascular invasion.

Distant Metastases

Breast cancers can disseminate widely to many organs, particularly the lungs, liver, ovaries, and adrenal glands, and the metastatic deposits occasionally mimic a primary neoplasm of lung, ovary, or other organs. The spine and pelvic bones are often involved, and the lesions may be osteolytic or osteoblastic (see Fig. 7.6**C**). Malignant pleural effusion and ascites are encountered in late cases of breast cancer. In such effusions, the neoplasm often form cell balls, a feature that points to the breast as the possible source of the cells.

The Contralateral Breast

Patients treated for primary carcinoma develop a new clinically apparent carcinoma in the contralateral breast at a cumulative rate of 1% per year. Bilateral carcinomas were also reported in about 50% of cases by the time these patients die. A disproportionately high number of these bilateral cancers were lobular (51, 52).

CYTOLOGIC DIAGNOSIS OF BREAST CANCER

Cytologic breast samples are obtained from nipple discharge or by aspiration of solid or cystic lesions. Carcinoma rarely presents as nipple discharge, and cytologic examination of a smear prepared from a small drop, gently expressed from the nipple, may establish the diagnosis (Fig. 7.27). Palpable solid masses are aspirated using thin (No. 22 or 23 gauge) needles; adequate samples are procured in the majority of cases (53–56). The development of newer imaging techniques and stereotaxic localization improved the ability to localize early and small lesions, thus enhancing the role of aspiration in the diagnosis of mammary carcinoma (57). Estrogen receptor assays have been successfully achieved using aspirated material (52, 58). The likelihood of complications is negligible; the technique is almost painless and allows sampling of more than one nodule at a time. Clinical follow-up, histologic, and survival rate studies of large series have not demonstrated any increase in the risk of spread of tumor cells along the fine-needle tract, as compared with that of open biopsies. Furthermore, the definitive surgical resection and/or radiotherapy fields include the needle tract (59–61).

Aspirates from adenocarcinomas are characterized by an abundance of epithelial cells,

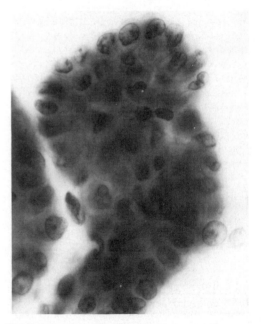

Figure 7.27. Nipple discharge from a papillary carcinoma showing malignant cells in papillary formation.

Table 7.8. Cytologic Features of Common Types of Breast Carcinoma

Feature	Infiltrative Ductal	Medullary	Infiltrative Lobular
Formations	Abundant aggregates, Loose and tight	Abundant clusters, Mostly loose	Rare clusters, Loose
Cellularity	Abundant	Abundant	Sparse
Cell size	Medium, 10–15 μm	Large, 15 μm	Small, 7–12 μm
Cytoplasm	Moderate amount	Abundant or scant	Scant, ill-defined
Nuclei	Large, pleomorphic	Large, some naked	Small uniform
Chromatin	Clumped	Prominent clumping	Bland
Nucleoli	Prominent, large	Prominent	Rare
Lymphocytes	Rare	Abundant	Rare
Positive diagnosis	In 70% of cases	In 85%	In 25%

many of which are isolated, although some appear as *small* clusters. Most carcinomas possess large hyperchromatic nuclei that vary in shape and have irregular contours, with thick nuclear membranes and clumped chromatin (Fig. 7.28). Necrosis, frequent mitotic figures, and an occasional calcific deposit may be present. The differentiation of in situ from invasive cancer is usually not feasible. Some infiltrating breast carcinomas consist of uniform cells with medium-sized nuclei that are deceptively bland. These nuclei, however, are more than double the size of those in normal ductal cells. Small cell tumors, particularly lobular carcinoma, are more difficult to differentiate cytologically, although their nuclei are still larger than those of lymphocytes. Mucinous carcinomas exhibit an abundance of mucicarmine-positive background material and signet-ring cells. The cytologic features of the common types of breast cancer are summarized in Table 7.8.

A distinction between a "positive" and a "highly suspicious but not conclusive" diagnosis is essential; the latter is a clear indication for an open biopsy or frozen section. False-negative diagnoses occur in an average of about 7% (62). Most cases result from inadequate sampling due to extensive fibrosis or sampling the wrong area. Using this technique, worries about suspicious lesions discovered during self-examination, or calcific deposits detected incidentally by mammography, can be alleviated. Patients with palpable and clinically operable lesions are allowed time for decision-making and for planning surgery, without the need for a second procedure. Metastatic workup or preoperative radiotherapy can be instituted with minimal hospital stay. Operative procedures for the sole purpose of diagnosis of inoperable tumors can be avoided, particularly since attempts for steroid receptor assays in aspirates appear to be feasible. Aspiration can also be used in poor-surgical-risk patients.

In conclusion, aspiration biopsy can play a significant role in the diagnosis of breast disease if its limitations are clearly understood by the clinician and the pathologist. A positive diagnosis should be as reliable as a frozen section, but a negative diagnosis must be followed by open biopsy if there is clinical suspicion of malignancy. The use of new stereotaxic imaging techniques with aspiration biopsy may

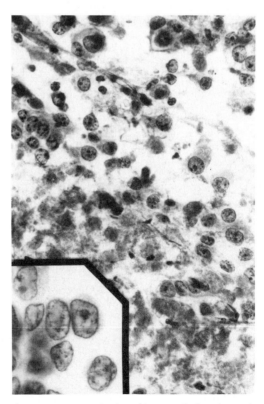

Figure 7.28. Aspiration biopsy of ductal carcinoma, showing malignant cells in small clusters. Note the necrosis, cellularity of the aspirate and the lack of cell cohesion, resulting in an abundance of isolated cells. *Inset* shows pleomorphic nuclei at higher magnification.

hold a promise for the future of early diagnosis of breast cancer by noninvasive but reliable procedures.

"Diagnosis by aspiration is as reliable as the combined intelligence of the clinician and the pathologist makes it"—Fred W. Stewart (63).

REFERENCES

1. Silverberg E, Lubera JA. Cancer statistics, 1988. CA 1988;38:5–22.
2. Azzopardi JG. Problems in breast pathology, vol 11. In: Bennington JL, ed. Major problems in pathology. Philadelphia: Saunders, 1979.
3. McDivitt RW, Stewart FW, Berg JW. Tumors of the breast. In: Atlas of tumor pathology, 2nd series, Fas. II. Washington, DC: Armed Forces Institute of Pathology, 1968.
4. World Health Organization. Histological typing of breast tumors. Tumori 1982;68:181.
5. Wellings SR, Jensen HM, Marcum RG. An atlas of subgross pathology of the human breast with special reference for possible precancerous lesions. J Natl Cancer Inst 1975;55:231–273.
6. Page DL, Dupont WD, Rogers LW, et al. Intraductal carcinoma of the breast: follow-up after biopsy only. Cancer 1982;49:751–758.
7. Lagios MD, Westdahl PR, Margolin FR, et al. Duct carcinoma in situ: relationship of extent of noninvasive disease to the frequency of occult invasion, multicentricity, lymph node metastases, and short-term treatment failures. Cancer 1982;50:1309–1314.
8. Ozello L. The behavior of basement membranes in intraductal carcinoma of the breast. Am J Pathol 1959;35:887–899.
9. Ozello L. Ultrastructure of human mammary carcinoma cells in vivo and in vitro. J Natl Cancer Inst 1972;48:1043–1050.
10. Murad TM, Contesso G, Mouriesse H. Papillary tumors of large lactiferous ducts. Cancer 1981;48:122–123.
11. Ohuchi N. Abe R, Kasai M. Possible cancerous change of intraductal papillomas of the breast: a 3-D reconstruction study of 25 cases. Cancer 1984;54:605–611.
12. Rosen PP, Scott M. Cystic hypersecretory duct carcinoma of the breast. Am J Surg Pathol 1984;8:31–41.
13. Barsky SH, Grotendorst GR, Liotta LA. Increased content of type V collagen in desmoplasia of human breast carcinoma. Am J Pathol 1982;108:276–283.
14. Robertson AJ, Brown RA, Cree I, et al. Prognostic value of measurement of elastosis in breast carcinoma. J Clin Pathol 1981;34:738–743.
15. Lwin KY, Zuccarini O, Sloane JP, et al. An immunohistological study of leucocyte localization in benign and malignant breast tissue. Int J Cancer 1985;
16. Gould VE, Miller J. Jao W: Ultrastructure of medullary, intraductal, tubular and adenocystic breast carcinomas. Comparative patterns of myoepithelial differentiation and basal lamina deposition. Am J Pathol 1975;78:401–416.
17. Sloane JP. Biopsy pathology of the breast. New York: John Wiley & Sons, 1985.
18. Ridolfi RL, Rosen PP, Port A, et al. Medullary carcinoma of the breast: a clinicopathologic study with 10-year follow up. Cancer 1977;40:1365–1385.
19. Wargotz ES, Silverberg SG. Medullary carcinoma of the breast: a clinicopathologic study with appraisal of current diagnostic criteria. Hum Pathol 1988;19:1340–1346.
20. Ahmed A. Ultrastructural aspects of human breast lesions. Pathol Annu 1980;15:411–443.
21. Droulias CA, Sewell CW, McSweeney MB, et al. Inflammatory carcinoma of the breast: a correlation of clinical, radiologic and pathologic findings. Ann Surg 1976;184:217–222.
22. Fisher ER, Gregorio RM, Fisher B, et al. The pathology of invasive breast cancer: a syllabus derived from findings of the National Surgical Adjuvant Breast Project (Protocol No. 4). Cancer 1975;36:1–84.
23. Paget J. On disease of the mammary areola preceding cancer of the mammary gland. St Barth Hosp Rep 10:87–89,1874. (Quoted by McDivitt et al., 3.)
24. McDivitt RW, Boyce W, Gersell D. Tubular carcinomas of the breast: clinical and pathological observations concerning 135 cases. Am J Surg Pathol 1982;6:401–411.
25. Oberman H. Tubular carcinoma of breast. Am J Surg Pathol 1979;3:387–395.
26. Fisher ER, Gregorio RM, Redmond C, et al. Tubulolobular invasive breast cancer: a variant of lobular invasive cancer. Hum Pathol 1977;8:679–683.
27. Deos PH, Norris HJ. Well-differentiated (tubular) carcinoma of the breast: a clinicopathologic study of 145 pure and mixed cases. Am J Clin Pathol 1982;78:1–7.
28. Wheeler JE, Enterline HT. Lobular carcinoma of the breast in situ and infiltrating. Pathol Annu 1976;11:161–188.
29. Rosen PP, Lieberman DH, Braun DW, et al: Lobular carcinoma in situ of the breast: detailed analysis of 99 patients with average follow-up of 24 years. Am J Surg Pathol 1978;2:225–251.
30. Martinez V. Azzopardi JG. Invasive lobular carcinoma of the breast: incidence and variants. Histopathology 1979;3:467–488.
31. Fechner RE. Histologic variants of infiltrating lobular carcinoma of the breast. Hum Pathol 1975;6:373–378.
32. Steinbrecher JS, Silverberg SG. Signet-ring cell carcinoma of the breast. The mucinous variant of infiltrating lobular carcinoma? Cancer 1976;37:828–840.
33. Gersell DJ, Katzenstein AA. Spindle cell carcinoma of the breast: a clinicopathologic and ultrastructural study. Hum Pathol 1981;12:550–561.
34. Eusebi V, Lamovec J, Cattani MG, et al. Acantholytic variant of squamous cell carcinoma of the breast. Am J Surg Pathol 1986;10:855–861.
35. Eggers JW, Chesney TM. Squamous cell carcinoma of the breast: a clinicopathologic analysis of eight cases and review of the literature. Hum Pathol 1984;15:526–531.

36. Galloway JR, Woolner LB, Clagett OT. Adenoid cystic carcinoma of the breast. Surg Gynecol Obstet 1966;122:1289–1294.

37. Page DL, Dixon JM, Anderson TJ, et al. Invasive cribriform carcinoma of the breast. Histopathology 1983;7:525–536.

38. Tavassoli FT, Norris HJ. Secretory carcinoma of the breast. Cancer 1980;45:2404–2413.

39. Aboumrad MH, Horn RC, Fine G. Lipid-secreting mammary carcinoma: report of a case associated with Paget's disease of the nipple. Cancer 1963;16:521–525.

40. Hood CI, Font RL, Zimmerman LE. Metastatic mammary carcinoma in the eyelid with histiocytoid appearance. Cancer 1973;31:793–800.

41. Rosen PP, Urban JA. Coexistent mammary carcinoma and cystosarcoma phyllodes. Breast 1975;1:9–15.

42. Stewart FW, Treves N. Lymphangiosarcoma in postmastectomy lymphedema. A report of six cases in elephantiasis chirurgica. Cancer 1948;1:64–81.

43. Mambo N, Butler J. Primary lymphoma of the breast. Cancer 1977;39:2033–2040.

44. Fisher ER, Gregorio RM, Redmond C, et al. Pathologic findings from the National Surgical Adjuvant Breast Project (Protocol No. 4): I. Observations concerning the multicentricity of mammary cancer. Cancer 1975;35:247–254.

45. Elston CW, Gresham GA, Rao GS, et al. The cancer research campaign (Kings/Cambridge) trial for early breast cancer: clinicopathological aspects. Br J Cancer 1982;45:655–669.

46. Gunduz N, Zheng S, Fisher B. Fluoresceinated estrone binding by cells from human breast cancers obtained by needle aspiration. Cancer 1983;52:1251–1256.

47. Bloom HJG, Richardson WW. Histologic grading and prognosis in breast cancer. A study of 1409 cases, of which 359 have been followed for 15 years. Br J Cancer 1957;11:359–377.

48. Dunn BH, Elrod BA. The selection of axillary lymph nodes in radical mastectomy specimens. Cancer 1957;10:687–689.

49. Thomas JM, Redding WH, Sloane JP. The spread of breast cancer: importance of the intrathoracic lymphatic route and its relevance to treatment. Br J Cancer 1979;40:540–547.

50. Rosen PP. Tumor emboli in intramammary lymphatics in breast carcinoma: pathologic criteria for diagnosis and clinical significance. Pathol Annu 1983;18:215–232.

51. Lewis TR, Casey J, Buerk CA, et al. Incidence of lobular carcinoma in bilateral breast cancer. Am J Surg 1982;114:635–638.

52. Robbins GF, Berg JW. Bilateral primary breast cancers: a prospective clinicopathological study. Cancer 1964;17:1501–1527.

53. Elston CW, Cotton RE, Davies CJ, et al. A comparison of the use of the "Tru-cut" needle and fine needle aspiration cytology in the pre-operative diagnosis of carcinoma of the breast. Histopathology 1978;2:239–254.

54. Frable WJ. Needle aspiration of the breast. Cancer 1984;53:671–676.

55. Kline TS, Kannan V, Kline IK. Appraisal and cytomorphologic analysis of common carcinomas of the breast. Diagn Cytopathol 1985;1:188–193.

56. Ramzy I. Clinical cytopathology and aspiration biopsy. Norwalk, CT, Appleton-Lange, 1990:261–271, 331–353.

57. Bolmgren J, Jacobson B, Nordenström B: Stereotaxic instrument for needle biopsy of the mamma. Am J Roentgenol Radium Ther Nucl Med 197;129:121–125.

58. Silfversward C, Humla S. Estrogen receptor analysis on needle aspirates from human mammary carcinoma. Acta Cytol 1980;24:54–57.

59. Ferrucci JT, Wittenberg J, Margolies MN, et al. Malignant seeding of the tract after thin-needle aspiration biopsy. Radiology 1979;130:345–346.

60. Sinner WN, Zajicek J. Implantation metastasis after percutaneous transthoracic needle aspiration biopsy. Acta Radiol 1976;17:473–479.

61. Zajdela A, Ghossein NA, Pilleron JP, et al. The value of aspiration cytology in the diagnosis of breast cancer: experience at the Foundation Curie. Cancer 1975;35:499–506.

62. Zajicek J. Aspiration biopsy cytology. Part I. Cytology of supradiaphragmatic organs. Monographs in clinical cytology. Basel, S. Karger, 1974:136–194.

63. Stewart F. The diagnosis of tumors by aspiration biopsy. Am J Pathol 1933;9:801–812.

64. Black MM, Opler SR, Speer FD. Survival in breast cancer cases in relation to the structure of the primary tumor and regional lymph nodes. Surg Gynecol Obstet 1955;100:543–551.

8

Introduction to Mammography

Lawrence W. Bassett
Richard H. Gold

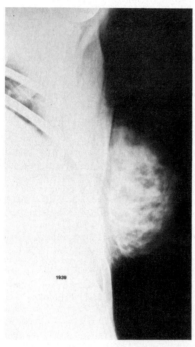

Figure 8.1. Mediolateral film mammogram by Stafford Warren in 1939. Although excellent for its time, there is loss of detail due to long exposure and lack of compression.

Mammography is the only proven method capable of detecting nonpalpable breast cancer. Early detection, the key to successful management of breast cancer, is the fundamental objective of x-ray mammography.

HISTORY

In 1913, Salomon (1), a German surgeon, performed radiographs of excised breasts, correlating radiographic, gross, and microscopic anatomy. In the United States, Stafford Warren

pioneered the clinical use of breast radiography when, in 1930, he reported a stereoscopic technique for mammography (Fig. 8.1). In his article (2), he described and classified the appearances of normal breasts, identifying fatty and glandular types, as well as illustrating the changes of pregnancy, mastitis, and benign and malignant tumors. However, for the next 20 years, mammography was not widely employed because of the techical difficulties of the examination.

It was not until the early 1950s that mammography began to gain recognition as a useful diagnostic procedure (3). Leborgne in Uruguay revitalized interest in mammography with the publication of a series of articles reporting plain mammography and duct injection. He used a nonscreen film system. Leborgne reported on carcinomatous microcalcifications that resembled "fine grains of salt." He identified such microcalcifications in about 30% of breast cancers (4). In the United States, Gershon-Cohen (5) reported extensively on the malignant and benign abnormalities identified on mammograms. Comparison of the mammographic findings with whole-breast histologic sections enabled investigators to recognize characteristic mammographic findings of benign and malignant disease and to establish reliable criteria for carcinoma (5).

The widespread adoption of mammography in the United States is primarily attributable to the work of Egan (6). He established a reproducible technique for nonscreen film mammography and reported excellent results in imaging the breasts of his first 1000 patients (6). Egan was largely responsible for the training of radiologists across the country in the performance and interpretation of mammograms.

Advances in technology through the years have led to a striking improvement in image quality and a dramatic reduction in radiation

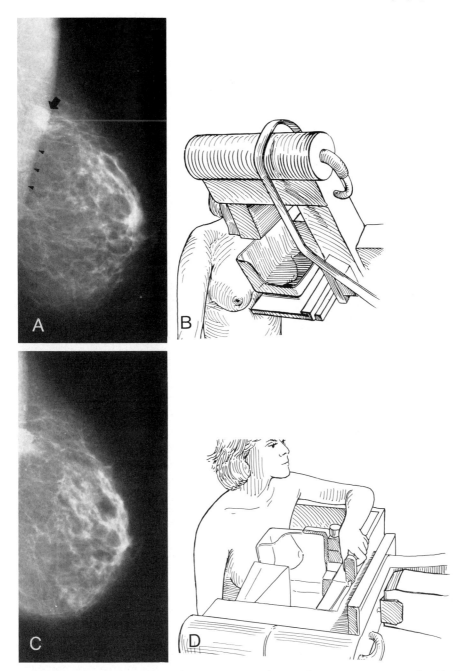

Figure 8.2. Film-screen mammogram and xeromammography. **A,** Film-screen mammography. Mediolateral oblique is optimal view because it includes the axillary tail. The pectoral muscles (*arrowheads*) are included in the image. A mass (*arrow*) is seen in the upper hemisphere. Biopsy revealed carcinoma. **B,** Postioning for the mediolateral-oblique film-screen view. The film holder lies under the breast, parallel to the pectoral muscle. Vigorous compression is applied, and dedicated mammography equipment must be used. (From Bassett LW, Gold RH. Breast radiography using the oblique projection. Radiology 1983;149:585–587.) **C,** Direct medio-lateral view, although showing less of the upper outer quadrant than oblique view, is needed to determine exact location of the mass. **D,** Positioning for the mediolateral view. (From Gormley L, Bassett LW, Gold RH. Positioning in film-screen mammography. Appl Radiol July 1988;35–37.)

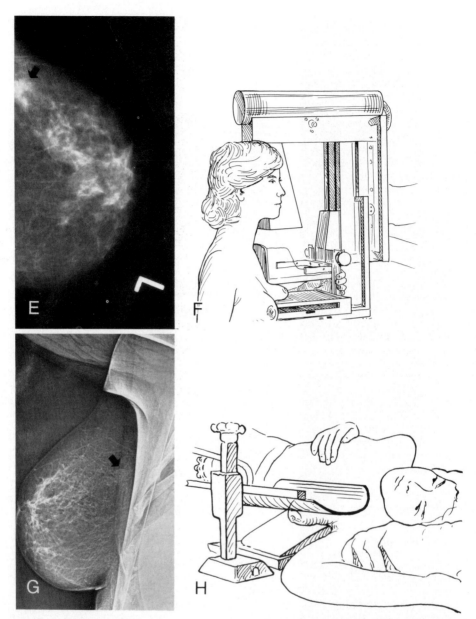

Figure 8.2. **E**, Craniocaudal view indicates that the mass (*arrow*) is in the outer hemisphere. **F**, Positioning for craniocaudal view. **G**, Xeromammogram. Mediolateral chest wall view of same breast. This projection includes juxtamammary chest wall structures. Although the mass (*arrow*) is easier to see in the high-contrast, film-screen image, the calcification in the center of the mass in shown better in the xeromammogram due to edge enhancement. **H**, Positioning for the chest wall xeromammogram. The patient lies on her side, the breast is elevated from the table with a sponge, only moderate compression is used, and dedicated mammography equipment is not required. (From Pagani JJ, Bassett LW, Gold RH, et al. Efficacy of combined film-screen xeromammography: Preliminary report. AJR 1980;135:141–146.)

dose. The first completely dedicated mammography unit was developed by Gros in France in the middle 1960s (7). A special x-ray target heightened the contrast between parenchyma, fat, and calcific densities, and a built-in compression device decreased scattered radiation and motion artifacts and separated breast structures.

In 1972 the introduction of a high-definition intensifying screen/single-emulsion film combination revolutionized film mammography (8). The new film-screen combination permitted rapid processing, an improved image, and a greatly reduced dosage.

The introduction of xeromammography in 1972 provided an alternative to film mammography that improved image quality by enhancing the edges of high-density structures, particularly calcifications (9, 10). Unfortunately, the aluminum filtration and negative-mode processing that was later required to reduce surface exposure to acceptable levels degraded the exquisite detail characterizing the images made with the original unfiltered positive-mode technique (11).

Clinical investigations have failed to reveal a significant difference in accuracy between film-screen mammography performed with dedicated equipment and xeromammography (12, 13). In 1979, Jans and associates (14) reported that film-screen units accounted for 45% of all mammography units in the United States, xeromammography for 45%, and direct-exposure (nonscreen) film mammography for 10%. A 1986 survey of mammography practices indicated that 54% of participating radiologists used film-screen mammography, 30% used xeromammography, 16% used combined film-screen and xeromammography, and less than 1% used direct film (15). The latter survey also reported that 71% of the mammography equipment had been purchased since 1983, that 72% of the surveyed radiologists had changed their method of mammography in the previous 10 years, and that the most frequently reported change (50%) was from xeromammography to film-screen mammography.

STATE OF THE ART

For optimal image quality, breast radiography should be performed only by film-screen or xeromammographic methods (Fig. 8.2). Film-screen mammography (Kodak Min-R screen/OM film) currently requires less radiation than xeromammography for the same two-view examination (for a 5-cm-thick breast BR12 breast phantom) an average glandular dose of 0.05 rad (no grid) to 0.1 rad (with grid) for film-screen (16) vs. 0.26 rad for negative-mode xeromammography and 0.13 rad for black liquid toner systems (17). In general, film-screen mammography offers higher image contrast, lower dose, and less equipment downtime. In comparison with earlier models, new dedicated units for film-screen mammography have smaller focal spots and longer distances between the x-ray source and the breast, resulting in better image resolution. They also have more effective compression devices, configura-

tions that allow easy and rapid positioning by permitting the patient to stand during exposures, and a microfocal spot x-ray target for magnification images. Used with the newest film-screen combinations, these x-ray systems provide greater image contrast and detail and require less dosage than ever before (18).

While film-screen mammography requires dedicated equipment, xeromammography can be performed with general purpose x-ray equipment. Xeromammography possesses two unique characteristics that improve visualization of breast pathology: wide recording latitude, which allows for good detail of both the chest wall and the thin peripheral portions of the breast, and edge enhancement, which accentuates the depiction of spiculations and calcifications (Fig. 8.3). The Xerox Corporation introduced a dedicated mammography unit suitable for xeromammography or film-screen mammography of a standing or recumbent patient. Xerox has also developed a new black liquid toner system that provides improved image resolution and broad area contrast, and a significant reduction in x-ray dose compared with their conventional blue powder-toner system. Nonetheless, declining sales resulted in an announcement by Xerox in February 1989 that they were discontinuing the production of xeromammography equipment.

PERFORMING THE EXAMINATION

A mammographic examination should consist of at least two views of each breast (19): a lateral or oblique and a craniocaudal view. For film-screen mammography, the mediolateral-oblique is the most efficient single radiographic view, because it depicts the greatest amount of breast tissue and includes the deeper structures in the upper-outer quadrant and axillary tail (Fig. 8.2A and B) (20, 21). A direct lateral projection (Fig. 8.2C), either mediolateral or lateromedial, in conjunction with a craniocaudal (Fig. 8.2D) is necessary to determine the exact location of a nonpalpable breast lesion. The "soft" x-ray beam used for film-screen examinations requires vigorous compression of the breast for adequate breast penetration. Although the chest wall is not included on the film-screen image, film-screen mammographers believe that when properly performed, the examination includes most or all of the breast parenchyma (22).

Breast compression improves resolution by bringing breast structures closer to the film and by preventing breast motion, it decreases the radiation dose by decreasing the thickness of the breast, it separates overlapping structures, and it aids in the differentiation of cystic and

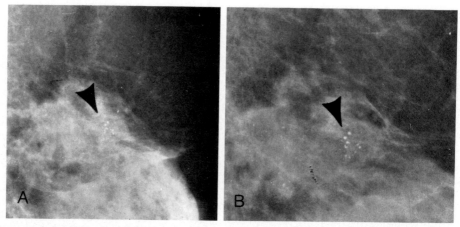

Figure 8.3.   Magnification view of microcalcifications. **A**, A small group of microcalcifications (*arrowhead*) is barely visible on this coned-down view. **B**, Microfocal spot magnification improves the depiction of the calcifications (*arrowhead*) which are numerous and vary in size and shape, features suggestive of malignancy. Biopsy revealed intraductal carcinoma.

solid masses. The vigorous compression required for film-screen mammography is acceptable to patients when they understand its importance.

Xeromammographers usually use a mediolateral chest wall view performed with the patient lying on her side (Fig. 8.2E). The chest wall view depicts the anterior chest wall structures as well as the breast. Some xeromammographers have claimed that 6 to 10% of carcinomas will be missed if the chest wall is not included in the image (23). Other xeromammographers prefer a mediolateral-oblique view obtained with dedicated xeromammography equipment. As with film-screen mammography, the lateral xeromammogram is supplemented by a craniocaudal view. The wider recording latitude and harder x-ray beam of xeromammography require less compression than film-screen mammography to ensure adequate image quality. As with film-screen mammography, however, greater compression allows a lower dose.

Additional views may be performed when an abnormality suggestive of cancer is identified. Modified craniocaudal views are needed when a lesion is identified on the oblique, lateral, or chest wall view but not on the standard craniocaudal view. The abnormality can usually be imaged in the craniocaudal view by turning the patient so as to move either the outer or inner aspect of the breast directly over the film holder or Xerox cassette.

Magnification views are used to enhance the depiction of microcalcifications (Fig. 8.3), masses, and equivocal findings (24). However, because magnification mammography requires considerably more radiation, its major role is to supplement standard mammography when the latter discloses equivocal findings (25). Magnification views can only be performed if the mammography equipment includes a microfocal spot x-ray target.

THE NORMAL BREAST

The breast contains 12 to 24 lobes of glandular tissue radiating from the nipple and located between the superficial and deep layers of the superficial fascia. The lobes drain through lactiferous (secretory) ducts and are separated from each other by sheaths of fibrous connective tissue. In adolescent women the breasts are composed almost entirely of fibroglandular tissue, resulting in a homogeneous radiopacity because they contain only a small amount of radiolucent fat. With advancing age or childbearing, the glandular tissue atrophies, undergoing transformation to fat, and the connective tissue sheaths then become visible in mammograms (Fig. 8.4). The breasts of older women are composed primarily of radiolucent fat (Fig. 8.5), enabling the detection of a cancer that is only a few millimeters in size.

The suspensory ligaments of Cooper are projections of breast parenchyma covered by fibrous connective tissue that extend from the skin to the deep layer of superficial fascia. The breast tissue is normally distributed in a bilaterally symmetrical pattern. Asymmetry may result from previous surgery, fibrocystic changes, or a desmoplastic response to carcinoma. Therefore, the mammograms should be arranged for viewing so that the right and left breasts appear to be mirror images of each other.

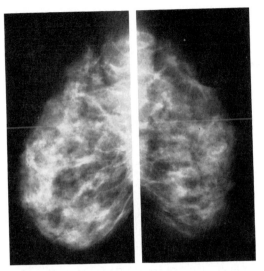

Figure 8.4. Normal bilateral film-screen mammograms of a 40-year-old woman show a mixture of radiodense fibroglandular tissue and radiolucent fat. The breasts, viewed side-by-side as mirror images, are bilaterally symmetrical.

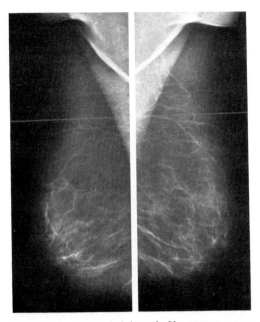

Figure 8.5. Normal bilateral film-screen mammograms of a 65-year-old woman show that the fibroglandular tissue has been completely replaced by radiolucent fat, an excellent background for the detection of small, nonpalpable cancers.

MAMMOGRAPHY FOR CANCER SCREENING

The first randomized controlled study to assess mammography in the periodic screening of asymptomatic women was that of the Health Insurance Plan of Greater New York (HIP). Beginning in 1963, enrolled women were offered annual screening by physical examination and mammography for 4 successive years. Evaluation after 7 years showed a 30% reduction in breast cancer mortality in the group offered screening compared with the control group. Fourteen years after the completion of screening, mortality was still reduced by 24% (26). Survival was greatest for women whose cancers had been detected by mammography alone. However, possibly because of the primitive state of the mammography, mortality was not reduced among the women who were under the age of 50.

In 1973, after the publication of the 7-year HIP results, the American Cancer Society and National Cancer Institute jointly initiated the Breast Cancer Detection Demonstration Project (BCDDP) (27). Five consecutive annual screening examinations were undertaken using physical examination and mammography. Thermography was also used for the first two or three annual screenings, but was abandoned when shown to be ineffective. Although the BCDDP was not a controlled study and the population was self-selected, the accumulated

data showed that mammography had undergone a striking technological advance since the HIP study and was far superior to physical examination in detecting cancer, especially early cancer. Mammography detected 91% of all cancers. The proportion of cancers detected by mammography alone was 42%, compared with 33% in the HIP study; while the proportion detected by physical examination alone was only 9%, compared with 44% in the HIP study. One-third of all cancers were noninfiltrating, or infiltrating but less than 1 cm in size; the majority of these cancers were detected by mammography alone (27, 28).

Three recent studies have confirmed the value of mammography for early breast cancer detection. In one Dutch study, all female residents age 35 and over in the city of Nijmegen were invited to participate in single-view mammography screening every other year starting in 1975. All deaths from breast cancer that occurred in the invited group between 1975 and 1982 were ascertained and a case-control study was conducted. The 48% relative risk of dying from breast cancer among the women who had been screened compared with those not screened implied a reduction in breast cancer mortality of 52% in the screened population (29).

A second Dutch study was conducted in the city of Utrecht, where all women ages 50 to 64 were invited to be screened by mammography and physical examination. Screening was repeated at 12-, 18-, and 24-month intervals. A case-control evaluation carried out in the same manner as in the Nijmegen project revealed a reduction in breast cancer mortality of 70% among women who were screened (30).

A Swedish screening study initiated in 1977 was designed as a randomized control prospective investigation. Of the enrolled women age 40 and over, one-half were offered screening at 24- and 33-month intervals by single-view mammography, while the other half served as controls. After 7 years, a reduction in breast cancer mortality of 31% occurred among the screened group compared with the control group. Although women under the age of 50 showed no mortality reduction, the number of deaths in that group was too small to give statistically significant results. The study showed that the rate of stage II and more advanced cancers was 25% lower among women who were screened than in the control group, while the rate of in situ and stage I cancers was much higher. Thus, the effectiveness of mammography in detecting cancer at an early stage was confirmed (31).

INDICATIONS FOR MAMMOGRAPHY

Mammography should be performed at any age when clinical findings lead a physician to suspect cancer. As useful as mammography is for examining a palpable breast lesion prior to biopsy, it is even more important to use mammography to evaluate both breasts for clinically occult cancer. Should the mammogram detect an abnormality in an area other than the one to be biopsied, a biopsy of each abnormal area should be obtained.

The American Cancer Society (ACS) provides the following guidelines for mammography in asymptomatic women (32, 33):

1. A single baseline mammogram should be performed between ages 35 and 40.
2. For women ages 40 to 49, mammography should be performed every 1 to 2 years, with frequency based on analysis of individual relative risk factors.
3. Women 50 years of age and older should have a mammogram every year.
4. Women with personal or strong family histories of breast cancer should consult their physicians about the need to begin mammography before age 40.

UNDERUTILIZATION OF MAMMOGRAPHY

Despite the gloomy statistics on the high incidence of breast cancer, the well-publicized guidelines for periodic screening mammography, and the overwhelming evidence that mammography can help detect breast cancer even before a physician or a woman feels a lump, most women do not undergo screening mammography. A survey of 257 Michigan women of a broad range of ages, education, and employment, disclosed reasonable rates of compliance for monthly breast self-examination (53 to 69%) and physical examination by a health professional (70 to 78%) (34). However, only 19% of the women age 35 to 49 and 25% of the women age 50 and older reported having undergone at least one mammogram. Of the women who had mammograms, 46% had them performed for abnormal clinical findings, and only 9% for health maintenance or cancer prevention. Twenty-six percent of the women who obtained a mammogram did so without knowing the specific reason ("doctor's advice"), and 48% planned to have future mammograms based solely on the advise of referring physicians. Contrary to commonly held belief, less than 1% of women who had or intended to have mammograms cited the influence of news media or the presence of breast cancer among friends or relatives in having the examination performed. The results of this study imply that the most important factor in the utilization of periodic screening mammography is the attitude of the referring physician.

In 1982, a mail survey of 509 family physicians in New York State indicated that although family physicians recognized that mammography could detect breast cancer in its early stages, most of the physicians did not recommend routine mammograms. In that study, the reason most commonly given for not recommending mammography was radiation risk (35).

In a 1984 survey of referral practices of Los Angeles physicians for screening mammography, 887 of the 4200 physicians queried returned a postage-paid questionnaire (36). Only 10.7% of respondents followed the ACS recommendation for annual mammographic screening of women over age 50, the least controversial of the guidelines. There was a significant difference in compliance between physicians less than 40 years old and those age 40 and older; the younger physicians were more apt to refer their asymptomatic patients for screening mammography. Physicians practicing in a group rather than in a solo practice also had a greater tendency to refer their patients for screening mammography. There was no significant difference in compliance between male and female physicians. Of those who did not refer asymptomatic women over 50 for annual screening, 54.5% gave high cost/low yield as the major reason, 17.3% were concerned about radiation risk, and 7.4% felt that other screening methods were adequate. A telephone survey by the ACS yielded similar results, and confirmed high cost as the major deterrent to ordering screening mammography (37).

OVERCOMING THE BARRIERS TO SCREENING

Ongoing efforts to increase the utilization of mammography for breast cancer screening include cost reduction, physician and patient education, and implementation of mandatory reimbursement for screening (38). In order to reduce costs, screening mammography, which is performed in asymptomatic women, should be performed differently than consultative mammography, which is performed on women with a breast problem, usually a lump. Whereas two standard views of each breast suffice for a screening examination, consultative mammography should be supervised on site by the radiologist and often includes special positioning techniques, coned-down and magnification views, correlative physical examination, and sonography.

One method for lowering costs is the establishment of screening clinics that perform only the basic test. Mobile vans are sometimes used for high-volume screening. These vans can be taken directly to the work place. Screening examinations can be performed by the technologist at a remote site and interpreted later by the radiologist in his or her office. Some screening facilities require that patients pay at the time they receive their examination, thus eliminating billing costs. Computerized standard dictations or checkoff lists for normal cases reduce the costs of report dictation and transcription. When abnormalities are identified, the patient can be referred for further diagnostic workup. Batch processing of the radiographs is a time-saving device by which mammograms made during the working day are processed later (39).

The ACS has played a major role in educating patients and physicians about the benefits of mammography screening to detect early breast cancer. ACS divisions across the United States have sponsored local low-cost screening projects intended to increase physician and public awareness about the value of mammography. In 1987, the ACS made a major national commitment to "breast cancer awareness." Ed-

ucational efforts were directed toward primary care physicians in order to increase their referrals for high-quality, low-dose screening mammography.

Consultative or diagnostic mammograms, performed to evaluate a suspicious condition such as a lump or nipple discharge, are generally covered by health insurance. However, screening mammography currently is not covered by most health insurance plans because such coverage does not conform to the basic mandate of insurance: to provide payment for illness and injury. In actual practice, many insurance plans do pay for mammography screening even though it may not be official policy to do so. In order to ensure reimbursement for screening mammography, some physicians have felt compelled to fabricate a diagnostic problem such as "fibrocystic disease" or "breast thickening." Unfortunately, this practice may lead to future difficulty for the patient should she apply for health insurance from another provider. The new provider may deny coverage for subsequent breast problems on the basis of a preexisting breast condition.

Unlike private insurance plans, health maintenance organizations tend to support mammographic screening. For example, the Kaiser hospitals in Los Angeles support periodic mammographic screening ordered by their physicians, and Cigna Health Plans of California encourage their physicians to comply with the ACS mammography screening guidelines.

Mary Rose Oakar, a congresswoman from Ohio, introduced a bill in the U.S. House of Representatives four years ago that has been viewed as the first step toward mandatory insurance coverage for screening mammography. Although passage of this bill still seems unlikely at this time, Representative Okur intends to reintroduce it in the future. Similar bills have already been passed by the Maryland, Texas, and California legislatures. The Maryland bill was passed largely due to the leadership of Rose Kushner and the National Alliance of Breast Cancer Organizations, a group that provides a telephone hotline and a periodic newsletter to directly influence issues such as research funding priorities, insurance reimbursement, and health care legislation.

FALSE-NEGATIVE MAMMOGRAMS

Although mammography is the most effective method for the early detection of breast cancer, even properly performed mammograms fail to disclose 10 to 15% of breast cancers. If a false-negative mammogram leads to a delay in biopsy, the prognosis may be adversely affected (40). In a 2-year period, 36 women with palpable breast cancers and negative mammograms were seen at the UCLA-Jonsson Comprehensive Cancer Center. Seventeen of these patients had had a biopsy performed within 2 months of the negative mammogram, and only 3 (17.6%) of the 17 were found to have extension of their disease to the axillary lymph nodes at operation. The remaining 19 patients had biopsy delays ranging from 3 to 24 months (mean delay of 12 months), and 11 of them (57.9%) had axillary node involvement at operation.

Dense parenchymal tissue is the major reason for false-negative interpretations. Other causes of a false-negative mammogram include faulty radiographic technique and errors in interpretation (41). The mammography report may be used to warn the referring physician against a delay in biopsy of a palpable mass when the mammogram is negative. This can be accomplished by adding a codicil to every report such as "Mammography is not a substitute for biopsy in the presence of clinical findings suggestive of carcinoma." Many radiologists and referring physicians object to the use of a routine codicil because it suggests indecisiveness. An alternative is the use of a warning only in those cases where a palpable abnormal mass is not identified on the mammogram. The radiologist may also report the presence of dense parenchymal tissue that limits the accuracy of the examination.

REFERENCES

1. Salomon A. Belträge zur pathologie und klinik der mammakarzinome. Arch Klin Chir 1913;101:573–668.
2. Warren SL. A roentgenologic study of the breast. Am J Roengenol Radium Ther 1930;24:113–124.
3. Bassett LW, Gold RH. The evolution of mammography. AJR 1988;150:493–498.
4. Leborgne R. Diagnosis of tumors of the breast by simple roentgenography; calcifications in carcinoma. Am J Roengenol Radium Ther 1951;65:1–11.
5. Gershon-Cohen J, Ingleby H. Roentgenography of cancer of the breast: a classified pathological basis for roentgenologic criteria. Am J Roentgenol Radium Ther Nucl Med 1952;68:1–7.
6. Egan RL. Experience with mammography in a tumor institution. Evaluation of 1000 cases. Radiology 1960;75:894–900.
7. Gros CM. Methodologie. J Radiol Electrol Med Nucl 1967;48:638–655.
8. Weiss JP, Wayrynen RE. Imaging system for low-dose mammography. J Appl Photogr Engr 1976;2:7–10.
9. Wolfe JN. Xerography of the breast. Radiology 1968;91:231–240.
10. Martin JE. Xeromammography—an improved diagnostic method: review of 250 biopsied cases. AJR 1973;117:90–96.
11. Sickles EA. Mammographic detectability of breast microcalcifications. AJR 1982;139:913–918.
12. Snyder RE, Kirch RL. Comparison study of xeromammography and low-dose mammography. In: Gallagher HS, ed. Early breast cancer detection and treatment. New York: Wiley & Sons, 1975: 199–204.
13. Pagani JJ, Bassett LW, Gold RH, et al. Efficacy of combined film-screen/xeromammography: preliminary report. AJR 1980;135:144–146.
14. Jans RG, Butler PF, McCrohan JL Jr, Thompson WE. The status of film/screen mammography. Results of the BENT study. Radiology 1979;132:197–100.
15. Bassett LW, Diamond JJ, Gold RH, McLelland R. Survey of mammography practices. AJR 1987;149:1149–1152.
16. Haus AG. Trends in screen-film mammography: grids, small focal spots, high-speed screen-film combination, controlled film processing, reduced radiation dose. Health Sciences Division, Eastman Kodak Company, 1986.
17. Speiser RC, Zanrosso EM, Jeromin LS. Dose comparison for mammographic systems. Med Phys 1986;13:667–673.
18. Logan WW, Janus JA. Performing the examination. In: Bassett LW, Gold RH, eds. Breast cancer detection. Orlando, Fl: Grune & Stratton, 1987; 75–87.
19. Bassett LW, Bunnell DH, Jahanshahi, Gold RH, Arndt RD, Linsman J. Breast cancer detection: one versus two views. Radiology 1987;165:95–97.
20. Lundgren B. The oblique view at mammography. Br J Radiol 1977;50:626–628.
21. Bassett LW, Gold RH. Breast radiography using the oblique projection. Radiology 1983;149:585–587.
22. Bassett LW, Pagani JJ, Gold RH. Pitfalls in mammography: demonstrating deep lesions. Radiology 1980;136:641–645.
23. Kalisher L. Factors influencing false-negative rates in xeromammography. Radiology 1979;133:297–301.
24. Sickles EA, Doi K, Genant HK. Magnification film mammography: Image quality and clinical studies. Radiology 1977;125:69–76.
25. Sickles EA. Microfocal spot magnification mammography using xeroradiographic and screen-film recording systems. Radiology 1979;131:743–749.
26. Shapiro S, Venet W, Strax P, Venet L, Roeser R. Ten- to fourteen-year effect of screening on breast cancer mortality. J Natl Cancer Inst 1982;69:349–355.
27. Baker LH. Breast Cancer Detection Demonstration Projects: Five-year summary report. CA 1983;33:255.
28. Bearhs OH, Shapiro S, Smart C. Report of the Working Group to Review the National Cancer Institute-American Cancer Society Breast Cancer Detection Demonstration Projects. J Natl Cancer Inst 1979;62:639–698.
29. Verbeck AL, Hendriks JH, Holland R, Mravunac M, Sturmans F. Reduction of breast

cancer mortality through mass screening with modern mammography. First results of the Nijmegen project, 1975–1981. Lancet 1984;1:1222–1224.

30. Collette HJ, Day NE, Rombach JJ, de Waard F. Evaluation of screening for breast cancer in a non-randomized study (the DOM project) by means of a case-controlled study. Lancet 1984;1:1224–1226.

31. Tabar L, Fagerberg CJ, Gad A, et al. Reduction in mortality from breast cancer after mass screening with mammography. Randomized trial from the Breast Cancer Screening Working Group of the Swedish National Board of Health and Welfare. Lancet 1985;1:829–832.

32. American Cancer Society Report on the Cancer-Related Health Checkup: cancer of the breast. CA 1980;30:224–229.

33. American Cancer Society Mammography guidelines 1983: Background statement and update of cancer-related checkup guidelines for breast cancer detection in asymptomatic women age 40 to 49. CA 1983;33:255.

34. Fox S, Baum JK, Kos DS, Tsou CV. Breast cancer screening: the underuse of mammography. Radiology 1985;156:607–611.

35. Cummings KM, Funch DP, Mettlin C, Jennings E. Family physician's beliefs about breast cancer screening by mammography. J Fam Pract 1983;17:1029–1034.

36. Bassett LW, Bunnell DH, Cerny JA, Gold RH. Screening mammography: referral practices of Los Angeles physicians. AJR 1986;147:689–692.

37. Survey of Physician's Attitudes and Practices in Early Cancer Detection. CA-A J Clin 1985;35:197–213.

38. Bassett LW, Gold RH. Screening mammography: overcoming the barriers. Admin Radiol 1987;5:13–16.

39. McLelland R. Mammography 1984: challenge to radiology. AJR 1984;143:1–4.

40. Mann BD, Giuliano AE, Bassett LW, Barber MS, Hallauer N, Mortoon DL. Delayed diagnosis of breast cancer as a result of normal mammograms. Arch Surg 1983;118:23–24.

41. Martin JE, Moskowitz M, Milbrath JR. Breast cancer missed by mammography. AJR 1979;132:737–739.

Mammographic Features of Benign Disease

Richard H. Gold

OBSTACLES TO MAMMOGRAPHIC DETECTION OF MASSES

The capability of a mammogram to reveal a mass largely depends on the presence of sufficient fat to serve as a contrasting radiolucent background. Mammography may disclose an obvious lesion only a few millimeters in diameter in a breast in which fibroglandular tissue has been replaced by fat. But in very dense breasts packed with radiopaque tissue, as those of young nulliparous, pregnant, or lactating women, and in breasts manifesting severe fibrocystic change, even a large mass may be obscured by the dense surrounding parenchyma. Therefore, in the evaluation of a breast manifesting such strikingly increased density, the physician must be aware that mammography is of limited value.

MARGIN OF LESION: BENIGN VS. MALIGNANT

The key mammographic feature distinguishing carcinoma from most benign breast masses is the irregular margin of carcinoma and the smooth margination of benign masses. The infiltrative character of most carcinomas is reflected in spicules of fibrous connective tissue and cords of tumor cells that aggressively infiltrate the surrounding parenchyma. Carcinomas that infiltrate less aggressively and grow more slowly, such as papillary, medullary, and mucinous carcinomas, tend to appear more circumscribed but still manifest irregular or indistinct margins. In contrast to the infiltrative, spiculated character of most carcinomas, the majority of benign masses—cysts and fibroadenomas—usually have smooth margins. Only rarely is a carcinoma so well-circumscribed as to resemble a benign mass. Metas-

tases to the breast from extramammary malignancies also are characteristically well-circumscribed and may mimic benign lesions.

MAMMOGRAPHIC FOLLOW-UP OF LESIONS THAT APPEAR PROBABLY BENIGN

While it might be considered prudent to perform needle aspiration, excision biopsy, or ultrasonograpy of *all* solitary breast masses regardless of their mammographic features (except in cases of typical "popcorn" calcifying fibroadenoma, which is described later), this is impractical because of their great numbers. Masses that are less than 1 to 1.5 cm in size with smooth margins and containing no microcalcifications are almost all benign and may be followed by documenting their stability with repeat mammography in 6 months and then yearly for a total of 2½ to 3 years (1). If a mass is greater than 1.5 cm in greatest diameter, sonography should be performed; the disclosure of echoes within the mass implies a solid lesion that must be excised. If the mass is not palpable, excision may be performed with prebiopsy needle localization.

The stability of a benign mass is most easily proven by comparison with previous mammograms. Because some cancers grow exceedingly slowly, if possible the comparison should be made with examinations dating back several years.

MULTIPLE DISCRETE MASSES

The presence in a breast of more than two discreet masses, each manifesting the same mammographic features as the others except for different size, implies that they are all benign. A rare exception would be multiple me-

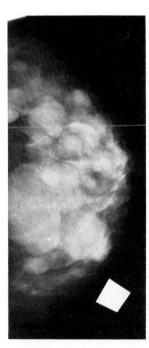

Figure 9.1. Multiple cysts. The margins of the cysts are smooth, a feature that is best seen where there is fat adjacent to the cyst wall.

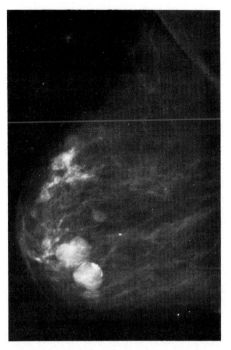

Figure 9.2. Multiple fibroadenomas. One of them contains characteristic coarse calcifications, and another has a typical lobulated shape. The masses have smooth margins.

tastases from an extramammary malignancy, which often have a benign appearance. Cysts are frequently multiple, and fibroadenomas are sometimes multiple (Figs. 9.1–2). Primary multicentric carcinoma of the breast usually does not appear as multiple discrete masses but as two or more foci of clustered microcalcifications or architectural distortion separated by at least 2 cm.

THE SOLID MASS

It is convenient to classify mammographic abnormalities that have proved to be solid by ultrasonography according to three types of options: (*a*) those that demand prompt histologic evaluation, (*b*) those that are clearly benign and of no clinical concern, and (*c*) those of such a high probability of being benign that they may be followed by mammography to demonstrate their stability (1). The mammographic follow-up of lesions in the third category consists of obtaining a repeat mammogram within 3 to 6 months of the initial examination, and thereafter at yearly intervals for a minimum of 2½ to 3 years before declaring the mass to be stable, thereby making the possibility of malignancy a remote consideration (2).

MAMMOGRAPHIC FOLLOW-UP OF CALCIFICATIONS THAT APPEAR PROBABLY BENIGN

The microcalcifications characteristic of benign conditions tend to be larger, rounder, fewer, and less variable in size than the calcifications associated with malignancy (Figs. 9.3 to 9.5). However, certain benign disorders—sclerosing adenosis, fat necrosis, and apocrine metaplasia—may manifest microcalcifications similar to those seen in malignancy. All clusters of calcifications suggestive of malignancy should be biopsied, with the aid of needle localization if the lesion is nonpalpable, even though some of the calcifications will be found to result from benign disease, usually sclerosing adenosis. For microcalcifications that appear probaby to be benign, but with minimal uncertainty as to their origin, the same type of mammographic follow-up schedule should be considered as for solid masses that are probably benign: repeat mammography in 3 to 6 months followed by mammograms at yearly intervals for a minimum of 2½ to 3 years total. During this time, an increase in the number of calcifications or a suspicious change in their character should prompt a biopsy.

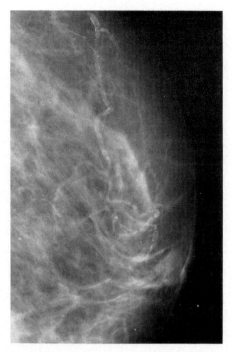

Figure 9.3. Calcified artery, signified by broken parallel lines of calcium in the wall of the vessel.

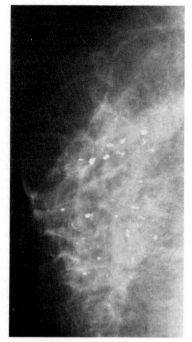

Figure 9.4. Secretory disease, characterized by typically benign-appearing, scattered, ring-shaped calcifications.

BENIGN DISORDERS

Intramammary Lymph Node

Normal intramammary lymph nodes are usually located in the upper-outer quadrant of the breast, near the chest wall, and are usually not palpable. They tend to be less than 1 cm in diameter, often have a bean or kidney shape with a distinctive hilar notch, often are partially replaced by fat, and, as most benign masses, they have a smooth outline. Should an intramammary lymph node enlarge and its fat content be replaced by inflammatory or neoplastic cells, the node may clinically and mammographically resemble a primary carcinoma (3).

Mole and Surgical Scar

A mole on the skin of the breast may simulate a well-circumscribed intramammary lesion in the mammogram.

A surgical scar, particularly of recent origin, may have radial spiculations that resemble those of carcinoma (4) (Fig. 9.6). Palpation is useful in excluding the possibility of carcinoma in the region of a known scar. A scar is usually only palpable as a minimal, vague thickening, while most infiltrating carcinomas feel two or three times larger than their mammographic images and are rock hard. Moreover, follow-up mammograms usually disclose a gradual decrease in the size and prominence of the scar.

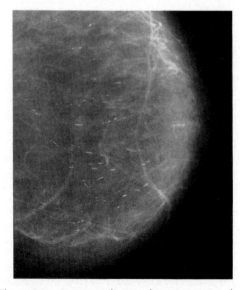

Figure 9.5. Secretory disease, featuring coarse, homogeneous rod-shaped calcifications.

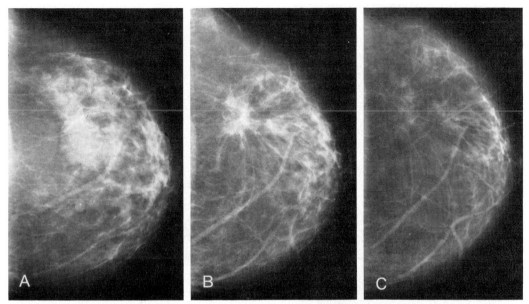

Figure 9.6. Evolution of a surgical scar. **A,** Prominent region of nodularity in the upper hemisphere was correlated with a palpable mass. Biopsy revealed fibrocystic changes. **B,** Follow-up examination 1 year later reveals new spiculated shadow. Palpation, however, revealed only a vague thickening rather than the expected rock-hard mass characteristic of carcinoma. On this basis, the mammographic diagnosis was "scar." **C,** One year later, the scar had completely and spontaneously resolved.

Cyst

Cysts result from dilatation of terminal ducts (Figs. 9.1 and 9.7). Because the fluid within a cyst is usually under tension, the wall of the cyst tends to be displaced equally in all directions. A cyst, therefore, has a smooth, sharp border and, as shown by air insufflation, a thin wall with a smooth lining. Although intracystic papillomas and papillary carcinomas may result in a bloody aspirate, this is not invariably the case. Therefore, some mammographers prefer to inject the aspirated cyst with air in order to seek irregularities in the normally smooth inner contour of the cyst wall that might imply an intracystic tumor. Insufflation also tends to reduce the chance of fluid reaccumulation (5). The injected air gradually and spontaneously resorbs within a few weeks.

Fibroadenoma

Fibroadenoma is the most common solid benign tumor of the breast. It consists of an encapsulated fibrous connective tissue stroma that envelops ramifying tubules lined with epithelium. While cysts are usually round or oval, fibroadenomas are often lobulated but still maintain a smooth margin (Fig. 9.2). With advancing age, a fibroadenoma may undergo hy-

alinization and develop characteristic coarse or popcorn-like calcifications (Fig. 9.8). Lipo-

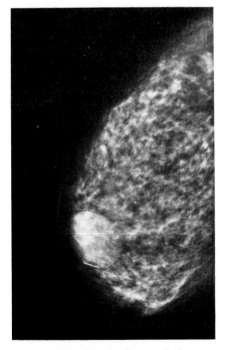

Figure 9.7. Cyst with curvilinear calcification in its wall. Calcification of a cyst wall is unusual. The oval configuration and smooth margin are characteristic.

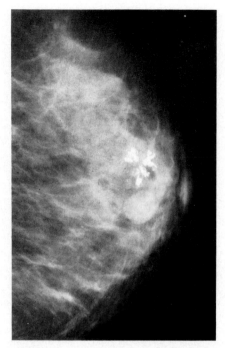

Figure 9.8. Two fibroadenomas. The upper mass has typical popcorn-like calcifications, but the border is obscured by surrounding dense parenchyma. The lower lesion, although uncalcified, has a typical smooth margin that is surrounded by sufficient fat to make it visible.

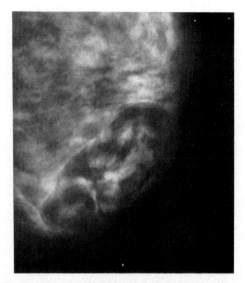

Figure 9.9. Lipofibroadenoma (hamartoma) featuring a well-circumscribed mass containing a mixture of fatty and fibroglandular tissues. The central cauliflower-like appearance is characteristic. The large amount of fat in this lesion made it difficult to palpate.

fibroadenoma is a rare fibroadenoma-like lesion that contains abundant fat and has a "cauliflower" appearance in the mammogram (Fig. 9.9). Its abundant fat content makes it difficult to palpate.

Cysts and fibroadenomas are often surrounded by a thin radiolucent halo. Rarely, well-circumscribed malignant masses may also be surrounded partly or entirely by a radiolucent halo (6). Thus, a radiolucent halo is suggestive but not pathognomonic of a benign mass. On the other hand, a lack of fat in surrounding dense parenchymal tissue may obscure the margin of a cyst or fibroadenoma, leading to a failure of detection or, more important, to a false-positive finding and misdiagnosis of infiltrating carcinoma.

Cystosarcoma Phyllodes

Cystosarcoma phyllodes is a rare tumor that bears pathologic similarities to fibroadenoma, except for a more cellular, hyperplastic stroma. Mammographically, it tends to be well-circumscribed but may invade the adjacent tissue to a limited extent. Rarely, it undergoes hematogenous metastasis. A wide margin of surrounding normal breast tissue is therefore excised

with the cystosarcoma. The tumor may contain cystic cavities filled with clear or semisolid bloody fluid and may have fatty elements as well. The histologic classification of a cystosarcoma as benign or malignant is based on the histology of its stroma. Mammographically, it sometimes manifests coarse calcifications similar to those of fibroadenoma.

Lipoma

When they are surrounded by fat of equivalent radiographic density, lipomas may be difficult to detect mammographically. They are characterized by a discrete radiolucent mass with a thin wall of fibrous connective tissue.

Sclerosing Adenosis

Sclerosing adenosis is the most commonly occurring benign disorder that mammographically may mimic malignancy. It is one of many conditions included in the spectrum of breast pathology known as fibrocystic changes. The latter probably result from an exaggeration and distortion of cyclic changes that normally occur during the menstrual cycle. At least four histologic patterns occur at different rates and with so much overlap that it is usually impossible to detect one pattern in the absence of the others: (a) cysts, (b) stromal fibrosis, (c) proliferation of duct epithelium, and (d) adenosis or lobular hyperplasia. Fibrocystic changes occur clini-

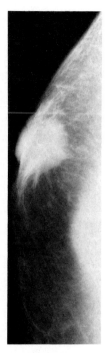

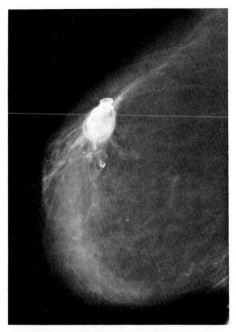

Figure 9.10. Retroareolar abscess in a male breast. Edema surrounding the abscess has lead to a slightly indistinct margin that mimics carcinoma.

Figure 9.11. Traumatic fat necrosis characterized by smoothly marginated lipid-filled cavity with densely calcifying wall.

cally in 50 to 80% and histologically in 90% of women. Seventy percent of women with fibrocystic changes have nonproliferative lesions that are not potentially precancerous. The remaining 30% have proliferative changes that double their risk for breast cancer as compared with the risk of other women in the general population. Women at highest risk are those with atypical ductal or lobular hyperplasia: their risk is up to five times that of women without such changes. Fortunately, only 4% of all women with histologic evidence of fibrocystic changes exhibit atypical hyperplasia (7).

Sclerosing adenosis evolves in two stages: an early stage of florid proliferation of epithelial cells and a late stage of stromal fibrosis with loss of lobular boundaries. The disorder usually appears mammograpically as an ill-defined, widespread, mottled, and nodular process, or, after coalescence of the nodules, as an extensive homogeneous soft-tissue density with indistinct margins (8). Flecks of calcium, which tend to be fewer, rounder, but similar in size to those found in association with carcinoma, may permeate the lesion, simulating carcinoma calcifications and resulting in the need for a biopsy to definitively exclude malignancy.

Breast Abscess

Breast abscess (Fig. 9.10) may cause diffuse thickening of the skin, a sign that may be misinterpreted as signifying lymphatic permeation by a carcinoma (9). Although carcinoma must always be suspected first among the causes of diffuse mammary skin thickening, breast abscess frequently can be excluded only by aspiration or biopsy. The abscess may be surrounded by intense edema, creating a mammographic and clinical appearance that simulates lymphatic carcinomatosis or inflammatory carcinoma. Calcifications are not a mammographic feature of breast abscess.

Traumatic Fat Necrosis

Traumatic fat necrosis is a nonsuppurative inflammatory process that may result in a variety of mammographic appearances, many of which may be confused with carcinoma. It can also mimic mammary carcinoma on clinical examination (8). Branching, rod-like, or angular microcalcifications identical to those of carcinoma may occasionally be seen (10). Other mammographic features may include a spiculated density indistinguishable from carcinoma; associated localized thickening and deformity of the skin that may further raise suspicions of carcinoma; and single or multiple benign-appearing, lipid-filled cavities with or without calcified walls (11) (Fig. 9.11). A location close to the skin or areola is a clue that the lesion may have resulted from blunt or surgical trauma. Traumatic fat necrosis is particularly common in women who have had reduction mammoplasties or lumpectomy with radiation therapy.

Skin Thickening: Differential Diagnosis

The thickness of the skin of normal breasts seldom exceeds 1.5 mm. The exception is the normally thicker skin of the inframammary crease. The skin of small, firm breasts may appear somewhat thickened in mammograms because of the difficulty in achieving optimal compression during the x-ray exposure; since the skin tangential to the x-rays is less closely apposed to the film than the skin of larger, flabby, more easily compressible breasts, the result may be roentgenographic magnification and, hence, apparent skin thickening.

Diffuse thickening of the skin suggests lymphatic permeation by the metastases of an underlying primary carcinoma. Although carcinoma must always be considered first, other causes, benign and malignant, are possible (9): abscess, fat necrosis, radiotherapy, subcutaneous extravasation of pleural fluid after thoracentesis, progressive systemic sclerosis (scleroderma), obstruction of the superior vena cava, pemphigus, nephrotic syndrome, lymphoma, and lymphatic extension from contralateral breast carcinoma. In a bedridden woman, congestive heart failure may lead to edematous skin of a dependent breast.

ROLE OF MAMMOGRAPHY IN EVALUATING THE BREAST BEFORE AND AFTER LUMPECTOMY AND RADIOTHERAPY

Breast-conserving therapy with lumpectomy and radiotherapy requires a coordinated effort among the surgeon, pathologist, diagnostic radiologist, and radiation oncologist. Contraindications to breast-conserving therapy include the following (12):

1. a primary tumor so large that it cannot be resected without major cosmetic deformity; although depending to some extent on breast size, a lesion more than 5 cm in greatest diameter would probably be a contraindication;
2. the presence of two or more widely separated ipsilateral primary tumors (i.e., both occupying more than one quadrant);

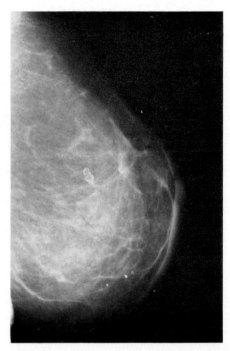

Figure 9.12. Breast 1 year after lumpectomy and radiotherapy. Lipid-filled cavities with calcified walls represent fat necrosis and are secondary to the trauma of the surgery, radiation, or both. Diffuse thickening of the skin and distortion of parenchymal architecture are other characteristic features that should not be misinterpreted as evidence of residual or recurrent tumor.

3. malignant microcalcifications occupying more than one quadrant; and, possibly,
4. extensive carcinoma in situ.

Mammograms are essential before treatment to delineate the extent of the primary tumor and to identify other possible foci of tumor in the ipsilateral and contralateral breast. If the resected tumor is associated with microcalcification, additional mammography is required prior to radiotherapy to ensure that all of the microcalcifications have been excised. However, mammography should not be performed until 2 to 4 weeks after lumpectomy. This delay is necessary to allow sufficient time for the incision to heal so that full and comfortable compression of the breast may be achieved during the x-ray exposure, and to allow any postoperative hematoma to resolve so that it is not misinterpreted as residual cancer.

Following radiotherapy, mammography and physical examination are of critical importance to seek local recurrent cancer that, if detected early, may be associated with a significant salvage rate. Because the interval between definitive therapy and recurrence may exceed

10 years (12), follow-up mammography is usually obtained at 6 months and 12 months posttreatment and then annually throughout life.

Findings suggestive of recurrent cancer include new microcalcifications that appear typical of malignancy, and a mass of architectural distortion, none of which were present in the posttreatment baseline mammograms. About two-thirds of recurrent cancers occur at the site of the primary tumor (13), and are usually treated by mastectomy. Comparison of the new mammogram with previous posttreatment mammograms is essential for their proper interpretation and to prevent the following benign posttreatment changes from being misinterpreted as evidence of recurrent tumor: skin thickening and retraction, parenchymal architectural distortion and increased density, benign-appearing dystrophic calcifications, and hematoma formation (Fig. 9.12). Fortunately, these benign changes usually diminish or stabilize by 6 to 12 months after therapy, as can be ascertained when the latest follow-up mammogram is compared with earlier ones (13).

REFERENCES

1. Homer MJ. Imaging features and management of characteristically benign and probably benign breast lesions. Radiol Clin North Am 1987;25:939–951.
2. Homer MJ. Nonpalpable mammographic abnormalities: timing the follow-up studies. AJR 1981;136:923–926.
3. Kopans DB, Meyer JE, Murphy GF. Benign lymph nodes associated with dermatitis presenting as breast masses. Radiology 1980;137:15–19.
4. Sickles EA, Herzog KA. Intramammary scar tissue: A mimic of the mammographic appearance of carcinoma. AJR 1980;135:349–352.
5. Tabár L, Pentek Z, Dean PB. The diagnostic and therapeutic value of breast cyst puncture and pneumocystography. Radiology 1981;141:659–663.
6. Swann CA, Kopans DB, Koerner FC, et al. The halo sign and malignant breast lesions. AJR 1987;149:1145–1147.
7. Hutter RVP. Goodbye to "fibrocystic disease." N Engl J Med 1985;312:179–181.
8. Gold RH, Montgomery CK, Rambo ON. Significance of margination of benign and malignant infiltrative mammary lesions. Roentgenologic-pathologic correlation. AJR 1973;118:881–894.
9. Gold RH, Montgomery CK, Minagi H, et al. The significance of mammary skin thickening in disorders other than primary carcinoma: Roentgenologic-pathologic correlation. AJR 1971;112:613–621.
10. Bassett LW, Gold RH, Cove HC. Mammographic spectrum of traumatic fat necrosis: the fallibility of "pathognomonic" signs of carcinoma. AJR 1978;130:119–122.
11. Bassett LW, Gold RH, Mirra JM. Non-neoplastic breast calcifications in lipid cysts: development after excision and primary irradiation. AJR 1982;138:335–338.
12. Hellman S, Harris JR. Breast cancer: considerations in local and regional treatment. Radiology 1986;164:593–598.
13. Stomper PC, Recht A, Berenberg AL, Jochelson MS, Harris JR. Mammographic detection of recurrent cancer in the irradiated breast. AJR 1987;148:39–43.

Mammographic Features of Malignancy

Lawrence W. Bassett

The features of breast carcinoma depicted on mammography can be primary, secondary, or indirect. The primary signs of malignancy include a mass and microcalcifications. Secondary signs include skin thickening and/or retraction, nipple retraction, and axillary node enlargement. Indirect signs include architectural distortion, unilateral duct prominence, or unilateral asymmetric density.

An early cancer is asymptomatic, too small to be palpated, and without regional or distant metastases. The prognosis for early breast cancer is good; however, the mammographic signs of early cancer may be subtle. Mammographic signs of early breast cancer include a small mass, calcifications, or more subtle indirect signs.

PRIMARY SIGNS

Mass

Mammographically, the majority of breast cancer masses are dense and have irregular margins.

Infiltrative Carcinomas

The nature of the tumor margin is the most important single criterion for the diagnosis of a malignant breast mass (1). Peripheral spiculations are an important feature of breast carcinomas, and, in general, the more highly infiltrative the lesion the more spiculated the margin will appear in the mammogram (Figs. 10.1 to 10.3) (2). Scirrhous carcinoma is named for the preponderance of fibrous tissue the tumor contains and may be of ductal or lobular origin. These tumors are typically rock hard on palpation. The radiating spicules of a scirrhous carcinoma may be sharp, dense, or composed of fine lines with variable length radiating in all directions (3). The larger the central tumor mass, the longer the spicules. Because of the edema and desmoplastic reaction these tumors elicit in the surrounding breast tissue, the size of the tumor is exaggerated on physical examination. The mammogram thus provides a more accurate estimate of the true size of the mass (Fig. 10.4).

Well-Circumscribed Carcinomas

Ductal carcinomas that infiltrate less aggressively are more sharply circumscribed but may still demonstrate knobby, irregular, or indistinct margins (Fig 10.5). Occasionally, a carcinoma is so well-circumscribed that it clinically and mammographically resembles a benign lesion. Examples of typically well-circumscribed tumors are papillary, medullary (Fig. 10.6), and colloid carcinomas. Because they incite little desmoplastic reaction, these carcinomas, like benign breast masses, tend to be the same size both at palpation and in the mammogram.

A papillary carcinoma may arise in a cyst or a lactiferous duct. It may develop by malignant degeneration of a benign papilloma or as a primary papillary carcinoma.

Medullary carcinoma grows predominately by producing cells from the center of the tumor; there is very little stroma. The tumor grows in an expansive as well as infiltrating fashion, so it may be smooth, lobulated, or poorly demarcated (4). There may be central necrosis and hemorrhage resulting in rapid enlargement of the tumor. Because of its shape, a medullary carcinoma may be mistaken mammographically for a cyst or fibroadenoma (Fig. 10.6).

Colloid, mucin-producing or mucinous carcinoma is a rare malignancy that usually

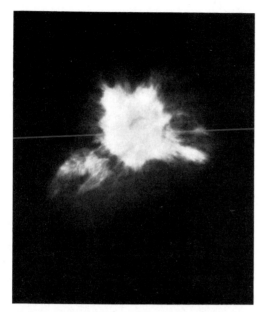

Figure 10.1. Specimen radiograph of scirrhous carcinoma. The mass is very dense, with spicules of varying thickness and length emanating from the surface of the tumor.

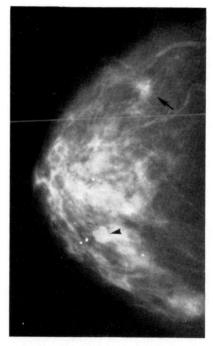

Figure 10.3. Cephalocaudal film-screen mammogram. Small scirrhous carcinoma (*arrow*) is contrasted with well-marginated fibroadenoma (*arrowhead*).

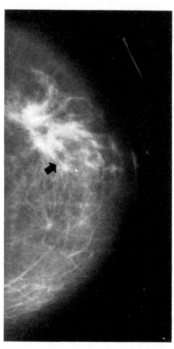

Figure 10.2. Cephalocaudal film-screen mammogram. Multifocal scirrhous carcinoma. There are two dense masses with radiating spicules (*arrow*).

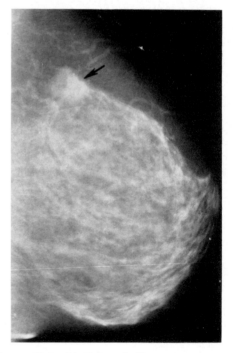

Figure 10.4. Mediolateral film-screen mammogram. Nonpalpable infiltrating ductal carcinoma (*arrow*) has dense center and poorly defined margins. Tumor measuring 2.5 cm in the mammogram was estimated to be 5 cm at palpation.

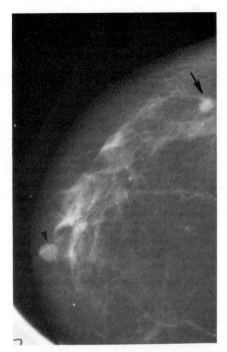

Figure 10.5. Outer breast from cephalocaudal film-screen mammogram. Nonpalpable ductal carcinoma (*arrow*) has moderately well-defined margins. The nipple (*arrowhead*) is not in profile.

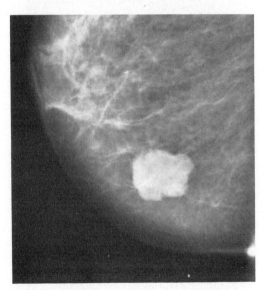

Figure 10.6. Mediolateral film-screen mammogram. Lobulated medullary carcinoma with smooth margins mimics a benign mass.

occurs in older women and has a relatively good prognosis. The tumor produces a large amount of mucous containing epithelial clusters. The tumor grows and expands slowly with little infiltra-

tion; thus, mammographically it is sharply separated from surrounding tissue.

Mammographically, well-circumscribed carcinomas may be confused for a benign lesion. There is no retraction of surrounding tissue and no associated architectural distortion. Therefore, regardless of mammographic features, needle aspiration, excisional biopsy, or ultrasonography of all solitary solid masses is recommended for women in the cancer age group. Benign-appearing solid masses less than 8 to 10 mm in diameter may be observed with follow-up mammograms rather than biopsied. However, if a solid, noncalcified mass shows an increase in size in serial mammographic examinations, a biopsy is indicated regardless of the size and mammographic appearance, it should be biopsied (Fig 10.7). These well-circumscribed cancers are less aggressive, grow more slowly, and metastasize later; thus, they have a more favorable prognosis than scirrhous or infiltrative lobular carcinomas.

Metastases

Metastatic disease to the breast from extramammary primary malignancies is unusual. The largest reported single source is melanoma, but a wide variety of other tumors may secondarily involve the breast (5). The autopsy incidence of metastasis to the breast from malignant neoplasms other than primary breast carcinoma varies from 1.7 to 6.6% (6). In contrast, the clinically observed rate ranges from only 0.5 to 1.3% (7, 8). Due to its late appearance in the course of the disease, a metastatic module is rarely the initial sign of malignancy. Metastatic foci to the breast appear in mammograms as circumscribed spheroid shadows with only slightly irregular margins and without evidence of microcalcifications, spiculations, or other signs of desmoplastic response that characterize many primary scirrhous carcinomas (Fig. 10.8) (9). While the presence of multiple mammographic lesions suggests the possibility of metastases, the majority of metastases to the breast are solitary.

Cystosarcoma Phyllodes

Cystosarcoma phyllodes is a rare tumor that bears pathologic similarities to fibroadenoma, except for a more cellular, hyperplastic stroma. The majority are benign. Mammographically, the tumor tends to be well-circumscribed and even when it abuts the skin it may not cause skin thickening (Fig 10.9). However, rarely, it may invade adjacent normal tissue to a limited extent and may then undergo hematogenous metastasis. The determination of malignancy is based on histologic criteria.

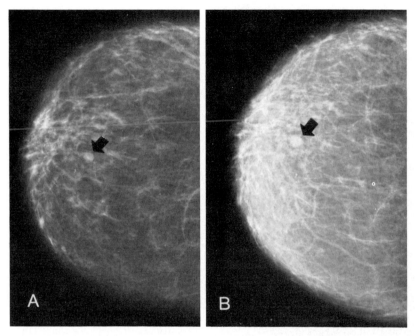

Figure 10.7. Well-defined ductal carcinoma. **A,** Cephalocaudal film-screen mammogram showed well-defined 5-mm mass (*arrow*). **B,** Mammogram 12 months later. Mass (*arrow*) grew to 8 mm. Biopsy was performed.

Calcifications

In the 1950s, Leborgne in Uruguay reported on the occurrence of mammographic carcinomatous calcifications, which, he said, resembled "fine grains of salt," and which he detected in about 30% of cancers (10). Gershon-Cohen (11) recognized calcifications as an early mammographic sign of carcinoma, especially ductal carcinoma, which could be present long before the tumor was palpable. Carcinoma calcifications may occur in association with an abnormal mass or independently, and one of the earliest mammographic signs of malignancy is the presence of microcalcifications not associated with a mass.

Microcalcifications can be reliably detected only by mammography. Although other imaging methods such as sonography, thermography, light scanning, and magnetic resonance imaging have been advocated for breast cancer detection, an important limitation of these modalities is their inability to depict calcifications in the breast.

Malignant Calcifications

Malignant calcifications typically are numerous and vary in size and shape, often appearing as casts of the ducts (Fig 10.10 to 10.12). Most of the calcifications that are visible on mammograms are larger than 50 μm. Carcinoma calcifications are often intraductal and

are found within the necrotic cells in the center of a tumor-filled duct (12). They may also occur in the lumen of small malignant glands without evidence of cell necrosis; it is also believed that malignant microcalcifications may occur as a result of an active secretory process (13).

In an excisional biopsy, tissue containing these calcifications does not feel different from adjacent tissue, and the fine calcifications are frequently shattered or dislodged during the preparation of histologic specimens. Therefore, it is important to radiograph biopsy specimens immediately after they are excised to verify the presence of calcifications (Fig 10.11).

Equivocal Calcifications

Nonspecific calcifications create the greatest dilemma. Such equivocal calcifications are not the fine-clustered, variable, and uncountable types characteristic of malignancy nor the coarse, scattered, dense, or amorphous types characteristic of benign conditions. Borderline types of calcifications result in a significant number of unavoidable false-positive biopsies.

Egan and associates have found the number, distribution, and variability of equivocal calcifications to be helpful in determining whether there is possible malignancy and, hence, if a biopsy should be performed. A cluster may be defined as three or more calcifications in a 0.5 × 0.5 cm area. The greater the

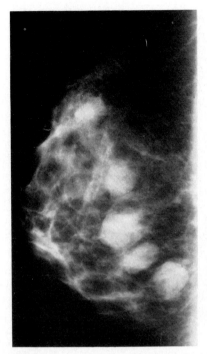

Figure 10.8. Mediolateral film-screen mammogram. Multiple metastases from alveolar rhabdomyosarcoma.

number of calcifications in a cluster, the greater the likelihood of malignancy. A cluster of greater than 10 calcifications is particularly

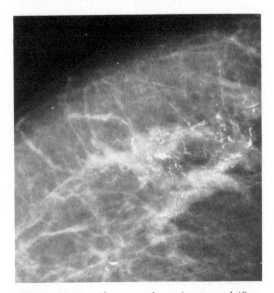

Figure 10.10. Close-up of carcinoma calcifications. Calcifications are numerous, varying in size and shape, and appear as casts of ducts. Vague increased tissue density is also present.

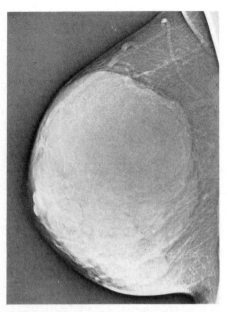

Figure 10.9. Mediolateral xeromammogram. Well-circumscribed cystosarcoma phyllodes fills most of the breast and abuts on skin without causing significant thickening.

likely to represent a malignancy. Variability in size and shape has also been found to be a feature of malignancy, although this finding may occur in some benign conditions such as epithelial hyperplasia. A pattern of scattered calcifications, without localized clusters, usually indicates a benign condition. However, in many cases calcifications are indeterminate and biopsy cannot be avoided.

Sickles (15) recommends magnification mammography as a valuable aid in the evaluation of microcalcifications. The superior images obtained with magnification can resolve some equivocal cases by improving the visualization of calcifications, which permits correct interpretation in a greater number of cases.

Management of Calcifications

The most common sign of early malignancy, and frequently the only sign, calcifications with mammographic features suggestive of malignancy, should always be biopsied (16).

When there is only a low suspicion of malignancy even after magnification techniques are applied, it is important to review all previous mammograms. If the calcifications have been stable for 2 to 3 years, a biopsy is not indicated. If the calcifications are new or have increased, biopsy is probably indicated. If previous mammograms have not been performed and calcifications are not strongly suspected to be malig-

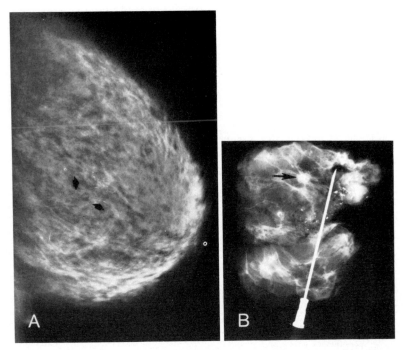

Figure 10.11. Nonpalpable carcinoma calcifications in asymptomatic woman referred for screening mammogram. **A,** Mediolateral film-screen mammogram. The breast is dense. Calcifications suggestive of carcinoma (*arrows*) are barely visible. **B,** Specimen radiograph following mammographically guided prebiopsy needle localization. The calcifications are readily visible around localization needle. The small mass (*arrow*) was not visualized in the original mammogram. Histologic diagnosis was ductal carcinoma.

nant, follow-up examinations may be recommended instead of biopsy. Such follow-up examinations are usually performed 4 to 6 months later, followed by annual bilateral studies for at least 2 years (17).

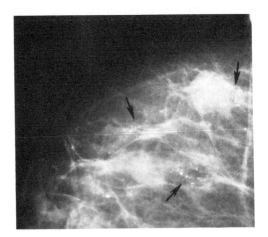

Figure 10.12. Multifocal duct carcinoma. Close-up shows multiple clusters of calcifications (*arrows*) and two masses. Only the larger mass was palpable.

SECONDARY SIGNS

Secondary mammographic features of malignancy include skin thickening and/or retraction, nipple retraction, and axillary node enlargement. These secondary signs are usually evidence of an advanced carcinoma, one for which the prognosis is poor.

Skin Thickening

The thickness of the skin is normally less than 1.5 mm, except for the region of the inframammary crease, which may be twice as thick. The desmoplastic response elicited by breast carcinoma may result in local fibrous connective tissue deposition in the skin. Localized skin thickening may also be due to previous surgery, regional abscess, fat necrosis, or dermatologic conditions.

Diffuse skin thickening suggests lymphatic permeation by metastases secondary to underlying carcinoma. Diffuse thickening may also be associated with abscess, progressive systemic sclerosis, obstruction of the superior vena cava, pemphigus, nephrotic syndrome, congestive heart failure, lymphoma, and lym-

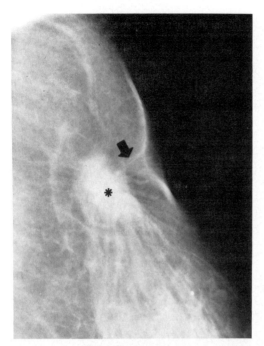

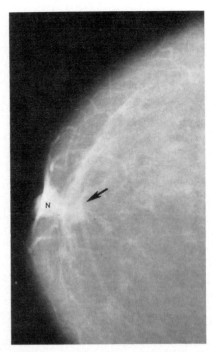

Figure 10.13. Skin retraction. Close-up of film-screen mammogram. Scirrhous carcinoma (*asterisk*) has thickened and shortened adjacent Cooper's ligaments (*arrow*) leading to skin retraction.

Figure 10.14. Nipple (*N*) is retracted secondary to underlying carcinoma (*arrow*).

phatic extension from contralateral breast carcinoma (18). One of the most difficult differential diagnoses is between abscess and carcinoma with lymphatic spread. In both conditions, the primary lesion may by completely obscured by surrounding edema, which makes mammographic detection impossible. In this situation, abscess may be excluded mammographically only if typical branching calcifications of carcinoma are present (19).

Skin and Nipple Retraction

Skin and nipple retraction associated with an underlying carcinoma may be observed on physical inspection of the breast. Skin retraction includes a spectrum of changes from a small local dimpling of the skin overlying a small tumor to shrinkage of the entire breast associated with a large, deeply located tumor. These changes are due to the fact that some neoplasms (scirrhous carcinomas) cause proliferation of fibroblasts not only within the tumor itself but also in the surrounding breast tissue. In time, the cicatrization, or scar formation, results in tissue contraction, and the normally loose, fatty tissues adjacent to the lesion may be pulled toward it by the shortening strands of fibroblasts. Skin retraction is a con-

sequence of such fibrotic changes involving the ligaments of Cooper, which are breast suspensory ligaments projected from breast parenchyma extending to the subcutaneous layer of superficial fascia. Cicatrization of the tissue around these ligaments causes the ligaments to thicken, shorten, and retract the adjacent skin. A similar process may occur with inflammation from bacterial infection or fat necrosis (20). When the x-ray beam is tangential to the involved breast surface, flattening of the breast contour or retraction will be depicted (Fig. 10.13). The retraction is sometimes exaggerated with the application of mammographic breast compression.

A similar phenomenon may affect the subareolar ducts, causing them to thicken and shorten; thus, the nipple area is first flattened and finally retracted (Fig. 10.14). Retraction of the skin or nipple may occur secondary to a previous surgical procedure. Thus, it is very important to be aware of the exact site of previous biopsies when viewing the mammograms.

Inversion of the nipple should be differentiated from retraction. Inversion is usually a long-standing process, often bilateral, which may occur in normal women. Nipple inversion can usually be reversed by applying manual pressure around the areola.

Axillary Lymph Nodes

Involvement of axillary lymph nodes is considered to be the most important factor in the prognosis of breast carcinoma. Routine use of the mediolateral oblique projection for film-screen mammography, or the noncontact mediolateral chest wall view for xeromammography, ensures that the lower axillary nodes are visualized. Radiographic features suggesting axillary node metastasis include absence of radiolucent fat within the node and a size greater than 2 cm (21). However, there are no radiographic criteria to definitely exclude early nodal involvement. Therefore, surgical exploration with histologic examination remains the most reliable method for evaluation of the axillary nodes (22).

INDIRECT SIGNS

Although the majority of early breast cancers are identified as small, poorly defined or spiculated masses or clustered calcifications, others show atypical and more subtle radiographic signs. The indirect mammographic signs of malignancy include a single dilated duct, localized architectural distortion, asymmetric density, and the developing density sign (23).

Single Dilated Duct

Dilatation of a single duct can be the only sign of an early intraductal carcinoma. However, the cause of a single dilated duct is more often benign than malignant. When this finding is identified on a mammogram, further workup is justified. Magnification views may disclose calcifications. If there is a discharge, ductography or aspiration cytology may be performed.

Localized Architectural Distortion

An abnormal arrangement of the ducts and ligaments of the breast is usually the result of a scirrhous carcinoma with fibrosis and distortion of the adjacent breast tissue. In a fatty breast a spiculated mass is usually easily identified, but in a dense breast an architectural distortion may be the only sign of the underlying malignancy (Fig. 10.15). Since an architectural distortion may be caused by a previous biopsy, it is important to be aware of the location of previous breast surgeries when the mammogram is interpreted.

Radial scars and benign radial sclerosing lesions may also cause architectural abnormalities that mimic those caused by malignancy. Unlike the spiculated density seen with scir-

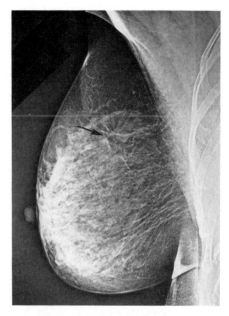

Figure 10.15. Architectural distortion. Radiating spicules (*arrow*) represent desmoplastic reaction of early scirrhous carcinoma.

rhous carcinomas, radial scars do not show a solid, dense, central tumor mass; radiolucent central regions may be seen in the radial scar (3). In addition, the spicules of the radial scar frequently lie in parallel with radiolucent linear structures between some of the spicules. Unlike carcinoma, the spicules are often more numerous and clumped in the central region. However, it is usually not possible to diagnose radial scars definitively with mammography. Therefore, biopsy is performed even when a radial scar is suspected.

Asymmetric Density

An asymmetric density may represent a carcinoma and is most likely to occur in a dense breast, where the asymmetric density represents the added density of a carcinoma to the surrounding parenchymal tissue. To detect mammographic asymmetry, the right and left mammograms are viewed side-by-side (Fig. 10.16). Since variations in the distribution of the parenchymal tissue normally occur, an unacceptably high rate of false-negative biopsies would result if all asymmetric densities were biopsied. Therefore, a biopsy is not indicated unless the asymmetric density is unusually extensive or has abnormal clinical or mammographic findings associated with it (24). Mammographic features mandating biopsy of an asymmetric density include associated architectural distortion, calcifications, and alterations in adjacent breast tissue. To

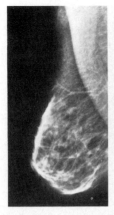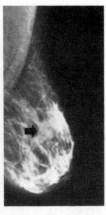

Figure 10.16. Asymmetric density. Bilateral medio-lateral oblique film-screen mammograms. The patient complained of left breast pain and intermittent inflammation of the nipple. At biopsy, asymmetric density (*arrow*), which was associated with architectural distortion, in left breast was found to represent fibrous tissue proliferation and inflammation associated with a noninvasive ductal carcinoma.

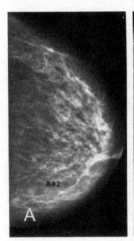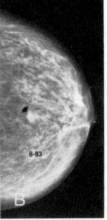

Figure 10.17. Neodensity. **A,** Cephalocaudal film-screen mammogram, 1982. **B,** Mammogram in 1983 later revealed poorly defined density (*arrowhead*) not present previously. Biopsy revealed infiltrating duct carcinoma.

localize an abnormal asymmetric density for biopsy, the radiologist must identify it on two right-angle mammographic projections, optimally lateral and cephalocaudal.

Developing Density Sign

Since the breasts in most women over age 40 should be undergoing involution, the appearance of a new density in the mammogram

should be considered a possible indirect sign of early breast cancer (Fig. 10.17) (25). To identify this developing density sign, the radiologist must have access to the patient's previous mammograms.

VALUE OF COMPARISON WITH PREVIOUS MAMMOGRAMS

Access to previous mammograms is essential in evaluating potential signs of malignancy. This is especially critical in the search for early breast cancers, which may be heralded only by subtle changes from earlier examinations (Fig. 10.6). In addition, unnecessary biopsies are often deferred on the basis that there are no significant changes in the mammographic findings when compared with previous examinations. It has been deemed so important to have previous mammograms available for comparison that the American College of Radiology has recommended that mammograms be retained longer than other radiographic examinations (26). Furthermore, if mammographic facilities cannot provide storage space for this purpose, they should consider allowing patients to retain their own mammograms.

REFERENCES

1. Gershon-Cohen J, Ingleby H. Roentgenography of cancer of the breast: a classified pathological basis for roentgenologic criteria. Am J Roentgenol Radium Ther Nucl Med 1952;68:1–7.
2. Gold RH, Montgomery CK, Rambo ON. Significance of margination of benign and malignant infiltrative mammary lesions: Roentgenologic-pathologic correlation. AJR 1973;118:881–894.
3. Tabár L, Dean PB. Teaching atlas of mammography. New York: Thieme-Stratton, 1983.
4. Barth V. Atlas of diseases of the breast. Stuttgart: Thieme, 1979;99.
5. Toombs BD, Kalisher L. Metastatic disease to the breast. Clinical, pathologic, and radiographic features. AJR 1977;129:673–676.
6. Abrams HL, Spiro R, Goldstein N. Metastases in carcinoma. Analysis of 1000 autopsied cases. Cancer 1950;3:74–85.
7. Sandison AT. Metastatic tumours in the breast. Br J Surg 1959;47:54–58.
8. Hajdu SI, Urban JA. Cancers metastatic to the breast. Cancer 1972;29:1691–1696.
9. Bohman LG, Bassett LW, Gold RH, Voet R. Breast metastases from extramammary malignancies. Radiology 1982;144:309–312.
10. Leborgne R. Diagnosis of tumors of the breast by simple roentgenography: calcifications in carcinomas. Am J Roentgenol Radium Ther Nucl Med 1951;65:1–11.
11. Gershon-Cohen J, Yiu LS, Berger SM. The diagnostic importance of calcareous patterns in roentgenography of breast cancer. Am J Roentgenol Ther Radium Nucl Med 1962;88:1117–1125.

12. Levitan LH, Witten DM, Harrison EG. Calcification in breast disease: mammographic-pathologic correlation. Am J Roentgenol Ther Radium Nucl Med 1964;92:29–39.

13. Ahmed A. Calcification in human breast carcinomas: ultrastructural observations. J Pathol 1975;117:247–251.

14. Egan RL, McSweeney MB, Sewell CW. Intramammary calcifications without an associated mass in benign and malignant diseases. Radiology 1980;137:1–7.

15. Sickles EA. Further experience with microfocal spot magnification mammography in the assessment of clustered breast microcalcifications. Radiology 1980;137:9–14.

16. Rodgers JV Jr, Powell RW. Mammographic indicators for biopsy of clinically normal breasts: correlated with pathologic findings in 72 cases. Am J Roentgenol Radium Ther Nucl Med 1972;115:799–800.

17. Homer MJ. Nonpalpable mammographic abnormalities: timing the follow-up studies. AJR 1981;136:923–926.

18. Gold RH, Montgomery CK, Minagi H, Annes GP. The significance of mammary skin thickening in disorders other than primary carcinoma: A roentgenologic-pathologic correlation. Am J Roentgenol Radium Ther Nucl Med 1971;112:613–621.

19. Gold RH. Secondary signs and other indications of breast cancer. In: Feig SA, ed. Syllabus for the Categorical Course on Mammography. Los Angeles: American College of Radiology, 1984;271–288.

20. Haagensen CD. Diseases of the breast. 3rd ed. Philadelphia: Saunders, 1986:527.

21. Kalisher L, Chu AM, Peyster RG. Clinicopathological correlation of xeroradiography in determining involvement of metastatic axillary nodes in female breast cancer. Radiology 1976;121:333–335.

22. Coopmans de Yoldi GF, Andreoli C, Costa A, Nessi R, Gilardoni L, Rasponi A. Lack of efficacy of xeroradiography to preoperatively detect axillary lymph node metastases in breast carcinoma. Breast Cancer Res Treat 1983;3:373–376.

23. Sickles EA. Mammographic features of "early" breast cancer. AJR 1984;142:461–464.

24. Kopans DB. Asymetric breast tissue. In: Feig SA, ed. Breast imaging categorical course syllabus. American Roentgen Ray Society, 1988:161.

25. Martin JE, Gallagher HS. Mammographic diagnosis of minimal breast cancer. Cancer 1971;28:1519–1526.

26. Statement of the Preservation of Mammograms. Prepared by the ACR Commission on Mammography and the Commission on Diagnostic Radiology. Reston, VA: American College of Radiology, 1988.

11

Prebiopsy Needle Localization, Ductography, and Pneumocystography

Lori S. Gormley
Lawrence W. Bassett

Several invasive techniques are used in conjunction with mammography. Mammographically guided needle localization facilitates the biopsy of nonpalpable lesions detected on mammograms. This method is extensively used to minimize the amount of breast tissue excised at biopsy. Ductography, injection of radiopaque fluid into the duct system, provides a method of visualizing intraductal lesions that cause nipple discharge. The value of ductography remains controversial. Pneumocystography, mammographically guided drainage of cysts followed by insufflation with air, may be both diagnostic and therapeutic. This technique is popular in Europe and is gaining in use in the United States.

PREBIOPSY NEEDLE LOCALIZATION

Early diagnosis of breast cancer is of major importance to successful treatment. Mammography is the only method proven to be effective for detection of early occult (nonpalpable) breast cancers (1). With high-resolution, low-dose film-screen and xeromammography, radiologists are finding earlier cancers and recommending more biopsies. Following detection of a nonpalpable abnormality, the lesion must be localized by the radiologist, excised by the surgeon, and evaluated by the pathologist. Prior to the advent of needle localization methods, the surgeon performed a biopsy guided only by written and verbal descriptions of the site of the lesion in the breast or surface markers taped to the skin. The latter method was often inaccurate because the mammograms were taken with the patient upright and the breast compressed, and the relationship of the lesion to surface landmarks invariably changed when the patient was placed supine for surgery. Frequently, the biopsy necessitated excision of a large specimen that had to be sliced like a loaf of bread and then radiographed to ensure that the pathologist examined the correct tissue. Since mammographic abnormalities are often benign, the acceptance of mammographic screening depends largely on the radiologist's ability to precisely localize abnormalities prior to biopsy, allowing for removal of smaller amounts of normal breast tissue. This has been accomplished through mammographically guided prebiopsy needle localization.

Needle localization is usually performed on an outpatient basis, either in a clinic or hospital operating room under local or general anesthesia. Multiple factors determine which arrangement is utilized: (*a*) location of the lesion; (*b*) size of the breast; (*c*) patient's ability to cooperate; and (*d*) preferences of the patient. The specimen is usually sent for permanent histologic sections, and any definitive surgery is performed later after consultation with the patient.

Indications

Any nonpalpable mammographic abnormality suggestive of carcinoma is an indication for prebiopsy needle localization. These abnormalities include calcifications, stellate lesions, dominant solid masses, distorted breast architecture in the absence of prior biopsy, and densities not present on previous mammograms.

Methods

Needle localization of occult breast abnormalities can be accomplished by direct needle, "spot," or needle-wire methods. Each of these begins with the placement of a needle into the breast so that the tip is as close as possible to the abnormality.

In *direct needle localization*, a hypodermic needle, spinal needle, or specially designed flat-hubbed needle is inserted into the breast until the tip is as close as possible to the lesion (2, 3). Following mammographic confirmation, the needle is taped in place and the patient is taken to surgery. The surgeon excises the tissue at the tip of the needle and sends it for histologic evaluation. A drawback to this method is that the needle may be accidentally displaced prior to biopsy.

In the *spot method*, 0.1 ml of methylene blue dye is injected through the properly positioned needle, and then the needle is removed. Sometimes a mixture of dye and radiopaque contrast medium is injected so that the position of the dye relative to the breast lesion can be demonstrated mammographically. Additional methylene blue may be injected in the tract as the needle is withdrawn to establish an easily visible route for the surgeon. At biopsy, the surgeon removes the breast tissue at the site of the dye spot. A drawback of the spot method is that dye may diffuse over a large area if biopsy is delayed.

Needle-wire methods are now widely used (4–7). The needle-wire apparatus should allow repositioning as needed until mammograms demonstrate adequate proximity to the suspected abnormality. Once this is accomplished, either a spring-hook barbed tip or retractable curved-end wire is afterloaded or advanced out of the shaft of the needle. The wire is anchored in place by either the barbed tip or curved end and the needle may be removed. There are a few reported problems with the needle-wire technique. The thin wire has been reported to migrate within the breast (8, 9). Another potential disadvantage is that most hook wires cannot be repositioned once inserted. If repositioning becomes necessary, a second wire must be placed, and then both wires must be removed at surgery. One J-shaped, curved-end retractable wire can be withdrawn into the needle and repositioned if incorrectly placed (7). However, this wire is not as well anchored as others, and it may be displaced if inadvertently tugged on during preparation for surgery.

Performing the Procedure

The procedure is scheduled to begin at least 1 hour prior to surgery. This allows sufficient time to perform the localization, which requires about 30 minutes, and to deal with any unforeseen difficulties. Patient cooperation is essential, and preoperative medications should be withheld until the localization has been completed. The authors routinely show the patient her mammograms, point out the area where the biopsy will be performed, and explain the procedure step by step. The patient is assured that the localization procedure is almost never painful. She is informed of the benefits of a precisely directed biopsy.

Generally, the lesion should be approached from the closest skin surface. A "hole plate" is used for the majority of our localizations (10, 11). This is a clear plastic mammography compression plate drilled with a grid system of holes that will be visible on the mammograms (Fig. 11.1**A**) The hole plate is applied to the breast surface closest to the lesion, in either a cephalocaudal or lateral direction. Moderate compression is applied, and a mammogram is made. Compression is maintained while the hole most directly over the lesion is determined fron the mammogram (Fig. 11.1**B**) The skin within this hole is then cleansed with Betadine, and a small amount of local anesthetic may be injected into the skin. The needle is directed through the hole and inserted up to the hub or until the tip is well beyond the lesion. Following this, another mammogram is done to confirm the location of the needle relative to the lesion. Compression is released, and a right-angle mammography is performed. The latter indicates the relative depth in the breast of needle tip and lesion. With the breast still compressed, the needle tip is pulled back to the lesion. Then the wire is introduced and the needle may be removed. The end of the wire is firmly taped to the skin. Mammograms indicate the proximity of the hooked end of wire to the lesion (Fig. 11.1**C**). The authors consider placement successful when the needle tip or wire hook is within 1 cm of the lesion in both cephalocaudal and mediolateral projections.

Specimen Radiography

Once the surgeon has excised the specimen it is radiographed. The purpose of the specimen radiograph is to verify that the mammographic abnormality is included in the excised tissue (Fig. 11.1**D**). Specimen radiographs can be performed with conventional mammography equipment. However, it is often convenient to use a smaller specimen x-ray unit so that patient examinations need not be interrupted. The authors perform specimen radiography for all mammographically guided biopsies. After specimen verification, a pin is of-

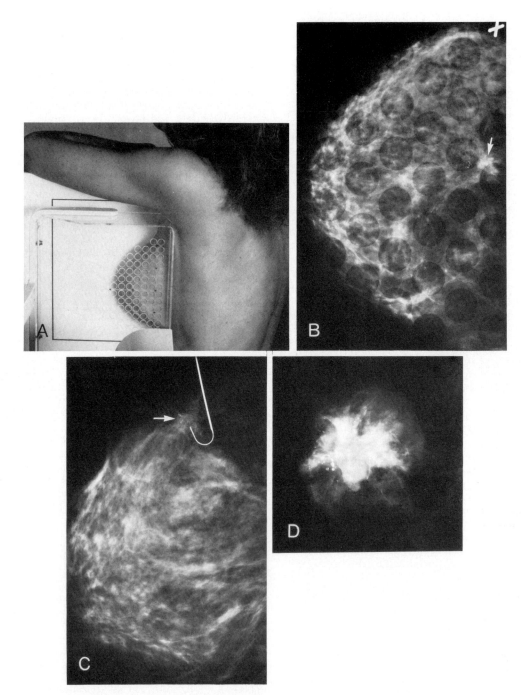

Figure 11.1.   Prebiopsy needle localization using hole plate. **A**, Hole plate is applied to breast surface closest to lesion. **B**, Cephalocaudal mammogram identifies hole overlying lesion, stellate mass (*arrow*) with calcifications. Radiopaque "*x*" taped on skin is used as a reference point when selecting hole for needle placement. **C**, Mammogram demonstrates relative positions of end of wire and lesion (*arrow*). **D**, Specimen radiograph verifies that lesion has been excised.

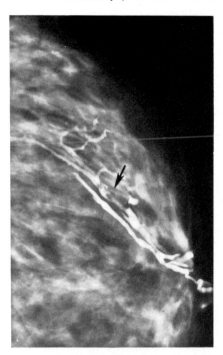

Figure 11.2. Ductogram. Elongate filling defect (*arrow*) proved to be intraductal papilloma and intraductal carcinoma.

ten placed into the specimen at the exact site of the lesion. The specimen and radiograph are taken to the pathologist for histologic examination. On occasion, abnormal densities or architectural distortions are difficult to appreciate in specimen radiographs; in this case, additional mammograms should be performed within approximately 2 months to ensure that the lesion has been removed.

There are only a few reported risks of needle localization: vasovagal reaction, minor bleeding-hematoma, allergic reaction to the local anesthetic, and infection. The most common complication is vasovagal reaction; the patient should be reassured that this is temporary, and, if necessary, atropine can be used to treat the reaction. The authors have not encountered any serious complications.

Results

What is the acceptable ratio of positive (malignant) to total biopsies for nonpalpable mammographic abnormalities? Published results vary from 11 to 36% true-positive rates (percent of needle-directed biopsies that prove to be cancers) (12). Some mammographers have advocated an aggressive approach in order to diagnose breast cancer at an early stage, asserting that positive biopsy rates as low as 10% (10 bi-

opsies for every cancer detected) would be acceptable for nonpalpable abnormalities (13). Today, most experienced mammographers strive for higher positive biopsy rates, thus minimizing the number of unnecessary biopsies without missing significant numbers of cancers.

Keys to Success

Successful prebiopsy needle localization requires a team approach. For radiologists and mammography technologists, the procedure is easier with experience. The radiologist should review the localization mammograms with the surgeon prior to biopsy. As the surgeon becomes more familiar with the procedure, the amount of tissue excised decreases. Operating room personnel must be educated not to move the needle or wire as the patient is prepared for surgery. Prebiopsy localization provides the pathologist with a manageable-size specimen, and pin placement in the suspicious area helps the pathologist to focus on the abnormal tissue.

DUCTOGRAPHY

Nipple discharge in nonlactating breasts indicates pathologic changes based on endocrinologic or local abnormalities. The majority of discharges have a benign etiology, with only 6 to 15% associated with cancer (14, 15). Bilateral discharge from multiple ducts is usually due to fibrocystic changes, duct ectasia, or endocrinologic imbalance. The most significant discharges are those that arise from a single duct and are serous, serosanguinous, or frankly bloody. There are usually no other localizing signs, and management is difficult. Surgery may result in unnecessary removal of a large amount of breast tissue if the exact origin of the abnormal discharge is not confirmed preoperatively. Ductography may be useful in evaluating the source of the discharge and in guiding the surgeon to the abnormal duct.

To perform ductography, the secreting duct is cannulated with a blunt-tipped needle, and a small amount of water-soluble contrast medium is injected until the patient experiences mild discomfort. Cephalocaudal and mediolateral mammograms are performed.

Just prior to surgical excision of an abnormality detected by a ductogram, the patient returns to the mammography suite, and a localization ductogram is performed. This consists of recannulating the abnormal duct, injecting contrast medium, and performing a mammogram to confirm that the correct duct has been injected. Methylene blue dye is injected into the abnormal duct. At surgery, a circumareolar incision is made; the duct contain-

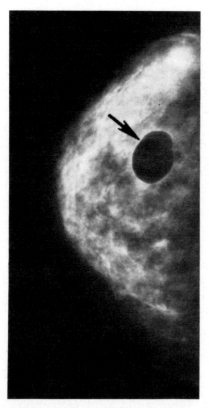

Figure 11.3. Pneumocystogram. Benign air-filled cyst (*arrow*) has smooth inner wall.

with room air. Following air injection, mammograms are obtained in the cephalocaudal and mediolateral projections. Air within the empty cyst provides radiolucent contrast with surrounding breast tissue, allowing assessment of the inner cyst wall (Fig. 11.3). A thick or irregular wall is suggestive of intracystic tumor and warrants biopsy.

In addition to its diagnostic aspect, pneumocystography may be therapeutic. Cyst recurrence is common following needle aspiration. However, it has been reported that fewer than 3 to 6% of simple cysts recur after air insufflation (17, 18). It is postulated that air dries out the cyst lining, inducing collapse and sclerosis.

Pneumocystography has had mixed acceptance in the United States. Many believe that breast sonography provides adequate evaluation of the inner cyst wall. Advantages of sonography include its facility in evaluating multiple cysts (common in cystic disease) and cysts smaller than 1 cm, which are difficult to evaluate by pneumocystography. It has not been proven that therapeutic interventions are necessary for all simple cysts. Further investigations comparing sonography and pneumocystography are indicated before either can be accepted as the method of choice for evaluation of solitary cysts larger than 1 cm.

ing the methylene blue dye is identified; and the duct is excised. Thus, the amount of normal breast tissue removed is minimized.

Benign causes of nipple discharge include ductal ectasia, which on ductograms exhibits dilated ducts with interspersed smooth segments of narrowing. In cystic breasts, there is opacification of multiple small cysts communicating with the ductal system (16). The most common cause of a filling defect is intraductal papilloma. Malignancy can present as a filling defect indistinguishable from papilloma (Fig. 11.2) or as multiple filling defects easily confused with epitheliosis. Malignancy may also result in irregular areas of stricture, distortion, or abrupt termination of a duct.

PNEUMOCYSTOGRAPHY

Breast cysts are most frequent in the perimenopausal years. They are the most common cause of palpable breast masses in this age group. Pneumocystography has been widely utilized in Europe for both diagnostic evaluation and treatment of cysts. Pneumocystography consists of cyst aspiration, followed immediately by insufflation of the cyst cavity

REFERENCES

1. Baker LH. Breast Cancer Detection Demonstration Project: Five-year summary report. CA 1982;132:194–225.
2. Threatt B, Appleman H, Dow R, O'Rourke T. Percutaneous needle localization of clustered mammary microcalcifications prior to biopsy. AJR 1974;121:839–842.
3. Kalisher L. An improved needle for localization of nonpalpable breast lesions. Radiology 1978;128:815–817.
4. Frank HA, Hall FM, Steer L. Preoperative localization of nonpalpable breast lesions demonstrated by mammography. N Engl J Med 1976;295:259–260.
5. Hall FM, Frank HA. Preoperative localization of nonpalpable breast lesions. AJR 1979;132:101–105.
6. Kopans DB, Meyer JE. Versatile spring hookwire breast lesion localizer. AJR 1982;138:586–587.
7. Homer MJ. Nonpalpable breast lesion localization using a curved-end retractable wire. Radiology 1985;157:259–260.
8. Bristol JB, Jones PA. Transgression of localizing wire into the pleural cavity prior to mammography. Br J Radiol 1981;54:139–140.
9. Bigelow R, Smith R, Goodman PA, Wilson GS. Needle localization of nonpalpable breast masses. Arch Surg 1985;120:565–569.
10. Goldberg RP, Hall FM, Simon M. Preoperative localization of nonpalpable breast lesions using a

wire marker and perforated mammographic grid. Radiology 1983;146:833–835.

11. Rasmussen OS, Seerup A. Properative radiographically guided wire marking of nonpalpable breast lesions. Acta Radiol [Diagn] (Stockh) 1984;25:13–16.

12. Hall FM, Storella JM, Silverstone DZ, Wyshak G. Nonpalpable breast lesions: recommendations for biopsy based on suspicion of carcinoma at mammography. Radiology 1988;167:353–358.

13. Moskowitz M. Minimal breast cancer redux. Radiol Clin North Am 1983;21:93–113.

14. Tabar L, Dean PB, Pentek Z. Galactography: the diagnostic procedure of choice for nipple discharge. Radiology 1983;149:31–38.

15. Philip J, Harris WG. The role of ductography in the management of patients with nipple discharge. Br J Clin Pract 1984;38:293–297.

16. Threatt B. Ductography. In: Bassett LW, Gold RH, eds. Breast cancer detection: Mammography and other methods in breast imaging. 2nd ed. Orlando, FL: Grune & Stratton, 1987:119–129.

17. Tabar L, Pentek Z, Dean PB. The diagnostic and therapeutic value of breast cyst puncture and pneumocystography. Radiology 1981;141:659–663.

18. Dyreborg U, Blichert-Toft M, Boegh L, Kiaer H. Needle puncture followed by pneumocystography of palpable breast cysts: A controlled clinical trial. Acta Radiol [Diagn] (Stockh) 1985;26:277–281.

12

Breast Sonography

Lawrence W. Bassett

The breast was one of the first organs examined with diagnostic sonography. In 1952, Wild and Reid (1) investigated the use of A-mode ultrasound methods for differentiating cysts from solid masses in the breast. Later, DeLand (2), Jellins et al. (3), Kobayashi (4), and Kelly-Fry (5) developed B-mode ultrasound equipment for breast imaging. For the last 10 years, the role of sonography in the evaluation of breast diseases has been the subject of scientific investigation and debate. This chapter presents basic technical aspects of breast sonography, the current uses of breast sonography, the normal sonographic appearance of the breast, and a spectrum of benign and malignant breast masses as depicted in sonograms.

TECHNICAL ASPECTS AND INSTRUMENTATION

Ultrasound examination of the breast presents several technical problems. Breast tissue is unusually heterogeneous, and the many sonic impedances of different breast tissue interfaces rapidly diminish the ultrasound beam amplitude. Extensive refractions of sound also contribute to beam defocusing (6). In response to these problems, manufacturers of breast ultrasound equipment have developed tightly focused, large-aperture, high-frequency transducers in order to ensure depiction of smaller breast structures. Abnormalities located in the superficial breast tissues may be distorted or entirely missed when imaged within the near field of the transducer. Therefore, adequate performance of breast ultrasound requires a fluid offset between the transducer and the breast, or a transducer with a built-in fluid offset, in order to produce images of superficial breast lesions (7). To accommodate visualization of superficial breast tissues, transducers for automated whole-breast scanners are positioned within a water bath. Hand-held units may have a fluid offset built into the transducer. Otherwise, it may be necessary to interpose a water-filled plastic bag or a commercially available fluid offset pad between the transducer and the breast in order to examine the superficial breast tissues.

The most important application of breast sonography, differentiation between cysts and solid masses, is also highly dependent on technical factors. For example, demonstrating an anechoic interior, the most reliable sign of a cyst, depends on appropriate gain or power settings and time gain compensation adjustment. Technical factors such as power settings or gains that are too high, cyst imaging within the near field of the transducer, inappropriate gray scale adjustment, or a faulty amplifier electrical board may cause artifactual echoes. Artifactual echoes from inappropriately high power settings occur first in the anterior perimeter of the cyst, a characteristic finding that may be useful in differentiating between a cyst and a solid mass. Demonstration of enhanced echoes posterior to cysts also depends on technical factors such as power, correct time gain compensation, appropriate gray scale levels, and cyst location in the breast. Since chest wall structures rapidly attenuate sound, enhanced sound transmission distal to a juxtathoracic breast cyst, especially with the transducer applied to the front of the breast, may be impossible to demonstrate. However, directing the ultrasound beam from the side of the breast can demonstrate increased sound transmission in the breast tissue projected beyond the cyst.

Breast sonography can be performed adequately with either automated whole-breast units or high-frequency hand-held instruments. Automated dedicated breast units are designed to produce sequential thin-section whole-breast images, allowing for more accu-

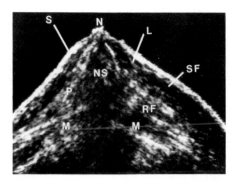

Figure 12.1. Normal breast anatomy, automated whole-breast image. *L*, suspensory ligament; *M*, pectoral muscle; *N*, nipple; *NS*, shadowing from nipple; *P*, parenchymal tissue; *RF*, retromammary fat; *S*, skin; *SF*, subcutaneous fat.

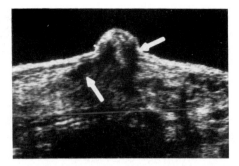

Figure 12.2. Normal sonolucent ducts (*arrows*) in subareolar region.

rate localization of abnormalities. Thus, automated whole-breast scanners are more appropriate for breast cancer screening examinations than hand-held units. In addition, automated units are less physician-dependent since the technologist can perform a complete breast survey that the radiologist can view later. Disadvantages of automated units include higher cost; greater space requirements; the need for specially trained technologists; and longer setup, performance, and review times.

Less expensive than automated units, hand-held units can also be used for sonographic examination of other organs. For breast imaging, the transducer should be 5 MHz or greater and should have a depth of focus of no more than 2 cm. Hand-held equipment can also be used for needle-guided biopsy.

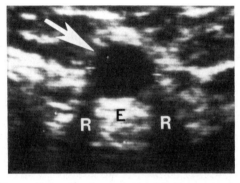

Figure 12.3. Cyst (*arrow*). Hand-held examination shows typical cyst features: sharp anterior and posterior margins, round shape, anechoic interior, enhanced posterior echoes (*E*), and lateral edge refraction (*R*).

CLINICAL APPLICATIONS

The most important clinical use of breast sonography is to differentiate between cysts and solid masses; in this endeavor studies report accuracy rates of 95 to 100% (8–11). For palpable lesions, needle aspiration of the mass may be more expedient. However, sonography is the best approach to determine whether a nonpalpable mass detected by mammography is cystic or solid. Sonography is also ideal for the evaluation and follow-up of patients with multiple cysts. Breast sonography has also been used as an adjunct to mammography when palpable masses have indeterminate mammographic features and when dense parenchymal tissue limits the mammographic evaluation of suspected breast abnormalities (12–15). Hand-held ultrasound-guided needle aspiration and prebiopsy needle localization are advocated for nonpalpable sonographically detected lesions (16).

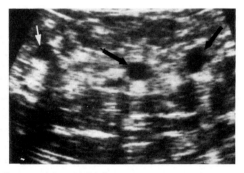

Figure 12.4. Multiple cysts (*arrows*). Note enhanced through-transmission of sound distal to cysts.

Automated whole-breast ultrasound has at various times in the past been advocated for

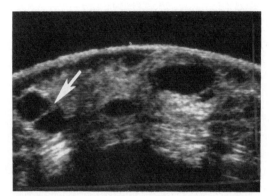

Figure 12.5. Multiple cysts. One contains a septum (*arrow*).

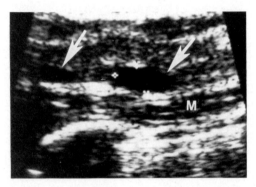

Figure 12.6. Cysts (*arrows*) are compressed against chest wall by transducer. *M*, pectoral muscle.

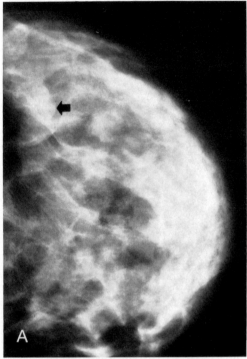

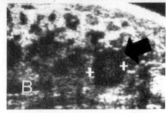

Figure 12.7. Fibroadenoma. Forty-year-old woman with palpable mass in upper hemisphere right breast. **A**, Film-screen mammogram. Mass (*arrow*) is barely visible due to dense breast tissue. **B**, Sonography. The mass (*arrow*) is well-defined and contains multiple, even echoes throughout, indicating it is solid.

breast cancer screening (17–19). However, the sensitivity and specificity of breast sonography to detect breast cancer is far lower than state-of-the-art mammography (15, 20, 21); the depiction of nonpalpable, mammographically negative cancers is so unusual that such reports are anecdotal. Sonography has the following limitations in the detection of breast cancer: (*a*) poor results in fatty breasts, (*b*) inability to detect microcalcifications, (*c*) inconsistent depiction of masses less than 1.5 cm in diameter, and (*d*) unreliable differentiation between benign and malignant solid masses.

A recent survey of American College of Radiology members indicated that 53% performed breast sonography (22). Ninety-three per cent of these radiologists used hand-held units for breast scanning; 7% used dedicated breast equipment. None of the radiologists surveyed used ultrasound for breast cancer screening.

THE NORMAL BREAST

The breast is composed of skin, fat, parenchymal tissue, ducts, connective tissue, and suspensory ligaments (Fig. 12.1). The amount of parenchymal tissue and fat varies with age and parity and between women of the same age and parity. The acoustic impedance of fat is the lowest; parenchymal tissue is intermediate; and connective tissue is the highest. The skin is highly refractive and is 0.5 to 2 mm thick. The nipple contains a large amount of connective tissue and, in combination with the subareolar ducts, causes acoustic shadowing. Subareolar ducts can be identified as 2- to 8-

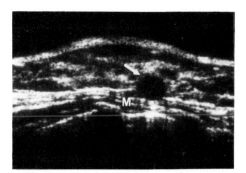

Figure 12.8. Fibroadenoma (*arrow*), with barely visible internal echoes, is adjacent to pectoral muscle (*M*) but is not flattened by the transducer.

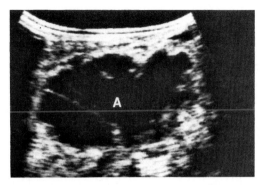

Figure 12.11. Abscess (*A*) is sonolucent and contains septations.

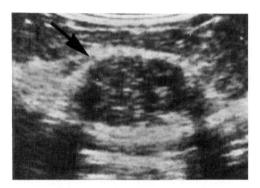

Figure 12.9. Cystosarcoma phyllodes (*arrow*) has thick capsule and contains several cystic areas. Round contour results in lateral edge refractions. There is distal echo enhancement.

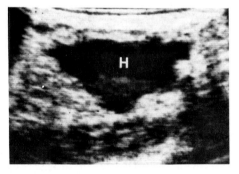

Figure 12.10. Two weeks following biopsy, post-surgical hematoma (*H*) contains anechoic fluid above the echoic sediment.

mm in diameter sonolucent tubules (Fig. 12.2). Subcutaneous fat causes weak echogenic reflections. The suspensory ligaments of the breast usually cause very high reflections, but the appropriate incident angle of the beam will produce marked shadowing from the ligaments due to refraction. Sonographic images of parenchymal tissue depend on the relative amounts of glandular tissue and fat (23).

In the fatty breast, fat lobules replace nearly all of the glandular tissue; well-suited to x-ray mammography, the fatty breast is poorly suited to ultrasound examination since fat transmits sound poorly and isolated fat lobules mimic sonolucent masses. Dense, fibrous breast contains abundant homogeneous echoes; although beam attenuation may be severe, sonolucent masses are easily identified. In these dense breasts, mammography is limited, and breast ultrasound is often a useful adjunct.

The retromammary fat layer is thinner than the subcutaneous fat layer. Visualization of the retromammary region ensures adequate ultrasound penetration of the breast. The pectoral muscle is easily identified due to the strongly echoic interphase between the retromammary fat and underlying pectoral muscle fascia.

BENIGN DISORDERS

Cysts

Cysts are the most frequent breast masses in women between the ages of 35 and 50. Cysts may be solitary or multiple, unilateral or bilateral. The most effective noninvasive method, sonography, detects cysts as small as 2 mm. Characteristic ultrasound features include well-circumscribed anterior and posterior boundaries, round or oval shapes, anechoic interiors, and enhanced echoes distal to the cyst (Fig. 12.3 and 12.4) (17, 24). Of these, the anechoic interior is the most reliable diagnostic feature, but artificial interior echoes can result from a number of technical and equipment-related factors. Debris within a cyst also appears as echoes, and gravity-dependent debris may lie

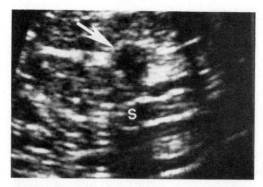

Figure 12.12. Scirrhous carcinoma (*arrow*). Hand-held sonography demonstrates relatively sharp anterior margin, poorly visualized posterior margin, irregular and weak internal echoes, and distal shadowing (*S*).

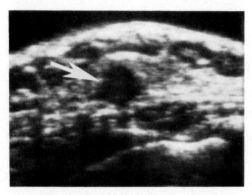

Figure 12.13. Infiltrating ductal carcinoma (*arrow*) has irregular margins and weak internal echoes.

on the bottom of a cyst. The curvature of the cyst may produce marked refraction of sound, which makes the lateral margins impossible to see (Fig. 12.1). Refraction results in echo attenuation distal to the lateral cyst margins. One or more septa are often seen within cysts (Fig. 12.5). With compression, cysts frequently flatten (Fig. 12.6). Enhancement of echoes distal to the cyst (tadpole sign) occurs because of the lower acoustic absorption coefficient of the cyst relative to surrounding parenchymal tissue.

Fibroadenoma

Fibroadenomas, the most frequent breast masses in women less than 25 years of age, may be solitary or multiple. This benign mass has smooth, well-circumscribed margins; round, oval or lobulated shape; and weak, uniform internal echoes (Fig. 12.7). Distal echoes may be unaffected, decreased, or increased.

During pregnancy, fibroadenomas may grow rapidly to a large size (Fig. 12.8).

Cystosarcoma Phyllodes

This fibroepithelial tumor, histologically similar to fibroadenoma, is usually benign but may rarely metastasize distally. The sonographic appearance (Fig. 12.9) is also similar to fibroadenoma, except that cystosarcoma may show interior cystic regions that produce enhanced posterior echoes (26).

Postsurgical Changes

A biopsy may create shadowing from skin thickening and retraction and architectural distortion in the parenchyma. A hematoma may develop and produce a mass that eventually liquefies, sometimes within hours after surgery. Later, the content of the hematoma may divide into fluid and cells (Fig. 12.10).

Abscess

Abscesses are most frequently located in the subareolar region. The patient may have fever, tenderness, and a palpable mass. The sonographic appearance may be similar to that of a cyst since the abscess usually contains fluid. The interior of an abscess may be hypoechoic or anechoic and may contain septa. (Fig. 12.11).

MALIGNANT LESIONS

Breast carcinomas have a variety of sonographic appearances, depending on the histology of the tumor.

Infiltrating, Poorly Circumscribed Carcinomas

The infiltrating, poorly circumscribed carcinoma is the most common type of breast malignancy; most of them are scirrhous carcinomas. Infiltrating scirrhous carcinomas histologically contain a preponderance of fibrous connective tissue and fewer epithelial tumor cells. Sonographically such carcinomas have irregular and moderately sharp anterior margins, and the posterior margins are not well visualized or are absent (Fig. 12.12). The internal echoes are uneven, inhomogeneous, and weak, as compared with the echoes of the parenchymal tissue surrounding the tumor. Distal echoes are usually attenuated (shadowing). The sonolucent tumor and posterior shadow may create a "keyhole" appearance (Fig. 12.12). Posterior shadowing occurs due to the high absorption of ultrasound waves by the tumor, and the degree of absorption relates directly to

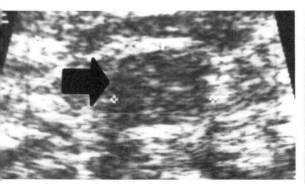

Figure 12.14. Well-circumscribed ductal carcinoma (*arrow*). "Benign" features include well-circumscribed margins, enhanced posterior echoes, and lateral edge refraction.

the tumor's fibrous connective tissue content. Posterior echo attenuation, while helpful, is not a consistent feature of cancers (Fig. 12.13). Of 33 cancers depicted with hand-held sonography, we found that 19 produced no discernible effect distally; 6 caused distal shadowing; and 8 resulted in distal echo enhancement (15).

Well-Circumscribed Carcinomas

About 10% of carcinomas are well-circumscribed and include well-differentiated ductal, medullary, papillary, and colloid carcinomas. Well-circumscribed cancers tend to show sonographic features that mimic benign solid masses, such as fibroadenomas. Features include smooth margins with sharp anterior and posterior boundaries, homogeneous internal echoes, and variable effect on echoes posterior to the tumor (Figs. 12.14 and 12.15). Therefore, biopsy is usually recommended for all solitary solid masses.

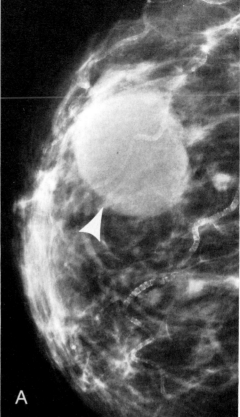

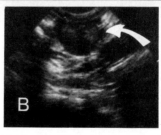

Figure 12.15. Papillary carcinoma. **A**, Mammogram shows well-circumscribed mass (*arrow*). **B**, Hand-held sonography demonstrates tumor (*arrow*) with smooth margins and enhanced distal echoes.

REFERENCES

1. Wild JJ, Reid JM. Further pilot echographic studies on the histologic structure of tumors of the living intact human breast. Am J Pathol 1952;28:839–861.
2. Deland FH. A modified technique of ultrasonography for the detection and differential diagnosis of breast lesions. Am J Roentgenol Radium Ther Nucl Med 1969;105:446–452.
3. Jellins J, Kossoff G, Buddee FW, Reeve TS. Ultrasonic visualization of the breast. Med J Aust 1971;1:305–307.
4. Kobayashi T. Review: ultrasonic diagnosis of breast cancer. Ultrasound Med Biol 1975;1:383–391.
5. Kelly-Fry E. Breast imaging. In: Sabbagha RE, ed. Diagnostic ultrasound applied to obstetrics and gynecology. New York: Harper & Row, 1980:327–350.
6. Kossoff G, Jellins J. The physics of breast echography. Semin Ultrasound 1982;3:5–12.
7. Kimme-Smith C, Hansen M, Bassett L, Sarti D, King W III. Ultrasound mammography: effects of focal zone placement. RadioGraphics 1985;955–970.
8. Rosner D, Weiss L, Norman M. Ultrasonography in the diagnosis of breast disease. J Surg Oncol 1980;14:83–96.
9. Sickles EA, Filly RA, Callen PW. Benign breast lesions: ultrasound detection and diagnosis. Radiology 1984;151:467–470.

10. Fleischer AC, Muhletaler CA, Reynolds VH, et al. Palpable breast masses: evaluation by high frequency, hand-held real-time sonography and xeromammography. Work in progress. Radiology 1983;148:813–817.

11. Hilton SV, Leopold GR, Olson LK, Willson SA. Real-time breast sonography: application in 300 consecutive patients. AJR 1986;147:479–486.

12. Rubin E, Miller VE, Berland LL, Han SY, Koehler RE, Stanley RJ. Hand-held real-time breast sonography. AJR 1985;144:623–627.

13. Fleischer AC, Thieme GA, Winfield AC, et al. Breast sonotomography and high-frequency, hand-held, real-time sonography: a clinical comparison. J Ultrasound Med 1985;4:577–581.

14. Cole-Beuglet C. Ultrasound. In: Bassett LW, Gold RH, eds. Mammography, thermography, and ultrasound in breast cancer detection. New York: Grune & Stratton, 1982:151–167.

15. Bassett LW, Kimme-Smith C, Sutherland LK, Gold RH, Sarti D, King W III. Automated and hand-held breast US: effect on patient management. Radiology 1987;165:103–108.

16. Kopans DB, Meyer JE, Lindfors KK, Bucchianeri SS. Breast sonography to guide cyst aspiration and wire localization of occult solid lesions. AJR 1984;143:489–492.

17. Kobayashi T, Takatani O, Hattori N, Kimura K. Differential diagnosis of breast tumors. The sensitivity graded method ultrasonotomography and clinical evaluation of its diagnostic accuracy. Cancer 1974;33:940–951.

18. De Vere C. Current status of ultrasonic breast scanning. Appl Radiol 1980;9:145–149.

19. Cole-Beuglet C, Goldberg BB, Kurtz AB, Rubin CS, Patchefsky AS, Shaber GS. Ultrasound mammography: a comparison with radiographic mammography. Radiology 1981;139:693–698.

20. Sickles EA, Filly FA, Callen PW. Breast cancer detection with sonography and mammography: comparison using state-of-the-art equipment. AJR 1983;140:843–845.

21. Kopans DB, Meyer JE, Lindfors KK. Whole-breast US imaging: four-year follow-up. Radiology 1985;157:505–507.

22. Bassett LW, Diamond JJ, Gold RH, McLelland R. Survey of mammography practices. AJR 1987;149:1149–1152.

23. Cole-Beuglet C, Schwartz G, Kurtz AB, Patchefsky AS, Goldberg BB. Ultrasound mammography for the augmented breast. Radiology 1983;146:737–742.

24. Jellins J, Kossoff G, Reeve TS. Detection and classification of liquid-filled masses in the breast by gray scale echography. Radiology 1977;125:205–212.

25. Jackson VP, Rothschild PA, Kreipke DL, Mail JT, Holden RW. The spectrum of sonographic findings of fibroadenoma of the breast. Invest Radiol 1986;21:34–40.

26. Cole-Beuglet C, Soriano RZ, Kurtz AB, Meyer JE, Kopans DB, Goldberg BB. Ultrasound, x-ray mammography, and histopathology of cystosarcoma phyllodes. Radiology 1983;146:481–486.

27. Cole-Beuglet C, Soriano RZ, Kurtz AB, Goldberg BB. Ultrasound analysis of 104 primary breast carcinomas classified according to histopathologic type. Radiology 1983;147:191–196.

13

Thermography, Transillumination Light Scanning, and Magnetic Resonance Imaging

Barbara Monsees

The three imaging modalities discussed in this chapter, thermography, light scanning, and magnetic resonance imaging, have no established role in the evaluation of patients with breast disease. These imaging methods fall within the realm of experimental techniques. Although there has been hope that these modalities may be useful for evaluating clinically or mammographically detected abnormalities, their tissue characterization capabilities fall short of accepted clinical utility. The lower sensitivities of these modalities compared with mammography in detecting breast carcinoma cannot justify their use for screening asymptomatic women.

Commercial units are available for all three modalities and are in use in some practices. The clinician and patient should be aware that these cannot be substituted for the current standards of care: mammography and physical examination for screening asymptomatic women, and mammography, physical examination and ultrasound for diagnostic purposes. Charging for the experimental techniques adds expense without any documented overall benefit.

THERMOGRAPHY

Technique

Thermography is a direct method of measuring temperature variations emanating from the skin surface. The two most thoroughly investigated methods are telethermography and liquid crystal thermography, but other techniques include computer-assisted, graphic stress, and microwave thermography (1).

Telethermography uses a photovoltaic detector to measure infrared radiation emanating from the skin. A thermal skin temperature map is created, displayed on a monitor, and then photographically recorded if desired. Liquid crystal thermography utilizes a system of cholesterol esters encapsulated in flexible mylar sheaths. When placed in direct contact with the skin of the breast, a unique color pattern appears that can also be photographically recorded. In computer-assisted thermography, sample thermal measurements are obtained at standardized locations from each breast and evaluated via a pattern recognition algorithm. The results are more objective than those that depend on observer pattern recognition, but the method is less sensitive to temperature differences. Graphic stress thermography is based on the theory that breast cancer detection is augmented with cold stress and compares temperature readings taken before and after the patient's hands are immersed in ice water for 15 seconds. Microwave thermography utilizes longer wavelength and naturally emitted radiation, and can theoretically detect abnormalities deeper in tissue. Its disadvantages include lower intensity of emission by nine to ten orders of magnitude compared with infrared irradiation (2).

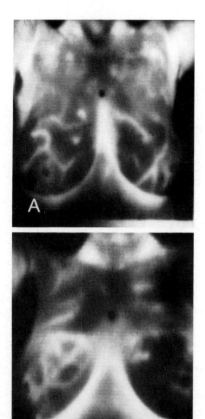

Figure 13.1. **A,** Normal thermograms. Breasts show relatively symmetrical infrared emission and normal breast contours. Lighter shades represent warmer areas; darker shades are cooler areas. **B,** Abnormal thermograms. Right breast shows asymmetric hypervascularity and some loss of normal round contour of its medial aspect associated with a carcinoma. (Courtesy of Dr. H. Isard.)

The ability of thermography to detect tumors is not well-understood. Increased blood perfusion and local heat from the tumor are theories as to the mechanism. The quality of the breast thermography image depends on ambient temperature; positioning of the patient; and sharpness, contrast, and brightness (3). Cooling the breasts accentuates abnormal heat patterns and the examination should be performed in a draft-free room. An abnormal thermogram is manifested by asymmetric qualitative differences in infrared radiation from opposite breasts; criteria of abnormality include diffuse or focal areas of increased heat, vascular discrepancy, the "edge sign," and occasionally a "cold" thermogram (3–5) (Fig. 13.1). Its features are nonspecific and inflam-

matory processes, benign tumors, fibrocystic breast changes, and other malignant tumors can all cause an abnormal thermogram. The location of the thermographic abnormality does not always reflect the site of the underlying lesion; therefore, if an abnormality is not seen on the patient's mammogram, it can be difficult to localize for surgery.

Breast Cancer Screening and Diagnosis

The largest study evaluating the ability of thermography for screening was the Breast Cancer Detection Demonstration Project (BCDDP) beginning in 1973 in which 280,000 women were screened utilizing mammography, physical examination, and thermography. In 1977 the use of thermography was discontinued in the project because thermography's role as a possible alternative to mammography was highly questionable (6). Abnormal thermography findings were reported for only 41% of the breast cancers detected through the first screening and the other 59% were normal or unknown. Thermography was not abnormal for two-thirds of the clinically occult cancers detected by mammography; therefore, thermography could not be used to select the group of women who should have mammograms.

Feig and associates (7) examined 16,000 women with thermography, mammography, and physical examination and detected 139 cancers. Mammography detected 78% of the cancers, physical examination 55%, and thermography 39%. For tumors larger than 3 cm, thermographic sensitivity was 83%, but if the tumor size was between 0.5 and 1 cm, its sensitivity was only 21%. Overall, 18% of the 16,000 women had positive thermograms, which reflected the nonspecific nature of the test.

Sterns and associates (8) compared telethermography and liquid crystal thermography in a study of 13 cancers diagnosed in a group of 502 women. The sensitivity of the two methods was comparable (33 and 36%) but low when compared with a 69% sensitivity of clinical examination. False-positive rates of 6 and 12% respectively were lower than in Feig's series. In addition, they reported inconsistency on readings between observers and "fewer than half of thermograms which were considered abnormal when the clinical data was known to the reporter, were interpreted in the same manner on another occasion without the clinical information" (8).

Isard and associates (9) studied 10,000 women with physical examination, thermography, and mammography and detected 306 cancers. Fifty-six percent of these women were symptomatic, and 36% of this symptomatic group had abnormal thermograms. They found 270 cancers in the symptomatic group. The sensitivity of clinical examination was 82%, mammography 85%, and thermography 72%. Of the 44% of women with no symptoms, 23% had abnormal thermograms. Of the 36 cancers in the asymptomatic group, only 61% were detectable on thermography, but 83% were detectable on mammography.

Moskowitz and associates (10) studied the thermograms of 42 patients with stage I or smaller carcinomas of the breast to see if thermography could identify patients with small cancers that were detectable by other means. To the group of patients with small cancers, they added 44 confounding cases and 64 randomly selected screening subjects. Patients with stage II carcinoma were excluded. The study was also designed to estimate a false-positive rate in a screening population and to compare the abilities of experienced and inexperienced thermographers. The true-positive call rate on the the same side as the cancer was less than the false-positive call rate, even in the hands of the expert thermographers. The false-positive rate for experienced readers was approximately 44% and for the inexperienced readers it was 47%. The true-positive rate was 24% for experienced readers and was 30% for the inexperienced readers.

Risk Indicator

Gautherie and Gros (11) reported that of 784 women with normal physical examinations, negative mammograms, and positive thermograms, within 10 years, 38% subsequently developed breast cancer. The more rapidly growing tumors with shorter doubling times showed progressive thermographic abnormalities. They concluded that thermography was useful as an indicator of risk and could also assess the more rapidly growing neoplasms. Moskowitz and associates (12) reviewed their own data of more than 10,000 patients enrolled in the Cincinnati BCDDP. In their hands, a patient with two or more positive thermograms over a 3-year period had no significant excess risk of later development of breast cancer in the study period when compared with patients who had normal thermograms.

Moskowitz and associates (13) assessed liquid crystal thermography (LCT) as a means of detecting proliferative disease of the breast. An international expert on thermography supervised and interpreted the studies blindly. The expert was unable to differentiate proliferative high-risk breast pathology at any greater rate than chance alone.

Summary

In summary, breast thermography is relatively insensitive and nonspecific and therefore cannot be used for screening or diagnosis at this time. Although thermography can be positive in occult lesions, its sensitivity is poorest in smaller lesions and there is no evidence that its addition to the clinical armamentarium of tests can result in diagnosis at an earlier stage.

In its professional and public policy statements, the American College of Radiology (1) states, "Because thermography does not employ ionizing radiation, some of its proponents consider the examination to be totally safe. However, lack of radiation risk from current reduced-dose mammography, utilization of thermography as a stand-alone test is seen to involve a much more serious risk, the risk does not justify the use of thermography. Indeed, when compared to the hypothetical risk that the false sense of security imparted by a 'normal' thermogram might preclude further study by mammography, the only procedure currently capable of detecting substantial numbers of pre-clinical breast cancers. The use of thermography in addition to physical examination and mammography involves no such risks. However, the addition of thermography to these established diagnostic examinations provides little clinically meaningful information, and substantially increases the cost of medical care."

TRANSILLUMINATION LIGHT SCANNING

Technique

As with thermography, transillumination light scanning (TLS) is a noninvasive alternative technique for breast imaging that relies on differential transmission by breast tissues of nonionizing radiation in the red and near-infrared range of the spectrum. Commercial video systems utilizing light in this spectal range are currently available. The transmitted light is detected by a vidicon tube sensitive to these wavelengths. Real time as well as static images can be recorded on video tape and floppy disk. Image processing functions allow display of infrared to red ratio data as well as total light transmission.

The mechanism for the ability of TLS to demonstrate carcinoma of the breast is not completely understood. It has been shown that the transmission of light in the red and near-infrared region is inhibited by hemoglobin (14). Thus, a possible explanation for differential transmission of some cancers as compared

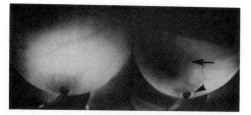

Figure 13.2. Light scan: carcinoma of left breast. Right breast is normal. Left breast shows large focal area of light absorption (*arrow*) in its medial aspect, which corresponds to a 3-cm palpable invasive carcinoma. Note thin light ring around left nipple (*arrowhead*), which is a light scan correlated of nipple retraction.

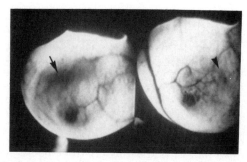

Figure 13.4. True-positive and false-positive light scan. Focal region of light absorption is seen in the right upper breast (*arrow*) corresponding to nonpalpable carcinoma. Smaller focal abnormality (*arrowhead*) in left breast had no mammographic or palpable correlate. (From Monsees B, Destouet JM, Gersell D. Light scan evaluation of nonpalpable breast lesions. Radiology 1987; 163:467–470.)

with glandular tissue may be related to higher hemoglobin content due to tumor vascularity.

Patient acceptance of the TLS examination is high because the examination takes approximately 10 minutes, and unlike mammography does not require aggressive breast compression. In a dark room the fiber-optic light source is placed against the breast and positioning as well as firm compression is performed by the operator. Numerous standard images are obtained with the light source and video camera at different positions about the breast surface in order to completely evaluate the patient. Comparable images are obtained of both breasts because symmetry can be important in the interpretation of the examination.

TLS is highly operator- and technique-dependent. An experienced technologist or physician must perform the examination with careful attention to uniform illumination of the breast, proper wavelength balance, and adequate breast positioning and compression.

TLS criteria for malignancy include the direct signs of focal areas of absorption or ratio changes in the amount of infrared to red light transmission (15) (Fig. 13.2). Indirect signs include abnormal vasculature (which may be manifested by change in course, caliber, and number or symmetry of vessels), asymmetric absorption or ratio values, and skin changes or

interval change between examinations. As with many other imaging techniques including mammography and thermography, the criteria are nonspecific. False-positive light scans can be attributed to fibrocystic changes, fat necrosis; inflammation; or a fibroadenoma, papilloma, or hematoma (Figs. 13.3 and 13.4). Cysts can be evident on TLS and have greater transmission of light through the fluid-filled structure (Fig. 13.5). Because the technique probably depends on differential absorption by hemoglobin content, after an attempted needle aspiration of the breast, TLS shows intense absorption at the site of the needle puncture. This iatrogenic abnormality can cause confusion in interpreting the examination by converting a normal light scan into an abnormal one, thus suggesting an underlying carcinoma.

Light Scanning vs. Mammography

Numerous studies of different experimental design have compared the sensitivities of light scanning and mammography in the evaluation of breast carcinoma (15–26) (Table 13.1). Except for the study by Dowle and associates (26) all

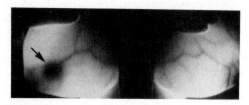

Figure 13.3. Light scan: fat necrosis. Intense focal absorption (*arrow*) is seen in medial aspect of right breast, which matches 1.5-cm mammographic abnormality that prompted biopsy. Pathologic diagnosis was fat necrosis.

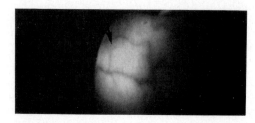

Figure 13.5. Light scan: cyst. Medial view of left breast shows focal region of greater light transmission (*arrow*), which corresponds to 3-cm palpable cyst.

Table 13.1. Sensitivity of Transillumination Light Scanning vs. Mammography[a]

	All Tumors		Tumors ≤1	
Author(s) (Ref)	TLS	Mam-mog-raphy	TLS	Mam-mog-raphy
McIntosh (16)	93	71		
Wallberg et al. (17)	85	86		
Bartrum and Crow (18)	76	94	44	89
Marshall et al. (19)	77	85		
Drexler et al. (20)	58	96		
Sickles (21)	53	96	19	90
Geslien et al. (22)	58	97	30	100
Greene et al. (23)	98	98	98	98
Merritt et al. (15)	77	76		
Gisvold et al. (24)	67	96		
Monsees et al. (25)	58	88	25	100
Dowle et al. (26)	87	83	60	100

[a]All values are percent.

the studies comparing the two modalities consist of more than 60% symptomatic patients, women with palpable masses. The larger, and therefore palpable, tumors were more consistently visible on TLS. When sensitivity by tumor size was evaluated, TLS often proved less sensitive with smaller tumors. For example, Dowle and associates found only a 60% sensitivity for TLS when invasive carcinomas smaller than a centimeter were evaluated, all of which could be detected by mammography. Bartrum and Crow (18) found that for tumors smaller than 1 cm, when evaluated blindly, the sensitivity of TLS was 44%, as compared with 89% for mammography. In the study by Sickles (21), only 19% of tumors smaller than 1 cm were detected by TLS, whereas 90% were detected by mammography. Comparable rates in the study by Geslien and associates (22) were 30% for TLS and 100% for mammography. The author's experience corroborates the same findings for both in situ tumors as well as small invasive tumors (25).

Results from studies currently underway may eventually determine whether another possible role for the use of TLS may be in a select group of patients, perhaps those with mammographically dense breasts. Several authors have reported that TLS could demonstrate carcinomas that were not discernible on mammograms. McIntosh (16) reported four such patients with dense breasts out of a total of 14 patients with carcinoma in his study group. Wallberg and associates (17) reported a series of 110 cancers, 7 of which were positive with TLS but negative with mammography; 5 of 7 of these patients had dense breasts.

A positive light scan in the presence of a negative mammogram and physical examination presents a difficult clinical problem. Although the specificity for light scanning by many of the above mentioned authors is the same or even better than that of mammography, false-positive light scans are not few. For example, Gisvold and associates (24) found 117 of 822 patients who had positive light scans and did not undergo biopsy. In the case of a positive light scan and a negative mammogram and physical examination, biopsy cannot be easily accomplished because three-dimensional localization cannot be performed. Alternatives include biopsy of a larger segment of the breast without mammographically guided needle localization or close clinical, TLS and mammographic follow-up.

Another possible adjunctive use for light scanning is in the evaluation of mammographically detected nonpalpable lesions. Since mammography is sensitive but not specific and many women undergo biopsy for benign lesions, a test that could differentiate benign from malignant without biopsy would be of great value. The author evaluated patients with nonpalpable mammographic abnormalities by TLS just prior to needle localization and biopsy of the breast (27, 28). TLS was performed by one of two radiologists well-trained in the technique and with full knowledge of the location and appearance of the mammographic abnormality. In one such study of 103 patients, TLS was positive in 58% of the patients with carcinoma (27). The second study, performed after an equipment change by the manufacturer, found that TLS was positive in only 30% of 23 patients with mammographically detected breast carcinoma (28). Both of these studies showed that the sensitivity of light scanning was proportional to tumor size. The author concluded that for suspicious lesions on mammograms, the need for breast biopsy cannot be eliminated on the basis of a negative light scan examination and that TLS is ineffective as a problem-solving or tissue characterization method. In addition, because the author's study was unable to demonstate a major fraction of carcinomas with TLS despite the directed nature of the examination, that TLS is also ineffective as a screening method.

Summary

Since the discrepancy between the sensitivities of mammography and light scanning is greatest in patients with better prognosis lesions (i.e., those with smaller and noninvasive tumors), then TLS cannot be utilized in lieu of mammography for screening. For diagnosis in a patient with a palpable mass, neither a negative

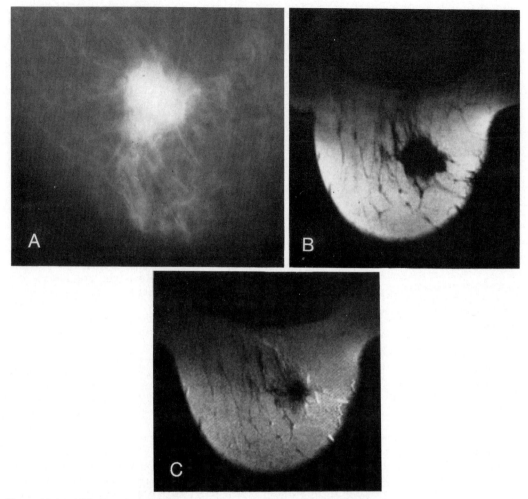

Figure 13.6.   MRI: invasive carcinoma. **A**, Mammogram shows large spiculated mass. **B**, T₁-weighted MRI. Mass has low signal intensity. **C**, T₂-weighted MRI. Mass has different signal intensities in center and periphery. (From Murphy WA, Gohagan JK. Magnetic resonance imaging of the breast. In: Stark DD, Bradley, WG Jr, eds: Magnetic resonance imaging. St. Louis: CV Mosby, 1988.)

light scan nor a negative mammogram can defer biopsy. When an indeterminate abnormality is detected on a screening mammogram, TLS cannot be used to determine if biopsy is necessary.

MAGNETIC RESONANCE IMAGING

Technique

Magnetic resonance (MRI) has received considerable attention as a possible tissue characterization technique (29–34). It is attractive as an imaging modality because of its ability at tissue differentiation. Instead of producing a summated image such as that produced with mammography, thermography, or transillumination, MRI produces a sectional image that can be further manipulated by using different sequencing pa-

rameters. Multiple pulse sequences must be performed to attempt tissue characterization. To those concerned with the potential risk of ionizing radiation, MRI is particularly attractive because of its lack of known adverse effects.

The examination is performed in a superconducting magnet. Better resolution for the breast can be achieved with use of a special coil made for breast imaging. The examination takes more than 30 minutes, during which the patient lies prone with her breast dependent within the coil. This position can be uncomfortable and therefore may result in poor patient acceptance. The site and equipment for MRI is expensive, and therefore examination costs are high. Patients with pacemakers, aneurysm clips, stimulators, or those who suffer from claustrophobia cannot be scanned.

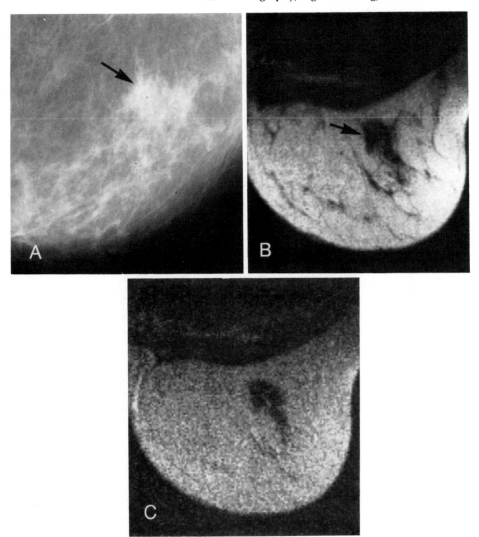

Figure 13.7. MRI: focal fibrosis. **A,** Mammogram shows dense focal area (*arrow*). **B,** T$_1$-weighted MRI shows similar low signal intensity region (*arrow*), **C,** T$_2$-weighted MRI shows low signal intensity in the region corresponding to dense collagenous tissue. (From Murphy WA, Gohagan JK. Magnetic resonance imaging of the breast. In: Stark DD, Bradley, WG Jr, eds: Magnetic resonance imaging. St. Louis: CV Mosby, 1988.)

Most of the information obtained is morphologic, and the images appear very similar to those obtained from a mammogram. In a prospective study of 30 patients with suspected abnormalities on mammography, El Yousef and associates (29) found that 10 patients with breast carcinoma were all "correctly diagnosed" by both mammography and MRI. In another study by Dash and associates (32) of 21 patients with carcinoma of the breast, MRI correctly identified 18 and mammography 19. Despite the hope that MRI might be tissue specific, there is significant overlap in signal intensity between normal and malignant tissue even with multiple pulse sequences (30, 35)

(Figs. 13.6 and 13.7). Cysts can be reliably differentiated from solid masses by use of different pulse sequences and have a characteristic low signal intensity on T$_1$-weighted images and very high signal intensity on T$_2$-weighted images (30) (Fig. 13.8). Fibroadenomas have a similar low signal intensity on T$_1$-weighted images, but because of variable histologic makeup of fibroadenomas this signal intensity can vary on T$_2$-weighted images. Therefore, they cannot be reliably differentiated from well-defined carcinomas (36) (Fig. 13.9).

MRI has no present application in screening for breast carcinoma. Small carcinomas, particularly if they are surrounded by glandular tis-

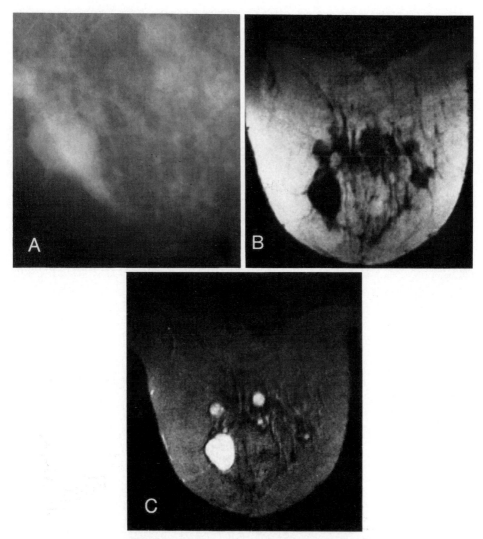

Figure 13.8.   MRI: cysts. **A,** Mammogram shows multiple round masses. **B,** T_1-weighted MRI. Masses have low signal intensity. **C,** T_2-weighted MRI. Cysts have high signal intensity compared with surrounding fat. (From Murphy WA, Gohagan JK. Magnetic resonance imaging of the breast. In: Stark DD, Bradley, WG Jr, eds: Magnetic resonance imaging. St. Louis: CV Mosby, 1988.)

sue rather than fat, may not be discernible. Because of dependence on morphology to depict abnormalities, MRI and mammography can more reliably detect carcinomas in fatty than in dense breast (30, 37). Heywang and associates (37) found that of 14 cancers in dense breasts, 10 could be seen on MRI and 11 on mammograms. Of 22 cancers in fatty breasts, MRI could distinguish 22 and mammography 21. Microcalcifications cannot be seen on MRI, another serious limitation of the test. For diagnostic purposes (i.e., characterization of mammographically detected or palpable abnormalities) MRI depends again on morphologic criteria, and with the exception of cystic

masses, is unable to supply tissue-specific answers. Enlarged axillary lymph nodes can be visualized, but micrometastases cannot be detected. Tumors deep within the breast that might involve the chest wall can be examined with a body scanner rather than a smaller breast coil. MRI may better visualize areas of breast parenchyma surrounding a silicone breast augmentation, which may be difficult to evaluate with mammography (37).

Because of the inability of MRI to provide tissue characterization despite the use of different pulse sequences, some have investigated the use of contrast agents that might alter proton relaxation times and result in improved

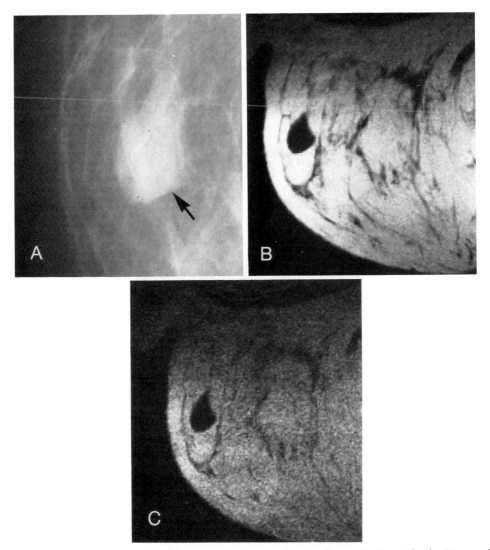

Figure 13.9. MRI: fibroadenoma. **A**, Mammogram shows well-defined mass. **B**, T$_1$-weighted MRI. Mass has low signal intensity. **C**, T$_2$-weighted MRI. Fibroadenoma maintains low signal intensity. (From Murphy WA, Gohagan JK. Magnetic resonance imaging of the breast. In: Stark DD, Bradley, WG Jr., eds: Magnetic resonance imaging. St. Louis: CV Mosby, 1988.)

sensitivity and specificity of MRI. Enhancement using these contrast agents has been seen in fibroadenomas and carcinomas, and their use may enable MRI to have a more definite role in the future (38). In particular patients with mammographically dense breasts might be better evaluated with the use of MRI and contrast enhancement.

Summary

Tissue characterization on the basis of tissue signal intensity even utilizing multiple pulse sequences is not specific. Although cysts may be reliably characterized using MRI, ultra-sound is more affordable and accessible. Further research utilizing contast agents may provide a role for MRI in the care of patients with diseases of the breast in the future.

CONCLUSION

The three breast imaging modalities discussed in this chapter have no established role in screening for carcinoma of the breast, or in the workup of a symptomatic patient or of a patient with an abnormal mammogram. None of these tests can be considered "a useful adjunct" to mammography because they do not dictate the next step in patient care (39).

REFERENCES

1. Digest of Official Council Actions of 1978–1987 and Bylaws. American College of Radiology, 1987:42–43.
2. Thermography for Breast Cancer Detection. Health Technology Assessment Reports, No. 22. U.S. Department of Health and Human Services, Public Health Service, Office of the Assistant Secretary for Health, 1983.
3. Isard HJ, Ostrum BJ. Breast thermography—the mammotherm. Radiol Clin North Am 1974;12:167–188.
4. Isard HJ. Thermographic "edge sign" in breast carcinoma. Cancer 1972;30:957–963.
5. Isard HJ. Cancer in the "cold" breast thermogram. AJR 1976;127:793–796.
6. Report of the working group to review the National Cancer Institute-American Cancer Society Breast Cancer Detection Demonstration Projects. J Natl Cancer Inst 1979;62:708.
7. Feig SA, Shaber GS, Gordon GF, et al. Thermography, mammography, and clinical examination in breast cancer screening. Radiology 1977;122:123–127.
8. Sterns EE, Curtis AC, Miller S, Hancock JR. Thermography in breast diagnosis. Cancer 1982;50:323–325.
9. Isard HJ, Becker W, Shilo R, Ostrum BJ. Breast thermography after four years and 10,000 studies. AJR 1972;115:811–821.
10. Moskowitz M, Milbrath J, Gartside P, Zermeno A, Mandel D. Lack of efficacy of thermography as a screening tool for minimal and stage I breast cancer. N Engl J Med 1976;295:249–252.
11. Gautherie M, Gros CM. Breast thermogaphy and cancer risk prediction. Cancer 1980;45:51–56.
12. Moskowitz M. Thermography as a risk indicator of breast cancer. Results of a study and a review of the recent literature. J Reprod Med 1985;30:451–459.
13. Moskowitz M, Fox SH, del Re RB, et al. The potential value of liquid-crystal thermography in detecting significant mastopathy. Radiology 1981;140:659–662.
14. Ertefai S, Profio AE. Spectral transmittance and contrast in breast diaphanography. Med Phys 1985;12:393–400.
15. Merritt CRB, Sullivan MA, Segaloff A, McKinnon WP. Real-time transillumination light scanning of the breast. RadioGraphics 1984;4:989–1009.
16. McIntosh DMF. Breast light scanning: A real-time breast-imaging modality. J Can Assoc Radiol 1983;34:288–290.
17. Wallberg H, Alveryd A, Bergvall U, Nasiell K, Sundelin P, Troell S. Diaphanography in breast carcinoma. Correlation with clinical examination, mammography, cytology and histology. Acta Radio [Diagn] Stockh 1985;26:33–44.
18. Bartrum RJ Jr, Crow HC. Transillumination light scanning to diagnose breast cancer: a feasibility study. AJR 1984;142:409–414.
19. Marshall V, Williams DC, Smith KD. Diaphanography as a means of detecting breast cancer. Radiology 1984;150:339–343.

20. Drexler B, Davis JL, Schofield G. Diaphanography in the diagnosis of breast cancer. Radiology 1985;157:41–44.
21. Sickles EA. Breast cancer detection with transillumination and mammography. AJR 1984;142:841–844.
22. Geslien GE, Fisher JR, DeLaney C. Transillumination in breast cancer detection: Screening failures and potential. AJR 1985;144:619–622.
23. Greene FL, Hicks C, Eddy V, Davis C. Mammography, sonomammography, and diaphanography (lightscanning). A prospective, comparative study with histologic correlation. Am Surgeon 1985;51:58–60.
24. Gisvold JJ, Brown LR, Swee RG, Raygor DJ, Dickerson N, Ranfranz MK. Comparison of mammography and transillumination light scanning in the detection of breast lesions. AJR 1986;147:191–194.
25. Monsees B, Destouet JM, Totty WG. Light scanning versus mammography in breast cancer detection. Radiology 1987;163:463–465.
26. Dowle CS, Caseldine J, Tew J, Manhire AR, Roebuck EJ, Blamey RW. An evaluation of transmission spectoscopy (lightscanning) in the diagnosis of symptomatic breast lesions. Clin Radiol 1987;38:375–377.
27. Monsees, B, Destouet JM. Gersell D. Light scan evaluation of nonpalpable breast lesions. Radiology 1987;163:467–470.
28. Monsees B, Destouet JM, Gersell D. Light scanning of nonpalpable breast lesions: reevaluation. Radiology 1988;167:352.
29. El Yousef SJ, O'Connell DM, Duchesneau RH, Smith MJ, Hubay CA, Guyton SP. Benign and malignant breast disease: magnetic resonance and radiofrequency pulse sequences. AJR 1985;145:1–8.
30. Alcorn FS, Turner DA, Clark JW, Charters JR, Petasnick JP, Shorey WD. Magnetic resonance imaging in the study of of the breast. RadioGraphics 1985;5:631–652.
31. El Yousef SJ, O'Connell DM. Magnetic resonance imaging of the breast. In: Kressell HY, ed. Magnetic resonance annual 1986. New York: Raven Press, 1986:177–194.
32. Dash N, Lupetin AR, Daffner RH, Sefczek RJ, Schapiro RL. Magnetic resonance imaging in the diagnosis of breast disease. AJR 1986;146:119–125.
33. Alcorn FS. Magnetic resonance imaging. In Bassett LW, Gold RH, eds. Breast cancer detection. Mammography and other methods in breast imaging. Orlando, FL: Grune & Stratton, 1987.
34. Murphy WA, Gohagan JK. Magnetic resonance imaging of the breast. In: Stark DD, Bradley, WG, Jr, eds: Magnetic resonance imaging. St. Louis, CV Mosby, 1988.
35. Wiener JI, Chako AC, Merten CW, Gross S, Coffey EL, Stein HL. Breast and axillary tissue MR imaging: correlation of signal intensitites and relaxation times with pathologic findings. Radiology 1986;160:299–305.
36. Stelling CB, Powell DE, Mattingly SS. Fibroadenomas: histopathologic and MR imaging features. Radiology 1987;162:399–407.

37. Heywang SH, Fenzl G, Hahn D. Krischke I, Edmaier M, Eiermann W, Bassermann R. MR imaging of the breast: comparison with mammography and ultrasound. J Comput Assist Tomogr 1986;10:615–620.

38. Heywang SH, Hahn D, Schmidt H, Krischke I, Eiermann W, Bassermann R, Lissner J. MR Imaging of the breast using Gadolinium-DTPA. J Comput Assist Tomogr 1986;10:199–204.

39. Kopans DB. What is a useful adjunct to mammography. Radiology 1986;161:560–561.

Diagnostic Imaging for Staging and Follow-up of Breast Cancer Patients

Lawrence W. Bassett
Armando E. Giuliano
Richard H. Gold

In addition to physical examination and routine laboratory studies, pretreatment evaluation and follow-up of the patient with breast carcinoma should include chest radiography and bilateral mammography. Other diagnostic imaging examinations should be limited to specific indications.

STAGING OF BREAST CARCINOMA

The TNM staging system of the American Joint Committee on Cancer has been widely accepted (1). This system is based on the size or local extent of the primary tumor (T), the status of the regional lymph nodes (N), and the presence or absence of distant metastases (M) (1).

Primary Tumor

Determination of tumor size and possible multifocality or bilaterality are important factors in selecting appropriate therapy. Most breast cancers cause a desmoplastic response that causes the tumor to feel larger at physical examination than it appears on mammograms. As a result, mammography is frequently more accurate than palpation in assessing tumor size. However, up to 10% of palpable breast carcinomas cannot be visualized in mammograms, and sonography may be used to determine tumor size in those cases that are able to be imaged (2).

Following breast-conserving surgery, mammography is the most effective method for revealing residual tumor and monitoring for local recurrence, especially when the tumor is associated with microcalcifications. In one series of 23 biopsy-proven recurrences, 8 were identified only on mammography, 9 only on physical examination, and 6 on both mammography and physical examination (3). Mammographic evidence of tumor recurrence includes calcifications, a mass, and architectural distortion (4, 5). However, mammograms performed after surgery and radiotherapy are frequently difficult to interpret. The following abnormalities in postoperative mammograms can result from surgery and may be mistaken for cancer: skin thickening or retraction, increased parenchymal density, architectural distortion, asymmetry, scarring, calcifications, and fat necrosis (6, 7). For this reason, postoperative mammograms should be interpreted with knowledge of previous surgery including the location of the excised primary tumor, and should make use of a comparison with previous preoperative and postoperative mammograms. Ideally, baseline mammograms should be performed at 6 and 12 months after surgery to exclude recurrent tumor and for evaluating subsequent examinations. Follow-up mammograms should thereafter be performed at least at yearly intervals.

Lymph Node Involvement

The breast lymphatics drain by three major regional routes: axillary, transpectoral, and internal mammary trunks. The status of the axillary lymph nodes is considered to be the most important prognostic factor. The axillary nodes are classified as free of disease, positive for cancer but freely movable, or positive and fixed. The mediolateral oblique projection for film-screen mammography and the noncontact mediolateral chest wall view for xeromammography allow visualization of the lower axillary nodes. Features suggesting axillary node metastasis include absence of radiolucent fat within the node, a change in the shape of the node from oval to spherical, and a diameter of 2.5 cm or greater (8). However, since there are no radiographic criteria to definitely exclude early nodal involvement, an axillary dissection biopsy is the only sure method for identifying nodal metastasis (9).

Involvement of the internal mammary lymph nodes can be determined by surgical biopsy or scintigraphy. Because the internal mammary chain is not readily accessible to the surgeon, some clinicians have found preoperative internal mammary lymphoscintigraphy a useful noninvasive method to evaluate the internal mammary lymph nodes for radiotherapy planning and to determine the need for systemic therapy (10). Radioisotope-labeled sulfur microcolloid is injected below the anterior rib cage, slightly off of the midline. Asymmetrically increased isotope accumulation in the internal mammary nodes indicates metastasis.

Extension to any other nodes, including the supraclavicular (1), is considered equivalent to distant metastases.

Metastases

The presence or absence of distant metastases is another important prognostic factor. Although breast carcinoma can metastasize to any remote organ, four most likely sites are bone, brain, liver, and lung. Diagnostic imaging is generally not useful to screen for metastatic disease. However, in specific circumstances, such as when there are abnormalities in serum chemistries or abnormal physical findings, diagnostic imaging may be used to confirm and evaluate the extent of clinically suspected metastases. Serial bone and liver imaging may be useful in high-risk patients.

EVALUATION OF THE SKELETON FOR METASTASES

Radionuclide bone scanning with technetium 99m diphosphonate is the most effective screening tool for bone metastases because of its high sensitivity and ability to show the entire skeleton in one examination. Indications for bone scanning include the following:

1. staging the high-risk asymptomatic patient;

2. evaluating persistent bone pain with negative radiographs;
3. determining extent of metastases when radiographs are abnormal;
4. evaluating areas difficult to study by conventional radiography;
5. identifying pathologic fractures by disclosing additional sites of osseous involvement;
6. planning radiotherapy;
7. monitoring treatment; and
8. periodically evaluating the asymptomatic high-risk patient (11).

False-positive scans arise from many common abnormalities including arthritis, healing fractures, bursitis, degenerative disk disease, Paget's disease, and benign lesions that increase the blood flow. For this reason, an abnormal bone scan must be correlated with radiographs before a diagnosis is made. False-negative bone scans are unusual. The role of preoperative bone scans in the asymptomatic patient with stage I or II breast carcinoma has not been clearly established. In one study of 205 patients with tumors smaller than 2 cm followed for 10 years, only 22 (15.6%) developed bone metastases (12). In another study of 10 patients with tumors smaller than 2 cm, none had abnormal scans at the time of mastectomy, and of 14 patients with tumors 2 to 4 cm in size, only one had an abnormal scan (13).

In a multicentered European study, 2450 patients with no symptoms underwent routine preoperative bone scans (14). Only 0.16% of 633 patients with T_1 tumors had metastases detected by bone scans, and only 1.18% of 189 patients with T_2 tumors had metastases detected by bone scans. The overall detection rate of metastatic disease was 0.9% (22 of 2450). Even the T_4 lesions were associated with only a 1.3% incidence of metastases detected by preoperative bone scans. However, there were 125 false-positive bone scans.

Currently, the authors do not perform routine bone scans on patients with stage I or stage II disease who have no symptoms of bone involvement and have a normal serum alkaline phosphatase level. Patients with more advanced disease undergo routine preoperative bone scans as do those who complain of bone pain or have an elevated serum level of alkaline phosphatase or calcium.

The value of routine postoperative bone scans is also controversial. The rate at which patients with initial negative scans develop positive scans varies with the stage of disease. One report indicated that 7% of patients with stage I disease eventually develop positive scans, whereas 45% of patients with stage II

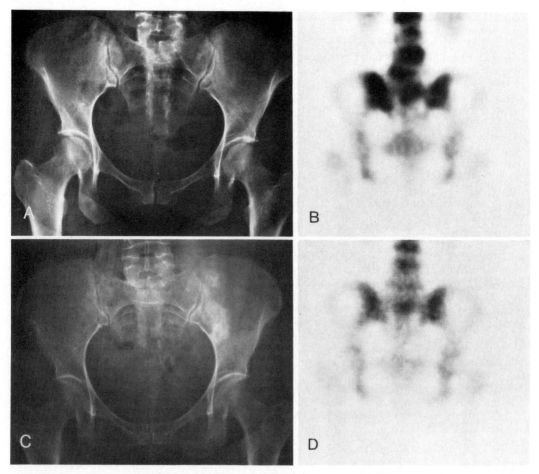

Figure 14.1. Radionuclide bone scan for detection of metastases and evaluation of treatment. The patient complained of pain in her back. **A**, Anteroposterior radiograph of pelvis from December 1984 was normal. **B**, Technetium diphosphonate bone scan revealed metastases (increased accumulations of isotope) in lumbar spine and around sacroiliac joints. Patient was treated with oophorectomy and chemotherapy. Radiograph from April 1986 (**C**), when she was asymptomatic, shows blastic bone formation in left ilium, but scan (**D**) has returned to normal indicating that radiographic bone formation represented inactive treated metastases.

and 58% of patients with stage III converted to positive scans (15).

Bone scans may be extremely useful to detect the healing of treated metastases. Healing metastases may show a temporary increase in scan intensity, and correlation of the bone scan with plain radiographs that show healing or no change will prevent a misinterpretation that the bone lesions have worsened (Fig. 14.1) (16). With continued healing, the activity of the metastases becomes less intense, and eventually may return to normal.

Conventional radiography is too insensitive to be used to screen for asymptomatic bone metastases. On the other hand, the nonspecificity of bone scans dictates that after a

scan depicts an abnormality, selected radiographs of the area should be obtained and correlated with the scan (17). Because the relatively high radionuclide activity in the bladder and sacro-iliac joints may obscure superimposed metastases, the authors always combine bone radionuclide examination with an anteroposterior radiograph of the pelvis. Solitary or unusual patterns of multiple foci of activity may be caused by a variety of benign conditions. Therefore, when the cause of an abnormal scan or clinical finding is not determined radiography, and sometimes conventional tomography, computed tomography (CT), magnetic resonance imaging (MRI), and/or biopsy, may be indicated.

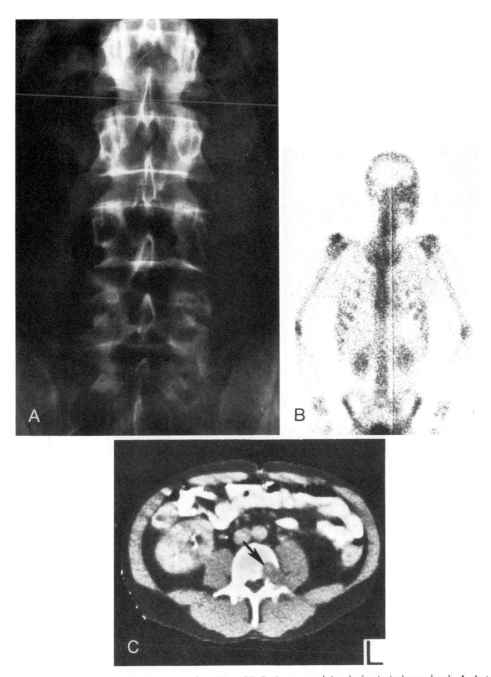

Figure 14.2.   False-negative bone scan and positive CT. Patient complained of pain in lower back. **A,** Anteroposterior radiograph was normal. **B,** Bone scan was also normal. **C,** CT scan performed same day shows low-density metastasis (*arrow*) in L4 body and pedicle.

Two indications for CT or MRI are (*a*) for the symptomatic patient with equivocal or negative standard radiographs and positive radionuclide bone scan (Fig. 14.2), and (*b*) for determining the extent of metastatic lesions when planning therapy.

Figure 14.3 shows an algorithmic workup for suspected bone metastases.

Workup for Bone Metastases

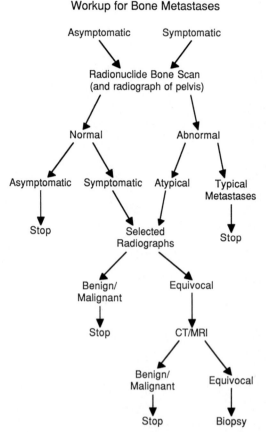

Figure 14.3. Algorithmic workup for suspected bone metastases.

EVALUATION OF THE BRAIN FOR METASTASES

Breast cancer is second in frequency only to lung cancer as a cause of cerebral and orbital metastases. Motor deficits, headaches, and changes in mental status are the most common presenting symptoms. Most patients already have clinical findings when brain metastases are found on CT; in one series, 16 of 17 patients with CT evidence of intracranial metastases already had abnormal clinical neurologic examinations (18).

CT and MRI are currently the most sensitive and accurate imaging modalities for the detection and evaluation of suspected brain metastases (19). In CT images, metastases may be either nodular or ring-shaped, single or multiple, and are usually associated with considerable edema in the surrounding tissues. Metastases show varying amounts of enhancement following intravenous injection of iodinated contrast agents. There are no specific morphologic CT criteria to distinguish the metastases of breast carcinoma from those of other primary neoplasms. MRI, due to its greater sensitivity, is expected to eventually replace CT as the diagnostic study of choice for the detection of brain lesions (20).

Despite its high sensitivity, however, MRI may fail to depict lesions smaller than 1 cm that do not exhibit peripheral edema or are obscured by the edema associated with adjacent metastases. Furthermore, false-positive MRI examinations may result when infarcts are misinterpreted as metastases. Intravenous gadolinium diethylenetriaminepentaacetic acid (Gd-DTPA)-enhanced MR imaging promises to further improve the detection of metastases by increasing the difference between their signal intensity and that of normal brain tissue (21, 22).

EVALUATION OF THE LIVER FOR METASTASES

Imaging examinations are not recommended as screening tests for liver metastases in asymptomatic patients due to low yield but should be reserved for patients with pertinent symptoms, abnormal liver chemistries, or hepatomegaly.

Technetium 99m sulfur colloid scans are relatively inexpensive and generally available, but most liver defects must be greater than 2 cm in diameter in order to be detected by this examination. Furthermore, false-positive scans are relatively common due to anatomic variations, defects caused by normal juxtahepatic structures, and alterations in reticuloendothelial cell activity or blood flow. In a study of 234 breast cancer patients who had routine preoperative liver scans, only 11 (5%) abnormal scans were obtained (23). Eight of the 11 abnormal scans were found to be false-positives, so that ultimately only 1% of the scans yielded metastatic disease.

Sonography is useful in the evaluation of intrahepatic metastases as small as 2 cm. Inexpensive, safe, and relatively simple to perform, sonography is also an excellent modality to follow the progress of metastases during treatment. Sonography can be used to localize larger lesions for biopsy or aspiration. Most investigators have found both sonography and CT to be more specific than radionuclide scans (24).

CT is generally considered to be the most effective method for detection of liver metastases. Intravenous injection of iodinated contrast material improves the CT detection of liver metastases (25). Although generally considered to be the most effective method for identifying liver metastases, CT scanning, even with the use of intravenous iodinated contrast agents, permits the detection of fewer than 50% of the metastases found at surgery (26). Ethiodized oil emulsion-13 (EOE-13), an intravenous CT contrast agent used specifically for scanning the liver and spleen, increases the CT detection rate for liver metastases to approximately 80% (27).

MRI is also being evaluated for liver scanning. With MRI, the inherent contrast between the signal intensities of normal and pathologic tissues can be accentuated by altering the pulse sequences. Most investigators have reported comparable results for CT and MRI in detecting focal hepatic lesions (28). Physiologic motion, currently a limiting factor in MRI of the upper abdomen, may eventually be solved by technologic improvements. In one study using short MRI pulse sequences, MRI was shown to reveal 14% more individual metastases than CT in 142 patients undergoing both examinations; MRI was also more specific (29). Another study of 20 patients with known liver metastases showed that EOE-13-enhanced CT and T_1-weighted MRI were overall the most sensitive and accurate methods for the detection of liver metastases (30).

EVALUATION OF THE LUNG FOR METASTASES

The expense and time used to search for pulmonary metastases should be predicated on whether or not their discovery will alter therapy. One large series of cases reports the incidence of pulmonary metastases from breast cancer as 4% at presentation and 60% at autopsy (31). Lung metastases usually occur by way of the pulmonary arteries and less often through lymphatic spread. Pulmonary metastases tend to be spherical, varying in size from miliary to 5 cm, are usually bilateral and multiple, and most often are located in the periphery of the lung bases (32). Lymphangitic metastases start out as an interstitial process that radiographically resembles early pulmonary venous hypertension; the fine linear septal lines eventually thicken and become associated with pleural effusions. Breast carcinoma rarely presents with endobronchial metastases manifested in radiographs by segmental atelectasis (33). Methods for detecting pulmonary metastases include conventional radiography, whole-lung tomography, and CT.

Posteroanterior and lateral chest projection using conventional radiography is the method of choice for preoperative evaluation and routine follow-up examinations. Conventional whole-lung tomography permits identification of smaller metastatic lesions than do plain radiographs.

CT is the most sensitive method for detecting pulmonary metastases and has replaced conventional tomography as the method of choice to evaluate equivocal radiographic findings or to identify additional metastatic nodules when metastases are found in plain films (34, 35). Contrast-enhanced CT provides accurate evaluation of both the lung and the mediastinum.

MRI shows promise for evaluating the mediastinum, but it is not useful for detecting lung nodules.

REFERENCES

1. American Joint Committee on Cancer. Manual for staging of cancer. Philadelphia: Lippincott, 1988:145–150.
2. Fornage BD, Toubas O, Morel M. Clinical, mammographic, and sonographic determination of preoperative breast carcinoma size. Cancer 1987;60:765–771.
3. Stomper PC, Recht A, Berenberg AL, Jochelson MS, Harris JR. Mammographic detection of recurrent cancer in the irradiated breast. AJR 1987;148:39–43.
4. Bloomer WD, Berenberg AL, Weissman BN. Mammography of the therapeutically irradiated breast. Radiology 1976;118:425–428.
5. Libshitz HI, Montague ED, Paulus DD. Calcifications and the therapeutically irradiated breast. AJR 1977;128:1021–1025.
6. Sickles EA, Herzog KA. Mammography of the postsurgical breast. AJR 1981;136:585–588.
7. Bassett LW, Gold RH, Mirra JM. Nonneoplastic breast calcifications in lipid cysts: development after excision and primary irradiation. AJR 1982;138:335–338.
8. Kalisher L, Chu AM, Peyster RG. Clinicopathological correlation of xeroradiography in determining involvement of metastatic axillary nodes in female breast carcinoma. Radiology 1976;121:333–335.
9. Coopmans de Yoldi Gf, Andreoli C, Costa A, Nessi R, Gilardoni L, Rasponi A. Lack of efficacy of xeroradiography to preoperatively detect axillary lymph node metastases in breast cancer. Breast Cancer Res Treat 1983;3:373–376.
10. Ege GN. Internal mammary lymphoscintigraphy. The rationale, technique, interpretation and clinical application. Radiology 1976;118:101–107.
11. O'Mara RE. Bone scanning in osseous metastatic disease. JAMA 1974;229:1915–1917.
12. Robbins GF, Knapper WH, Barrie J, Kripalani I, Lawrence J. Metastatic bone disease developing in patients with potentially curable breast cancer. Cancer 1972;29:1702–1704.
13. El-Dormeiri AA, Shroff S. Role of preoperative bone scan in carcinoma of the breast. Surg Gynecol Obstet 1976;142:722–724.

14. Ciatto S, Pacini P, Azzini V, et al. Preoperative staging of primary breast cancer. A multicentric study. Cancer 1988;61:1038–1040.
15. McNeill BJ, Gerber FH, Goodrey JJ, et al. The efficacy of preoperative and postoperative bone scans. N Engl J Med 1977;29:300–303.
16. Alexander JL, Gilespie PJ, Edelstyn GA. Serial bone scanning using technetium 99m diphosphonate in patients undergoing cyclical combination chemotherapy of advanced breast cancer. Clin Nuc Med 1976;1:13–17.
17. Bassett LW, Gold RH, Webber MM. Radionuclide bone imaging. Radiol Clin North Am 1981;19:675–702.
18. Weisberg LA. The computed tomographic findings in intracranial metastases due to breast carcinoma. Comput Radiol 1986;10:297–306.
19. Bentson JR, Steckel RJ, Kagan AR. Diagnostic imaging in clinical cancer management: brain metastases. Invest Radiol 1988;23:335–341.
20. Brant-Zawadzski M. MR imaging of the brain. Radiology 1988;166:1–10.
21. Russell EJ, Geremia GK, Johnson CE, et al. Multiple cerebral metastases: detectability with Gd-DTPA-enhanced MR imaging. Radiology 1987;165:609–617.
22. Healy ME, Hesselink JR, Press GA, Middleton MS. Increased detection of intracranial metastases with intravenous Gd-DTPA. Radiology 1987;165:619–624.
23. Weiner SN, Sachs SH. An assessment of positive liver scanning in patients with breast cancer. Arch Surg 1978;113:126–127.
24. Yeh H, Rabinowitz JG. Ultrasonography and computed tomography of the liver. Radiol Clin North Am 1980;18:321–338.
25. Foley WD, Berland LL, Lawson TL, Smith DF, Thorsen MK. Contrast enhancement technique for dynamic hepatic computed tomographic scanning. Radiology 1983;147:797–803.
26. Bernardino ME. The liver anatomy and examination techniques. In: Taveras JM, Ferrucci JT, eds. Radiology, vol 4. New York: Lippincott, 1986:1–6.
27. Sugarbaker PH, Vermess M, Doppman JL, Miller DL, Simon R. Improved detection of focal lesions with computerized tomographic examination of the liver using ethiodized oil emulsion (EOE-13) liver contrast. Cancer 1984;54:1489–1495.
28. Moss AA, Goldberg HI, Stark DB, et al. Hepatic tumors: magnetic resonance and CT appearance. Radiology 1984;150:141–147.
29. Ferrucci JT. Leo G. Rigler lecture. MR imaging of the liver. AJR 1986;147:1103–1116.
30. Reinig JW, Dwyer AJ, Miller DL, et al. Liver metastasis detection: comparative sensitivities of MR imaging and CT scanning. Radiology 1987;162:43–47.
31. Gilbert HA, Kagan AR. Metastases: incidence, detection, and evaluation without histologic confirmation. In: Weiss L, ed. Fundamental aspects of metastasis. Amsterdam: North-Holland, 1976:385–405.
32. Willis RA. Secondary tumors of the lung. In: Willis RA, ed. The spread of tumors in the human body. London: Butterworth, 1973:167–174.
33. Braman SS, Whitcomb ME. Endobronchial metastasis. Arch Intern Med 1975;135:543–547.
34. Schaner EG, Chang AE, Doppman JL, Conkle DM, Flye MW, Rosenberg SA. Comparison of computed and conventional whole-lung tomography in detecting pulmonary nodules: a prospective radiologic-pathologic study. AJR 1978;131:51–54.
35. Mintzer RA, Malave SR, Neiman HL, Michaelis LL, Vanecko RM, Sanders JH. Computed vs. conventional tomography in evaluation of primary and secondary pulmonary neoplasms. Radiology 1979;132:653–659.

15

Medical Management of Benign Breast Disease

Martin Farber
Geeta Chhibber
Guy Hewlett

Cystic disease of the breast, the most common lesion of the breast, was first described by Sir Astley Cooper and Benjamin Brodie in the mid-19th century. Reclus and Brissaud published comprehensive clinical and pathologic descriptions of the disease in the 1880s and were succeeded by Konig who, in the 1890s, coined the term chronic cystic mastitis when he concluded that the histologic changes were inflammatory in origin.

Over the past 100 years a myriad of alternative terms have been used for the diagnosis, including fibrocystic mastopathy, chronic cystic mastitis, mammary dysplasia, benign mastopathy, Reclus' disease, Schimmelbusch's disease, cystiphorous desquamative epithelial hyperplasia, and cystic disease of the breast. The latter term is divided into two subsets: gross disease when the cysts are >2 to 3 mm and microscopic disease when the lesions are smaller (1).

Histologically, a large spectrum of changes have been found. Gross cysts are lined by a single layer of flattened epithelium and, similarly, microcysts are lined by one or two layers of flattened epithelial cells. Blunt duct adenosis exists when terminal breast ducts end blindly as microcysts with tall or flattened epithelium. The epithelium of the ducts may be heaped up to totally or partially occlude the lumen or may form papillary projections. Cuboidal epithelium of the breast duct may be transformed into columnar epithelium, apocrine metaplasia of duct epithelium. Adenosis exists as small foci of benign proliferations of acini and ducts in a lobular pattern, and there is a variable amount of fibrosis present (see Chapter 6).

The prevalence of cystic disease of the breast is not known, although in several series some histologic characteristics of the disease were found in 100% of autopsies performed on women who died of a disease not related to the breast. Furthermore, different terms are used by different investigators to describe the same histologic changes found in excised specimens (2). To date, the etiology of this ubiquitous lesion is not known, and the cause of the constant or cyclically recurrent pain sometimes associated with the disease has not been found. Data concerning serum estradiol, progesterone, androgens, and gonadotrophin levels are all inconclusive (3).

There is a consensus that there are three main reasons to medically treat cystic breast disease after the diagnosis has been established: (a) the alleviation of breast pain (constant or cyclic); (b) the reduction or complete eradication of breast nodularity; and (c) prophylaxis for the development of breast cancer. The latter reason remains controversial, and not all histologic changes categorized as cystic breast disease appear to place a woman at increased risk for breast cancer. Those that do are reported to be multiple intraductal papillomas and atypical lobular and ductal epithelial hyperplasia (4).

As might be anticipated, the suggested modalities for the treatment of a lesion that is ubiquitous, whose etiology is unknown, whose associated symptoms are poorly understood, and whose prognostic implications are controversial, form a long list (Table 15.1). Although many of the enumerated therapies are of historical interest, only the most recent ones will be discussed in this chapter.

179

Table 15.1. Treatment for Benign Breast Disease

Hormonal
Estrogens
  Estriol
  Tamoxifen (nonsteroidal)
Progestins
  17-Hydroxyprogesterone caproate
  Norethisterone
  Norethynodrel
  Lynestrenol
  Mastodynon
Estrogen and progestin
  Norethynodrel and mestranol
  Lynestrenol and mestranol
Androgens
  Testosterone
  Furazabol (synthetic androgen)
  Orgasteron (nonsteroidal androgen)
  Danazol
Human chorionic gonadotrophin
Nonhormonal
Vitamins
  Vitamin A
  Vitamin B_1
  Vitamin E
Iodide preparations
  Iodine
  Potassium iodide
Diuretics
Bromocriptine
Abstention from methylxanthines

METHYLXANTHINES

Caffeine, theophylline, and theobromine belong to a class of chemicals collectively called methylxanthines and are found in common foods such as coffee, tea, cola, and chocolate. Ten years ago an undetailed and uncontrolled clinical study of 47 women with cystic breast disease raised the suspicion that methylxanthine consumption might be associated with an increased risk for the development of the disease and (implicit in the data) an increased risk for the development of breast cancer. Thirteen of 20 women who discontinued ingestion of foods containing methylxanthines experienced resolution of signs and symptoms of cystic breast disease, while only 1 of 27 women who continued methylxanthine consumption experienced a similarly favorable result (5).

Methylxanthines inhibit phosphodiesterase resulting in inhibition of the conversion of cyclic adenosine monophosphate (cAMP) to 5'-adenosine monophosphate (5'-AMP) and inhibition of the conversion of cyclic guanine monophosphate (cGMP) to 5'-guanine monophosphate (5'-GMP). It was postulated that the presumed increased intracellular concentration of cyclic nucleotides stimulated protein kinases, which affected protein synthesis of the breast cells and resulted in the proliferation of cystic breast tissue. Indeed, assays of the cyclic nucleotides in excised breast tissue demonstrated concentration of cAMP and cGMP increased in cystic disease, as compared with those in controls, and significantly increased in breast cancer (6).

By inference, the specter raised by these data is perturbing. Methylxanthines are contained in many foods and beverages consumed in this country, and caffeine has long been known to adversely affect human physiology. Acute ingestion of caffeine increases heart rate, blood pressure, stroke volume, and cardiac output. Catecholamine levels (epinephrine and norepinephrine) are elevated, and the respiratory rate increases. The metabolic rate increases; gastric acid and pepsin levels increase; and decreased sodium and water resorption by the renal tubules results in diuresis. There is a deleterious effect on fine motor coordination and on sleep (7). The addition of a causal relationship between methylxanthines and cystic breast disease and breast cancer would have serious implications for public health policy.

However, the significance of the data was seriously questioned by a prospective clinical study that demonstrated a natural tendency for cystic breast disease to change with time, despite the constant ingestion of methylxanthines. In a group of 72 women observed for 6 months in whom cystic disease of the breast was diagnosed clinically, and in whom methylxanthine consumption did not significantly change, 15% of the breasts examined demonstrated complete disappearance of the lesions; 33% of the breasts demonstrated disappearance and then reappearance of the lesions; and 87% of all breasts examined demonstrated some change in position or number of the lesions. There was no correlation between pain from fibrocystic disease and the quantity of methylxanthine consumption (8).

Furthermore, data from the study of an age- and race-matched cohort of approximately 3000 women who were part of the Breast Cancer Detection Demonstration Project from 1973 to 1980 sponsored jointly by the National Cancer Institute and the American Cancer Society demonstrated no association between methylxanthine consumption and benign breast disease categorically, and specifically no association between methylxanthine consumption and cystic disease or benign neoplasm (fibroadenoma). There was no association between methylxanthine consumption and specific types of cystic disease, including those with atypia, hyperplasia, sclerosing adenosis, and macrocysts. No age-specific increased association of methylxanthine consumption and benign breast disease was found, and there was no association between menstrual breast tenderness and methylxanthine consumption in premenopausal women with fibrocystic disease or in controls (9). In vitro human mammary carcinoma cells and normal mouse breast epithelial cells were not shown to contain significantly increased levels of cAMP upon exposure to caffeine (10). Caffeine administered to Wistar rats in the drinking water for 78 weeks resulted in no increased incidence of cancer, when compared to the rates for controls (11). An age-matched, retrospective, case-controlled study of 616 women with histologically confirmed breast cancer demonstrated no increased risk of breast cancer in women who consumed coffee. In fact, the relative risk for breast cancer was higher in women who drank 2 to 3 cups of coffee per day, as compared with those who drank greater than 4 cups of coffee per day (12).

Recently, retrospective data from 90 pairs of twins discordant for a history of biopsy-proven benign breast disease demonstrated the twin with the lesion to be significantly more likely to consume more coffee than the unaffected twin (13). Another recent retrospective age-matched, case-controlled study of women with histologically proven cystic breast disease demonstrated not only a significantly positive association between caffeine ingestion and cystic breast disease in general, but also the strongest associations were with atypical lobular hyperplasia and sclerosing adenosis with papillomatosis or papillary hyperplasia (both of which are thought to place a woman at increased risk for breast cancer). The odds ratios varied directly with the daily caffeine consumption (14).

At the present time, there is no conclusive scientific data to support the contention that methylxanthines cause benign or malignant breast disease. A woman should make well-informed dietary decisions concerning all aspects of health (including health of the breasts) based on easily understood and readily available information offered to her by all members of the health care team.

VITAMIN E

A favorable response from the administration of vitamin E (α-tocopherol) to patients with clinically demonstrable cystic breast disease was reported in an uncontrolled study 25 years ago (15). A prospective double-blind crossover study of the efficacy of α-tocopherol

(300 IU b.i.d.) vs. placebo administered for 2 successive months to 12 patients with clinical evidence of fibrocystic disease demonstrated a significantly favorable response from the drug in 10 of them (16, 17). Subsequently, a larger series of 26 premenopausal patients with biopsy-proven cystic breast disease and 8 premenopausal controls were given a placebo for 4 weeks followed by α-tocopherol (vitamin E, 600 IU/day) for 8 weeks. Twenty-two patients had a good or fair response to the drug, as determined clinically by the disappearance of cysts and the amelioration of breast tenderness. Serum levels of estradiol and progesterone did not significantly differ between patients and controls and were not affected by α-tocopherol. Serum levels of dehydroepiandrosterone (DHEA) were significantly higher in responders to the drug prior to therapy and were depressed to levels not significantly different from those of controls at the completion of therapy. DHEA levels in nonresponders prior to therapy were the same as controls but were significantly depressed to levels lower than those of controls when therapy was completed. The significance of these changes in androgen levels was not understood (18).

Results from in vitro and in vivo investigations suggest that vitamin E may have an inhibitory effect on tumorigenesis. It has significant intracellular antioxidant activity and in tissue culture inhibits glioma and neuroblastoma tumor cell growth (19). In cell-free systems prepared from these tumors, α-tocopherol has been demonstrated to bind to the cytosol, nuclear, and chromatin fractions (20), and it is presumed to exert its inhibition of mutagenesis by reducing DNA replication. It has been shown to depress the mutagenic activity of nitrosoguanidine (a carcinogen) on *Escherichia coli* cells and inhibits mutagenesis induced by 3,2'-dimethyl-4-aminobiphenyl (DMAB), as demonstrated by the Ames test (21).

Vitamin E accumulates significantly in fat when administered to rodents. In the vitamin E–supplemented rodent there is a decrease in the development of neoplasia and a demonstrably increased mean life span (22). In rats fed a high polyunsaturated fat diet, vitamin E and selenium inhibited dimethylbenzanthracene (DMBA)-induced mammary cancers (23).

In the human α-tocopherol inhibits endogenous nitrosation reflected by a decreased excretion of N-nitrosoproline (a putative carcinogen) in the urine (24). Ingested in doses as high as 800 IU/day, vitamin E has not been shown to produce toxic side effects (25). However, to date there are no conclusive data to suggest that the ingestion of vitamin E reduces the risk of cancer in humans (26).

DANAZOL

Danazol, an attenuated androgen, is a 2,3-isoxazol derivative of 17-α-ethynyl testosterone (ethisterone). At doses of 100 mg/day it usually inhibits the midcycle surge of luteinizing hormone (LH). Women in the reproductive age range treated with the drug have levels of LH and follicle-stimulating hormone (FSH) measured in peripheral venous blood in the normal range. When gonadotrophin-releasing hormone (GnRH) is administered to Danazol-treated women there is a normal gonadotrophin response, demonstrating a normal gonadotrophin reserve of the pituitary gland.

Ovarian enzymatic activity is suppressed by Danazol, including 3-β-hydroxysteroid dehydrogenase, 17-α-hydroxylase, and 17,20-lyase. Inhibition of these enzymes required for ovarian steroidogenesis accounts for the slightly depressed levels of estradiol and progesterone sometimes observed during therapy with the drug. Other studies have reported normal levels of these steroid hormones (27).

At multiple tissue sites Danazol binds to androgen and progesterone cytoplasmic receptors, after which the steroid-cytoplasmic receptor is translocated to the nucleus (28). In castrated rats it binds to hypothalamic and pituitary cytosol estradiol receptors and competitively inhibits the binding of estradiol in those tissues.

Adverse side effects reported from the drug are irregular menses or amenorrhea, muscle cramps, acne, oily hair, hot flushes, and weight gain.

Danazol has many therapeutic applications and was first used to treat fibrocystic disease of the breast in 1971 (29). Early uncontrolled studies reported administration of the drug to women with cystic breast disease in doses ranging from 100 to 800 mg/day for 3 to 6 months. Incremental doses were given depending on the severity of the syndrome. At the 100-mg dose 98% of the patients witnessed partial or complete elimination of the disease after 6 months. At both the 200- and 400-mg doses all patients experienced complete or partial resolution of the disease in 6 months. After 4 years a significant number of patients from each dosage group who remained in the study remained free of signs and symptoms of the disease (30, 31).

A double-blind crossover study comparing Danazol at two-doses (200 and 400 mg/day) with placebo for the treatment of cystic breast disease demonstrated a significant therapeutic effect from the active agent that persisted subsequent to discontinuation of the drug for 3 months. At the higher dose of Danazol, the favorable clinical response was more rapid in onset (32). Cyclic breast pain from midcycle to the onset of menses has been demonstrated to be ameliorated by Danazol (400 mg/day), and the favorable effect persisted in 17% of women for 9 months subsequent to discontinuation of the drug (33). Compared with bromocriptine, Danazol was found to have a significantly more favorable effect on midcycle breast pain, heaviness, and tenderness (34). A recent report of a recurrent periareolar abscess responsive to Danazol therapy (35) was followed by a communication suggesting that a periareolar abscess be drained and the chronic fistulous tract be excised (36).

BROMOCRIPTINE

Bromocriptine inhibits pituitary lactomorphs and causes decreased prolactin secretion. A double-blind crossover study of a group of women with cyclic pain and nodularity of the breast whose mean serum prolactin was normal revealed them to have a significantly favorable response to bromocriptine (5 mg/day) administered for 6 months. The mean serum prolactin of the group was significantly decreased by the drug. Another group of women with noncyclic breast pain and nodularity whose mean serum prolactin was normal was unaffected by the drug, and the mean serum prolactin did not significantly change (37).

TAMOXIFEN

Tamoxifen, a nonsteroidal triphenylethylene derivative, is an estrogen agonist-antagonist. It competitively inhibits the action of estradiol on the mammary gland and is therefore used to treat some estrogen receptor–positive breast cancers. Administration of the drug has been proposed for the prevention of breast cancer (38), especially to women age 40 to 49 at increased risk for the disease; i.e., increased premenopausal weight, early age at menarche, nulliparity, late age at first term delivery, family history of breast cancer. It has been suggested that Tamoxifen (20 mg/day for 2 to 4 years) be administered to this high-risk group and that they be studied for the potentially prophylactic effect of the drug (39).

Tamoxifen is not inherently oncogenic. Administered to women with breast cancer, they have no increased incidence of other primary tumors. Neither thromboembolism nor adverse ocular effects have been observed. Patients do complain of hot flushes and, occasionally, leukorrhea. Theoretically there may be a loss of bone density in premenopausal women, although this has not been established. Tamoxifen is contraindicated in pregnancy (40).

An uncontrolled prospective study of Tamoxifen administration (20 mg/day for 10 to 20 days per menstrual cycle for 2 to 6 cycles) reported a favorable effect on cystic breast disease and fibroadenomata. A favorable response was observed in 93% of the women with palpatory and mammographic evidence of fibroadenomata when their lesions were documented to significantly decrease in size. In 88% of women with a clinical diagnosis of fibrocystic breast disease the lesions regressed after Tamoxifen was administered. In 71% of patients breast pain disappeared, and the symptom was ameliorated in 27% of them. In general, improvement was noted within two treatment cycles (41). Corroboration of the favorable effect of Tamoxifen on cyclic and noncyclic breast pain was reported in a double-blind-controlled study of Tamoxifen (20 mg/day), given for 3 months. A significant decrease in breast pain was noted in the Tamoxifen-treated patients as compared with the placebo-treated controls (42).

ESTROGEN-PROGESTIN

Oral contraceptive agents usually contain an alkylated estrogenic steroid in combination with a 19-nortestosterone compound (Progestin). Women who use these drugs were found to have a decreased rate of hospitalization for benign breast disease, and the decrement varied directly with longevity of drug ingestion (43). Although it was attractive to infer from these data that combined oral contraceptive agents be used for the treatment of benign breast disease, a series of subsequent retrospective case-controlled studies of women with breast cancer and a history of fibrocystic breast disease suggested that their utilization of birth control pills conferred on them a relative risk for breast cancer from 2.5 to 9.2 (44–47).

Recent epidemiologic analysis of voluminous current information concerning this topic of major concern to women's health suggests that the reported increased relative risk is erroneous. As mentioned previously, only a few specific histologic types of fibrocystic breast disease appear to place a woman at increased risk for breast cancer. Oral contraceptives decrease the risk of fibrocystic disease with little or no atypia and do not decrease the risk of fibrocystic disease with marked atypia. The previously reported increased risk of breast cancer in women on oral contraceptives or in recent users with biopsy-proven fibrocystic disease is factitious. The apparent increased risk of breast cancer in these women represents the selective effect of oral contraceptives to prevent only a subset of fibrocystic breast disease that has no greater potential for malignant degeneration than normal breast tissue (48).

Postmenopausal women are commonly treated with a sequential estrogen-progestin regimen for the amelioration of their symptoms. A large retrospective study reported a significantly decreased incidence of breast cancer in the treated group, as compared with the results of a group to whom the steroid hormones had not been administered (49). It had been previously reported that a history of anovulation and progesterone deficiency conferred an increased risk on premenopausal and postmenopausal women for breast cancer (50, 51). It is suggested that a progestin be sequentially added to all estrogen replacement regimens in premenopausal and postmenopausal women.

REFERENCES

1. Haagensen CD, Bodian C, Haagensen DE. Breast carcinoma: risk and detection. Philadelphia: Saunders, 1981.
2. Mansel RE. Benign breast disease and cancer risk: new perspectives. Ann NY Acad Sci 1986;464:364–366.
3. Golinger RC. Hormones and the pathophysiology of fibrocystic mastopathy. Surg Gynecol Obstet 1978;146:273–285.
4. Berkowitz GS, Kase NG, Berkowitz RL, eds. Risk factors. In: Contemporary issues in obstetrics and gynecology, 1st ed. New York: Churchhill Livingstone, 1986:13–43.
5. Minton JP, Foecking MK, Webster DJT, Matthews RH. Response of fibrocystic disease to caffeine withdrawal and correlation of cyclic nucleotides with breast disease. Am J Obstet Gynecol 1979;135:157–158.
6. Minton JP, Foecking MK, Webster DJT, Matthews RH. Caffeine, cyclic nucleotides, and breast disease. Surgery 1979;86:105–108.
7. Curatolo PW, Robertson D. The health consequences of caffeine. An Intern Med 1983;98:641–653.
8. Heyden S, Muhlbaser LH. Prospective study of "fibrocystic breast disease" and caffeine consumption. Surgery 1984;96:479–483.
9. Schairer C, Brinton LA, Hoover RN. Methylxanthines and benign breast disease. Am J Epidemiol 1986;124:603–611.
10. Barber R, Goka TJ, Butcher RW. Hormone and methylxanthine action on breast cells. Life Sci 1984;34:2467–2476.
11. Takayama S, Kuwabara N. Long term study on the effect of caffeine in Wistar rats. Gann 1982;73:365–371.
12. La Veechia C, Talamini R, Decarli A, Franceschi S, Parazzini F, Tognoni G. Coffee consumption and the risk of breast cancer. Surgery 1986;100:477–481.

13. Odenheimer DJ, Zunzunegui MV, King MC, Shipler CP, Friedman GD. Risk factors for benign breast disease: a case control study of discordant twins. Am J Epidemiol 1984;120:585–591.

14. Boyle CA, Berkowitz GS, LiVolsi VA, et al. Caffeine consumption and fibrocystic disease. a case-control epidemiologic study. J Natl Cancer Inst 1984;72:1015–1019.

15. Abrams AA. Use of vitamin E in chronic cystic mastitis. N Engl J Med 1965;272:1080–1081.

16. London RS, Solomon DM, London ED, Strummer D, Bankoski J, Nair PP. Mammary dysplasia: clinical response and urinary excretion of 11 deoxy 17 ketosteroids and pregnanediol following α-tocopherol therapy. Breast Dis Breast 1978;4:19–22.

17. Gonzalez ER. Vitamin E relieves most cystic breast disease: may alter lipids, hormones. JAMA 1980;244:1077–1078.

18. London RS, Sundaram GS, Manimekalai S, et al. Mammary dysplasia: endocrine parameters and tocopherol therapy. Nutr Res 1982;2:243–247.

19. London RS, Murphy L, Kitlowski KE. Hypothesis: breast cancer prevention by supplemental vitamin E. J Coll Nutr 1985;4:559–564.

20. Prasard KN, Gaudreau D, Brown J. Binding of vitamin E in mammalian tumor cells in culture (41041). Proc Soc Exp Biol Med 1981;166:167–174.

21. Reddy BS, Hanson D, Mathews L, Sharma C. Effect of micronutrients and related compounds on the mutagenicity of 3,2′-dimethyl-4-aminobiphenyl, a colon and breast carcinogen. Food Chem Toxicol 1982;21:129–132.

22. Porta EA, Keopuhiwa L, Joun NS, Nitta RT. Effects of the type of dietary fat at two levels of vitamin E in Wistar male rats during development and aging. III. Biochemical and morphometric parameters of the liver. Mech Aging Dev 1981;15:297–335.

23. Horvath PM, Ip C. Synergistic effect of vitamin E and selenium in the chemoprevention of mammary carcinogenesis in rats. Cancer Res 1983;43:5335–5341.

24. Ohshima H, Bartsch H. Quantitative estimation of endogenous nitrosation in humans by monitoring N-nitrosoproline excreted in the urine. Cancer Res 1981;41:3658–3661.

25. Farrell PM, Bieri JG. Megavitamin E supplementation in man. Am J Clin Nutr 1975;28:1381–1386.

26. Willett WC, Polk BF, Underwood BA, et al. Relation of serum vitamins A and E and carotenoids to the risk of cancer. N Engl J Med 1984;310:430–434.

27. Madanes AE, Farber M. Danazol. Ann Intern Med 1982;96:625–630.

28. Chambers GC, Asch RH, Pauerstien CJ. Danazol binding and translocation of steroid receptors. Am J Obstet Gynecol 1980;136:426–429.

29. Greenblatt RB, Dmowski WP, Mahesh VB, Scholer HFL. Clinical studies with an antigonadotropin—danazol. Fertil Steril 1971;22:102–112.

30. Aksu MF, Tzingounis VA, Greenblatt RB. Treatment of benign breast disease with danazol: a follow-up report. J Reprod Med 1978;21:181–184.

31. Nezhat C, Asch RH, Greenblatt RB. Danazol for benign breast disease. Am J Obstet Gynecol 1980;137:604–607.

32. Mansel RE, Wisbey JR, Hughes LE. Controlled trial of the antigonadotropin danazol in painful nodular benign breast disease. Lancet 1984;1:928–931.

33. Sutton GLJ, O'Malley UP. Treatment of cyclical mastalgia with low-dose short-term danazol. Br J Clin Pract 1986;40:68–70.

34. Hinton CP, Bishop HM, Holliday HW, Doyle PJ, Blamey RW. A double blind controlled trial of danazol and bromocriptine in the management of severe cyclical breast pain. Br J Clin Pract 1986;40:326–330.

35. Grajower MM, Sas N. Danazol therapy for periareolar abscess. N Engl J Med 1986;314:923.

36. Love S. More on danazol therapy for periareolar abscess. N Engl J Med 1986;315:835.

37. Mansel RE, Preece PE, Hughes LE. A double-blind trial of the prolactin inhibitor bromocriptine in painful benign breast disease. Br J Surg 1978;65:724–727.

38. Tamoxifen for benign breast disease (Editorial). Lancet 1986;1:305.

39. Gazet JC. Tamoxifen prophylaxis for women at high risk of breast cancer. Lancet 1985;2:1119.

40. Diver JMJ, Jackson IM, Fitzgerald JD. Tamoxifen and non-malignant indication. Lancet 1986;1:733.

41. Cupceancu B. Short term tamoxifen treatment in benign breast diseases. Rev Roum Med-Endocrinol 1985;23:169–177.

42. Fentiman IS, Calefi M, Brame K, Chaudary MA, Hayward JL. Double-blind-controlled trial of tamoxifen therapy for mastalgia. Lancet 1986;1:287.

43. Ory H, Cole P, MacMahom B, Hoover R. Oral contraceptives and reduced risk of benign breast diseases. N Engl J Med 1976;294:419–422.

44. Fasal E, Faffenbarger RS. Oral contraception as related to cancer and benign lesions of the breast. J Natl Cancer Inst 1975;55: 767–773.

45. Paffenbarger RS, Fasal E, Simmons ME, Kampert J. Cancer risk as related to use of oral contraceptives during fertile years. Cancer 1977;39:1887–1891.

46. Paffenbarger RS, Kampert JB, Chang HG. Characteristics that predict risk of breast cancer before and after the menopause. Am J Epidemiol 1980;112:258–268.

47. Lees AW, Burns PE, Grace M. Oral contraceptives and breast disease in premenopausal Northern Albertan women. Int J Cancer 1978;22:700–707.

48. Stadel BV, Schlesselman JJ. Oral contraceptive use and the risk of breast cancer in women with a "prior" history of benign breast disease. Am J Epidemiol 1986;123:373–382.

49. Gambrell RD. Role of progestogens in the prevention of breast cancer. Maturitas 1986;8:169–176.

50. Cowan LD, Gordis L, Tonascia JA, Jones GS. Breast cancer incidence in women with a history of progesterone deficiency. Am J Epidemiol 1981;114:209–217.

51. Gonzalez ER. Chronic anovulation may increase postmenopausal breast cancer risk. JAMA 1983;249:445–446.

16

Ambulatory Surgery for Diagnosis and Treatment

George W. Mitchell, Jr.

Discrete lumps and dominant projections from areas of fibrocystic change and mammographic abnormalities considered suggestive of cancer must be further evaluated by a surgical procedure. Radiographic findings of clustered calcifications, areas of increased density, distorted breast architecture, and stellate shaped shadows, often not palpable, are becoming increasingly common as mammographic techniques improve and as minimal breast lesions, presumably having a better prognosis, are more carefully sought. In most instances, fine-needle aspiration is the procedure of choice, with the use of manual proprioception when the lesion is easily palpable and ultrasonic or x-ray guidance when it is not. Palpable lesions, 1 cm or smaller, near the skin surface are usually better excised. Well-circumscribed lesions—thought to be cystic on the basis of the patient's history, the physical examination, or ultrasonic evaluation—should be aspirated. Prior to any first breast surgery, mammography is indicated, but a palpable lesion must be investigated even if the mammogram is negative.

ASPIRATION OF CYST

For aspiration procedures the patient is placed on the table stripped to the waist, with the ipsilateral shoulder elevated either by a pillow or by rotation of the operating table and the arm extended at right angles to the trunk. This stretches the pectoral muscles and flattens the breast. The area of the proposed puncture site is carefully cleansed. Local anesthesia is usually unnecessary, and the injection of a large amount of fluid can obscure the lesion and make accurate penetration by the needle more difficult. The lump is stabilized between the thumb and the first two fingers of the left

hand, and a No. 20 or No. 22 needle attached to a 20-ml syringe is passed tangentially into the lesion, while suction is maintained (Fig. 16.1). A direct downward thrust of the needle may penetrate the pleural cavity and cause pneumothorax. If the lesion is cystic, a clear or slightly turbid brownish fluid flows into the syringe, and its withdrawal causes the cyst to collapse. Although the fluid is often acellular and nondiagnostic, it should be sent to the laboratory for cytologic interpretation; the occasional intracystic malignant growth may be revealed (1). Cysts smaller than 1 cm in diameter are dif-

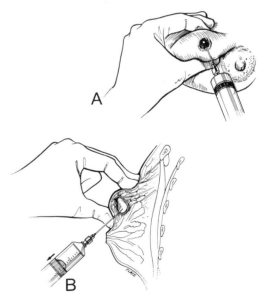

Figure 16.1. Needle aspiration of cyst. **A**, One hand stabilizes the cyst as the needle is passed into it. The path of the needle is tangential to the chest wall. **B**, Suction is maintained throughout, and the cyst is emptied as soon as the needle enters it.

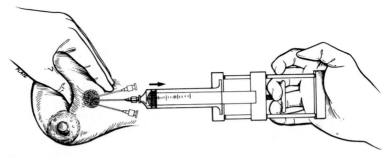

Figure 16.2. Fine-needle aspiration of solid mass. The needle is passed into the mass and withdrawn at different angles and in different places at least five times as suction on the syringe is maintained by a syringe holder.

ficult to aspirate; when no fluid is obtained after several attempts, the contents of the needle should be blown on a slide, fixed, and sent to the laboratory. If no diagnostic material is found, open biopsy is indicated, especially if this is the first such lesion. When the diagnosis of fibrocystic change has been made by previous biopsy and the histology has shown no risk factors, the decision to perform another biopsy depends on experience and judgment. Data have been compiled to suggest an association between frequent biopsies and the subsequent development of carcinoma but have not been statistically refined to show a cause-and-effect relationship.

FINE-NEEDLE ASPIRATION OF SOLID LESIONS

When a palpable mass is thought to be solid because of its contour, ultrasonic evaluation, or previous failure to aspirate fluid, fine-needle aspiration is indicated. Although introduced in the 1930s (2, 3), this method has gained acceptance only since the accuracy of cytologic interpretation of the aspirated material improved. This technique is preferred over open biopsy also because of the ease of obtaining the specimen, the low morbidity, and the low cost (3a). Before proceeding, the surgeon must supply the patient with all pertinent information concerning the reasons, risks, and possible results.

With the patient positioned as noted above, a 1½- to 3-inch No. 22 needle, attached to a syringe, with a syringe holder to facilitate forceful constant suction, is inserted at an angle tangential to the chest wall (Fig. 16.2). It is often possible to tell when the lesion is entered because of the difference in its consistency from that of the surrounding tissue. The needle is passed forward and back through the lesion in different planes four or five times in as short a period of time as possible; longer intervals tend to contaminate the specimen with blood cells

and clots, making interpretation more difficult. When suctioned material enters the hub of the needle, the vacuum should be released and the needle withdrawn. The syringe is then taken from the needle and 5 to 10 ml of air are aspirated. The syringe is then reattached to the needle and gently pushed until drops of the aspirated material from the needle are placed on at least two slides in as uniform a manner as possible. The material is then spread evenly over each slide with another slide or cover slip, by drawing them quickly apart in the manner used to prepare a blood smear (4). It is most helpful to have an expert cytologist on hand to prepare the material in the manner most suitable for his or her laboratory. Some experts prefer the use of frosted or albumin-coated slides to hold the cellular material, but the present trend is to use clear slides with a small sand-blasted end (4). Since Papanicolaou stains are most commonly used, the material on the slide should be fixed with 95% alcohol, either by spray or by immersion; the same fixative is appropriate if hematoxylin and eosin are to be applied. Occasionally, a modification of the Giemsa stain (Romanovsky) is used, and, if this is the case, air drying of the material is necessary (4, 5). If insufficient material is obtained in the first attempt, the procedure should be repeated, passing the needle through a different track to avoid the previously traumatized area. The technique is acceptable to most patients, easily performed in the office, and has a minimal complication rate (6). Considerable experience is necessary, however, before the operator can obtain specimens that are consistently reliable.

The sensitivity for the diagnosis of breast cancer with this technique was 89% in a large series, while specificity for the absence of breast cancer was 97% (7). In another series, the predictive value was 100% for positive findings and 97% for negative findings, with a specificity of 93% (7), a great increase in accuracy from earlier statistics (2, 8). False-negative values are most often ascribable to poor technique or insufficient material rather than to difficulty in interpretation.

Although the samples obtained by aspiration biopsy are considered to be cytologic, tissue patterns are thought to be as important as nuclear and cytoplasmic criteria (4). Aspiration specimens taken from mammographically abnormal areas, palpable thickenings, or even from presumably normal breast tissue can therefore be read with a high-degree of accuracy, and blind fine-needle aspirations of the upper-outer quadrants have been recommended for screening and follow-up (7). Negative needle aspirations have been used as a basis for following patients without biopsy (7, 9); the only disadvantage is that the lump may still be there. In some institutions, positive needle aspiration smears are used for final diagnosis prior to definitive treatment for breast cancer (D. J. Marchant, personal communication). It must be emphasized, however, that this is possible only in institutions where cytologic technology is highly developed. Even though percutaneous fine-needle aspiration approaches open biopsy in accuracy in terms of false positives, the incidence of false negatives remains somewhat higher. For this reason, when the diagnosis of malignancy is suspected on the basis of physical examination or adjunctive diagnostic aids, biopsy must follow a negative fine-needle aspiration.

In addition to the cytologic diagnosis of malignancy, fine-needle aspirates from the human breast are useful for the analysis of estrogen receptors. The results of estrogen receptor analysis in fine-needle aspirates by means of immunocytochemistry were concordant with receptor analyses in histologic specimens in 88% of the samples (10). In this series there were no false-positive estrogen receptor determinations in tumor aspirates. In another series the sensitivity, specificity, and predictive value of a positive test, and the efficiency of estrogen receptor analysis in cytologic material as compared with histologic material was 96%, 83%, 96%, and 93%, respectively (11). A method of using flow cytometry to evaluate the nuclei of tumor cells obtained by fine-needle aspiration for ploidy determination has also been developed. Ninety-two percent of the aspirates produced enough material for this assessment. It was concluded that DNA histograms derived from flow cytometry of fine-needle aspirate samples could be a valuable tool in the management of breast cancer (12).

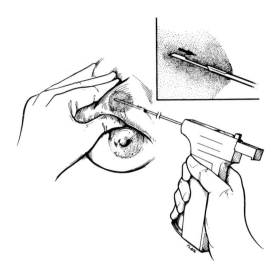

Figure 16.3. Needle biopsy. Under local anesthesia, the trocar is passed into the mass to its far side, and the trigger mechanism of the gun pulls the reverse cutting edge back into the cannula (*inset*).

CUTTING NEEDLE BIOPSY

Percutaneous cutting needle biopsy is an alternative to fine-needle aspiration but is seldom necessary in institutions where cytologic evaluation is advanced (13). It is less invasive than open biopsy and valuable when a tissue section is required for final diagnosis. A variety of instruments is available for this purpose, all based on the principle of a trocar with a reverse cutting edge sliding in a canula of small caliber. The instrument requires only the dominant hand for manipulation of the cutting edge. Because of the size of the trocar and sheath to be introduced, local anesthesia is recommended. A small intradermal weal is made over the lesion and small amounts of 1% lidocaine are injected around it. Meticulous sterile technique is used throughout. A small incision in the skin with a No. 15 scalpel allows introduction of the trocar, which is passed through the lesion to its far side. The trocar is advanced slightly and then retracted into the sheath by its trigger mechanism, bringing with it a small core of tissue (Fig. 16.3). Such a specimen improves diagnostic accuracy in many routine pathologic laboratories, but a negative report does not exclude the possibility of malignancy. If the lesion is clinically suspicious for malignancy, open biopsy is indicated.

OPEN BIOPSY

For nearly 100 years the diagnosis and treatment of breast cancer was performed in a two-stage single operation, consisting of open biopsy and radical mastectomy, when the lesion was proved by frozen section to be malignant (14). Although some surgeons still adhere to this formula, it has been largely discredited both in the medical and in the lay press as a result of new data indicating that more conservative approaches are applicable to the problem of breast malignancy (15). In the 1970s, it became apparent that a reasonable interval between diagnosis by biopsy and definitive treatment by mastectomy did not unfavorably alter the prognosis when the lesion was malignant (16, 17). It was also recognized that the systemic spread of malignant breast disease rather than local recurrence of the primary tumor was the principal risk to the patient, and more conservative types of surgery came into vogue.

The advantages to the patient of deferring definitive operation after biopsy are cogent:

1. The biopsy can be done with local anesthesia, and the patient is fully aware of what is happening.
2. The patient escapes the risks of general anesthesia and does not have to wake up wondering whether she still has her breast.
3. The pathologic diagnosis does not depend on frozen but on permanent sections, which are presumably more accurate.
4. The patient can discuss the situation at leisure with family and friends and possibly obtain a second opinion.
5. Full discussion of the problem between the biopsy and definitive treatment might obviate future claims of malpractice.
6. There is more efficient use of facilities and diagnostic studies. In some states full explanation of all of the modalities of treatment for breast cancer is required by law.

Certain disadvantages have also been recognized but are thought to be less significant. These include an improperly placed skin incision that might interfere with the incision of subsequent mastectomy, a hematoma, seroma or infection that might delay or increase the morbidity of subsequent surgery, and the possibility of having the biopsy and the definitive operation performed by two different surgeons in two different areas, increasing the chance of communication failure and inappropriate surgery (18).

More conservative primary operations for breast cancer had been proposed by McWhirter (19) and Crile (20, 21), either in the form of simple mastectomy or lumpectomy followed by irradiation, but their observations were largely discounted by the traditionalists. In 1985, Fisher and associates (15) published the five-

year results from the National Surgical Adjuvant Breast and Bowel Project, showing that, in cases carefully selected for primary tumor size, segmental mastectomy with or without irradiation was equal or superior to total mastectomy. T_1 lesions (less than 5 cm) were arbitrarily selected for this modified operation. The implication of this and subsequent reports has drastically affected the attitudes of the medical profession and the public, encouraging the more frequent use of breast-conserving surgery and even extending its application to lesions larger than those recommended. The elderly, the medically debilitated, and those with known distant metastases were also relegated to the category to be treated by conservative operations.

The recognized benefits of adjunctive chemotherapy for patients with nodal (N+) disease (see Chapter 21) require the resection of axillary lymph nodes for surgical staging. When radical or modified radical mastectomies were done, removal of the axillary contents was a standard part of the procedure. With the advent of segmental mastectomy and tylectomy, it became necessary to perform a separate axillary dissection when biopsy showed the lesion to be malignant. If the original biopsy is performed by a surgeon unskilled in the axillary approach, the patient must be referred to a surgeon adequately trained in this procedure, leading to possible delay and breakdown in communication. When the lesion is likely to be malignant, the patient's best interests are served by employing a surgeon prepared to proceed to the second operation, should the preliminary diagnosis be corroborated. Under these circumstances, general anesthesia, either as a primary method or at the onset of the second-stage procedure, is indicated. If the trend toward expanding the application of adjunctive chemotherapy to all patients with breast cancer continues, including those whose nodes are negative, axillary lymph node sampling will determine staging and provide a clue to prognosis but will not affect treatment.

It is evident that staging depends on three factors: careful measurement of the primary lesion, the results of preliminary x-rays, scans and blood chemistries to determine the presence of distant metastases, and the presence or absence of positive lymph nodes in the axilla. The TNM (tumor size, nodes, metastases) taxonomy has officially replaced the old staging system. How they correlate is shown in Table 16.1.

Routine use of physical examination, mammography, and fine-needle aspiration should serve to establish the diagnosis of cancer or no cancer in the majority of cases. Final judgment

Table 16.1.   Staging of Breast Cancer[a]

Primary Tumor	Involved Lymph Nodes	Distant Metastases	Stage
T is (in situ)	N0	M0	0
T_1 (<2 cm)	N0	M0	I
T_0 (no primary found)	N1	M0	
T_1	N1	M0	IIA
T_2 (<5 cm)	N0	M0	
T_2	N1 (movable)	M0	IIB
T_3 (>5 cm)	N0	M0	
T_0	N2 (fixed)	M0	
T_1	N2	M0	
T_2	N2	M0	IIIA
T_3	N1 or 2	M0	
T_4 (any size fixed to chest wall and/or skin, or inflammatory carcinoma)	Any N	M0	
Any T	N3 (internal mammary)	M0	IIIB
Any T	Any N	M1	IV

NOTE: 1. Metastases include ipsilateral supraclavicular lymph nodes.
2. If more than one ipsilateral primary, T is measured for the largest.
3. If bilateral primaries, each is staged separately.
4. Paget's disease of the nipple without underlying tumor is staged T.
5. Skin or nipple retraction without direct involvement may be T_1, T_2 or T_3.
6. Chest wall includes more than the pectoral muscle alone.

[a]From Manual for staging of cancer. 3rd ed. American Joint Committee on Cancer. Philadelphia: Lippincott, 1988.

depends on experience and consultation with the radiologist and pathologist. When the tumor is thought to be benign, as in the case of a fibroadenoma or primary cyst, the excision can be done in a suite designed for ambulatory surgery. The patient should have had nothing by mouth since midnight the night before and should be accompanied by an interested second party for support prior to the operation and to accompany her home. Analgesia is helpful if the patient is nervous; drugs such as meperidine and diazepam may be given intravenously a few minutes before operation.

The patient is placed supine on the operating table with the arm ipsilateral to the breast lesion at right angles to the body, stretching the pectoral muscles and making the lesion more accessible. That side can be further elevated by rotating the operating table. Circumareolar incisions are used when the lesion is beneath the areola or within 3 to 4 cm of its outer margin, but are not carried more than one-half of the way around the circumference of the areola to avoid compromising its blood supply (Fig. 16.4A). For lesions more peripheral, curvilinear incisions 3-4 cm long are made parallel to the areolar margin and immediately above the lesion (Fig. 16.4A) (6, 22). An attempt should be made to avoid placing the incision in an area that might compromise a subsequent mastectomy incision, which is usually transverse. If the decision has been made to perform total resection in the event that malignancy is discovered, the incision should be placed to achieve the best exposure and cosmetic effect. Radial incisions, especially in the upper half of the breast, are likely to be unsightly.

Using 1% lidocaine, an intradermal weal is made 1 cm below the lower pole of the proposed incision and carried upward to a point 1 cm beyond the upper pole (Fig. 16.4A). Through this weal, a 1½-inch No. 22 needle is passed downward on both sides of the lesion, depositing small amounts of anesthetic sufficient to encompass the area of probable dissection. When an intraductal papilloma is suspected, the major ductal system beneath the nipple is infiltrated. With incisions further toward the periphery, it is helpful to delineate the incision with a marking pen before injecting the anesthetic. Heavy infiltration tends to conceal the lesion and distort the anatomy, making dissection difficult; more local anesthetic can be added later, if necessary.

A No. 15 scalpel is used to incise the skin and subcutaneous fat down to the lobular tissue (Fig. 16.4B). Fine hooks retract the margins of the incision while the area of the lesion is explored with the forefinger. The consistency, symmetry, and mobility of the lesion and the condition of the surrounding tissue can further confirm or deny the original diagnosis. Since breast tissue is very dense, sharp dissection is necessary (Fig. 16.4C). Hemostasis is best achieved by cautery, except in

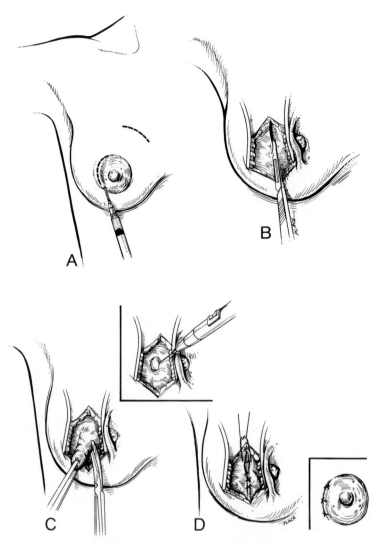

Figure 16.4. Open biopsy. **A**, Anesthetic weal for circumareolar incision (*dotted line*). Alternative peripheral incision for mass in upper inner quadrant. **B**, Self-retaining retractor in place as incision is made in breast tissue. **C**, Mass being enucleated with envelope of surrounding tissue. Bleeding controlled with needle cautery (*inset*). **D**, Lobular defect closed with interrupted absorbable sutures. (This step is omitted by some surgeons.) Skin closed with fine interrupted nonabsorbable sutures (*inset*).

the case of larger vessels (Fig. 16.4C *inset*). Fine absorbable suture material is used in the deeper structures. Repetitive finger exploration is indicated to direct the dissection to the lesion and around it. When within a few millimeters of the lesion, the tissue surrounding it is grasped with forceps and traction maintained, while the tumor is enucleated with a surrounding margin of normal tissue. This implies excising all or a portion of the lobule from which the tumor arises as well as the connective tissue.

The excised specimen is sent to the pathology laboratory, which should be adjacent to the operating room or connected to it by telephone so that the pathologist and surgeon can confer. The false-positive rate is so small as to be negligible, but the surgeon should see the microscopic sections with the pathologist before proceeding to further surgery and should seek a second opinion when the diagnosis is equivocal. The false-negative rate approximates 1% (5). When a frozen-section report of benign disease is returned, the incision is closed. There are pronounced differences of opinion regarding the best method of closure; some believe that the skin should be closed without drainage once hemostasis has been

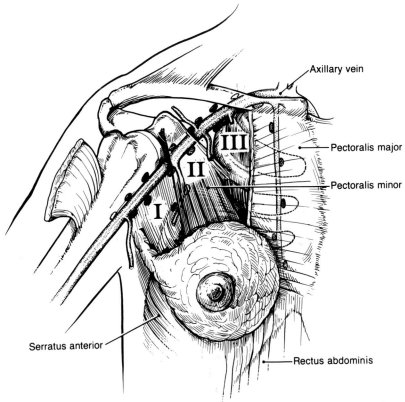

Figure 16.5. Lymphatics of axilla. The insertion of the pectoralis major has been severed and the muscle retracted, exposing the intact pectoralis minor, which can be retracted or cut to expose the underlying lymph nodes. All lymph node containing tissue beneath the axillary vein at levels I and II is removed.

achieved, others prefer to drain the so-called dead space, and still others prefer to close the lobular tissue and obliterate the dead space before closing the skin. The author's preference is for the latter technique, but it is important to avoid causing skin retraction when apposing the deeper tissues (Fig. 16.4D). Fine absorbable suture material is used for these ligatures, and the skin is closed either with a subcuticular stitch or with fine interrupted nylon (Fig. 16.4D *inset*). A pressure dressing for the first 24 hours is helpful in preventing accumulation of fluid in the deeper tissues. The sutures should be removed in 4 to 5 days and steri-strips applied to prevent permanent suture scars around the incision.

There are few complications of excision biopsy if proper technique is followed. Ecchymoses in the skin are fairly common, but acute hemorrhage and hematoma formation are very rare (23). Seromas can be treated with aspiration and pressure, and the occasional infection with drainage. Skin separation can be reapproximated with steri-strips.

When the workup strongly suggests that the disease is malignant and needle aspiration is inconclusive, the possibility that the open biopsy may also be the final surgical treatment must be kept clearly in mind. For this reason, a generous incision directly over the lesion should be used to facilitate total resection. Although the operation can be performed by a single surgeon, an assistant is very helpful in providing retraction, keeping the field clear, and assisting with hemostasis. In the absence of an assistant, self-retaining rake retractors are available (Fig. 16.4C, D). Traction is maintained on the tissue to be resected while the surgeon enucleates it with curved scissors (Fig. 16.4C). Frequent pauses and manual exploration assure the scope of the dissection and avoid cutting into the lesion. The clamps holding the lesion are shifted around its periphery as the dissection progresses to provide better exposure of the underside. It is not possible to quantitate exactly the amount of surrounding tissue that should be removed during the resection, but a margin of at least 5 mm of surrounding tissue is desirable. The pathologist

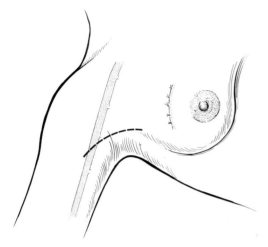

Figure 16.6. Axillary dissection A. Breast incision has been closed following total excision of lesion. Proposed axillary incision for staging has been outlined.

maintained on the insertion of the pectoralis major and to the pectoralis minor, the lymph nodes of levels I and II are resected (Fig. 16.6.) Some surgeons prefer to cut the insertion of the pectoralis minor to achieve better exposure and wider dissection. Since the nodes at level III are positive in only 2% of the cases, when the nodes at I and II are negative (24) and are difficult to reach, attempting a more complete removal is unproductive on balance. In the vital area, however, the so-called sampling or "berry picking" of lymph nodes is unacceptable. The final count from pathology should reveal the presence of not less than 12 to 15 nodes. The wound can be closed without drainage once hemostasis has been achieved, but the use of a small suction drain is often safer. If the operation has been performed early in the day and has not been protracted, the patient may be discharged the same evening with an underarm dry dressing; otherwise, an overnight stay is indicated.

can usually tell grossly whether the cancer has penetrated the surrounding envelope, but, if not, the histology provides the final answer. Further removal of breast tissue is required when the margins are not clear. When only the permanent sections show evidence of incomplete removal, a second operation is required and more breast tissue is removed. If the malignant tumor is larger than expected preoperatively and beyond a reasonable limit for local removal, a V-shaped wedge of tissue from the edge of the lesion may be taken for diagnosis or a needle may be used to obtain a representative specimen. Mastectomy will be needed and, unless permission has been obtained, must be postponed to a later date.

If the disease is thought to be malignant, it is desirable but not essential to perform axillary dissection at the time of biopsy, provided that permission to do so has been obtained. This is done under general anesthesia, which is preferably administered before biopsy but can be started for the second stage (18).

AXILLARY LYMPH NODE DISSECTION

A separate diagonal incision is made across the base of the axilla, ascending from the lateral edge of the pectoralis major to the medial edge of the latissimus dorsi (Fig. 16.5). The costocoracoid fascia overlying the axillary vein is opened, exposing the underlying fat pad containing the lymphatics to be removed. The undersurface of the vein is cleaned of nodes, fat, and connective tissue, ligating such venous tributaries as may be necessary in the process (Fig. 16.5). While strong medial retraction is

RESECTION OF INTRADUCTAL LESIONS

When a nipple discharge contains red blood cells, suggesting the presence of an intraductal papilloma or ductal malignancy, exploration of the ductal system is indicated, regardless of negative findings on physical examination, mammography, or fine-needle aspiration. A circumareolar incision is made in the breast quadrant most likely to be the source of the bleeding. Occasionally this can be predicted by noting the amount of discharge produced by manual pressure over different areas. Dissection is carried medially to the main ducts as they enter the subareolar reservoir. These are placed on traction with a small hook and the duct system is followed downward and outward until the lesion is encountered, usually not more than 3 or 4 cm from the surface. Papillomas are dark and often multiple; because they are soft they are difficult to palpate. A large portion of the duct system around the diseased area is resected with the lesion and the severed ends ligated (Fig. 16.7). Frequently, only a small amount of tissue need be resected, and the residual defect makes closure of the deeper structures unnecessary. If deep closure is attempted, a later problem can be nipple retraction. When an intraductal or paraductal lesion is malignant, the same principles apply as elsewhere in the breast.

NEEDLE LOCALIZATION AND BIOPSY OF NONPALPABLE LESIONS

Nonpalpable lesions noted by mammography and considered suggestive of cancer

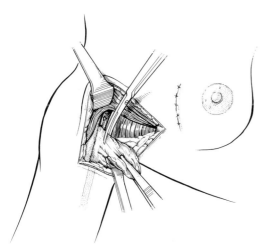

Figure 16.7. Axillary dissection B. Pectoral muscles are retracted as axillary lymphatics, fat and connective tissue are dissected from undersurface of axillary vein.

have been found to be malignant in at least 20% of the cases (25). Such lesions obviously require further investigation, regardless of the results of physical examination, and an attempt may be made to determine their pathogenicity by ultrasound- or x-ray-directed, fine-needle aspiration. Should this prove negative, the area in question must be excised; localizing instruments are available for this purpose (26). The

procedure must be done in cooperation with the mammographer, who inserts a hollow needle under continuous visualization until the tip is in proximity to the lesion (Fig. 16.8**A**). A fine wire with a flexible J hook on the end is passed through and out of the needle until the hook reverses and engages near the lesion. The needle is then withdrawn leaving the wire hook in situ, stabilized at the skin level with tape (Fig. 16.9). The patient is then removed to the operating room for excision of the lesion, which can be done either with local or general anesthesia; the former is satisfactory in most instances (25). A curvilinear incision is made near the entrance of the wire into the skin and carried down through subcutaneous and lobular tissue to the hooked end. A volume of tissue at least 3 cm in diameter around the hook is removed and sent to the radiologist (Fig. 16.8**B**), who radiographs it again to determine whether the suspected abnormality originally noted is present in the specimen. If not, more tissue must be removed until the original mammographic abnormality is recognized. When the lesion is found, it is forwarded to the pathologist for appropriate histologic and receptor studies. The defect is treated as noted previously.

SUMMARY

Breast biopsies are based on specific criteria, including risk factors, the patient's history, the

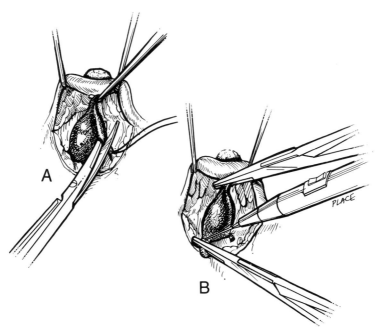

Figure 16.8. Excision of intraductal lesion. **A**, Traction on main duct and central dissection to expose ductal system. **B**, Identification and removal of ductal mass.

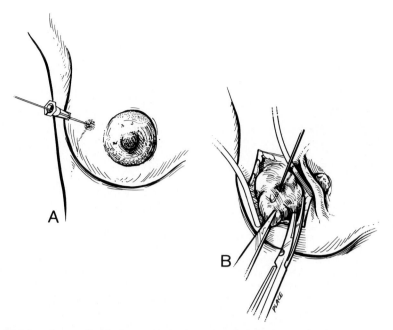

Figure 16.9. Excision of nonpalpable lesion. **A**, Needle containing wire marker has been inserted under x-ray guidance. **B**, The tissue surrounding the wire hook is excised en bloc.

physical examination, and adjunctive diagnostic aids. The surgeon's experience and judgment are of great importance when the indications are equivocal. In the younger age groups many biopsies are done for variants of fibrocystic change in the breasts, but repetitive resection of cysts and fibroadenomas may be unnecessary unless performed for cosmetic reasons or the presence of atypical hyperplasia (see Chapter 6) in previous specimens. The primary function of breast biopsy is the identification of breast cancer, but a secondary function may, in some instances, be therapeutic. For this reason, biopsies should be excisional unless additional surgery is planned. When the evidence suggests the presence of cancer, that diagnosis should be found to be correct in at least 20% of the biopsies. If the ratio is less than that, the indications for the operation may be too liberal, and vice versa.

The possibility of harboring breast cancer is an abiding fear among all women, and the recommendation to undergo biopsy causes acute anxiety, regardless of the good face some may put upon it. Such patients need, and should be given, all possible support until the ordeal is over. Compassionate care may alleviate the natural hostility that arises when malignancy is found and assist in the decision-making process that must ensue.

REFERENCES

1. McSwain GR, Valiecenti JF Jr, O'Brien PH. Cytologic evaluation of breast cysts. Obstet Gynecol 1978;51:921–925.
2. Martin HE, Ellis EB. Biopsy by needle punction and aspiration. Ann Surg 1930;92:169–181.
3. Stewart FW. The diagnosis of tumors by aspiration biopsy. Am J Pathol 1933;9:801–812.
3a. Hindle WH, Navin J. Breast aspiration cytology: a neglected gynecologic procedure. Am J Obstet Gynecol 1983;146:482–487.
4. Rosenthal DL. Breast lesions diagnosed by fine needle aspiration. Pathol Res Pract 1986;181:645–656.
5. Goodson WH, Mailman R, Miller TH. Three year follow-up of benign fine-needle aspiration biopsies of the breast. Am J Surg 1987;154:58–61.
6. Hunt TK, Crass RA. Breast biopsies on outpatients. Surg Gynecol Obstet 1975;141:591–594.
7. Frable WJ. Needle aspiration of the breast. Cancer 1984;53:671–676.
8. Kern WH. The diagnosis of breast cancer by fine-needle aspiration smears. JAMA 1979;241:1125–1127.
9. Griffith CN, Kern WH, Mikkelson WP. Needle aspiration cytologic examination in the management of suspicious lesions of the breast. Surg Gynecol Obstet 1986;162:142–144.
10. Reiner A, Spona J, Reiner G, et al. Estrogen receptor analysis on biopsies and fine-needle aspirates from human breast carcinoma. Correlation of biochemical and immunohistochemical methods using monoclonal antireceptor antibodies. Am J Pathol 1986;125:443–449.

11. Weintraub J, Weintraub D, Redard M, Vassilakos P. Evaluation of estrogen receptors by immunocytochemistry on fine-needle aspiration biopsy specimens from breast tumors. Cancer 1987;60:1163–1172.

12. Remvikos Y, Magdelenat H, Zajdela A. DNA flow cytometry applied to fine needle sampling of human breast cancer. Cancer 1988;61:1629–1634.

13. Elston CW, Cotton RE, Davies CJ. A comparative use of the "Tru-cut" needle and fine needle aspiration cytology in the pre-operative diagnosis of carcinoma of the breast. Histopathology 1978;2:239–254.

14. Halsted WS. The results of operations for the cure of cancer of the breast performed at Johns Hopkins Hospital from June 1889 to January 1894. Ann Surg 1894;20:497–555.

15. Fisher B, Bauer M, Poisson R, et al. Five-year results from the NSABP trial comparing total mastectomy to segmental mastectomy with and without radiation in the treatment of breast cancer. N Engl J Med 1985;312:665–673.

16. Baker RR. Out-patient breast biopsies. Ann Surg 1977;185(5):543–547.

17. Caffee HH, Benfield JR. Data favoring biopsy of the breast under local anesthesia. Surg Gynecol Obstet 1975;140:88–90.

18. Fisher B. Reappraisal of breast biopsy prompted by the use of lumpectomy (Commentary). Surgical strategy. JAMA 1985;253:3585–3588.

19. McWhirter R. Simple mastectomy and radiotherapy in the treatment of breast cancer. Br J Radiol 1955;28:128–139.

20. Crile G. How much surgery for breast cancer? Modern Medicine June 11, 1973;32–37.

21. Crile G, Jr. Rationale of simple mastectomy for clinical stage I cancer of the breast. Surg Gynecol Obstet 1965;120:975–982.

22. Walker GM, Foster RS, McKegney CP, McKegney FP. Breast biopsy. Arch Surg 1978;113:942–946.

23. Mitchell GW, Homer MJ. Outpatient breast biopsies on a gynecologic service. Am J Obstet Gynecol 1982;144:127–130.

24. Schwartz GF, D'Ugo DM, Rosenberg AL. Extent of axillary dissection preceding irradiation for carcinoma of the breast. Arch Surg 1986;121:1395–1398.

25. Homer MJ, Smith TJ, Marchant DJ. Outpatient needle localization and biopsy for nonpalpable breast lesions. JAMA 1984;252:2452–2454.

26. Leis HP, Jr., Cammarata A, LaRaja RD, Higgins H. Breast biopsy and guidance for occult lesions. Int Surg 1985;70(2):115–118.

Plastic Surgery of the Breast

W. David McInnis

A. BREAST AUGMENTATION

Augmentation mammoplasty is a very common procedure in our country, second in popularity only to suction-assisted lipectomy. It is a straightforward surgical procedure that corrects an easily discernible problem. Patient satisfaction is high as evidenced by the fact that even patients who have complications rarely want the implants removed.

The typical patient seeking breast augmentation is a married woman of 30 with two children, whose husband feels that she is fine the way she is. However, she liked the size of her breasts during pregnancy and now that they have lost volume wishes to regain that appearance. These patients normally have a good self-image and are bright and articulate.

In the past, there was a feeling that women seeking breast augmentation had psychiatric problems (1), but this is no longer true. Patients requesting breast augmentation realize that our society emphasizes the female breast as symbolic of an individual's total femininity (see Chapter 5). Women seeking breast augmentation recognize that the procedure will not salvage a broken marriage nor return a wayward husband. The goal of breast augmentation is to enhance self-image by increasing the size and improving the shape of the breast.

HISTORY

The first reported augmentation mammoplasty dates to 1895, when a German surgeon named Czerny (2) used a lipoma from a patient's back to replace breast tissue that had been removed for a benign tumor (2). The volume in the breast was not maintained because the transplanted fat was resorbed. In the 1890s, paraffin was injected into the breast to increase volume, but this procedure caused severe complications, including multiple, hard foreign body reactions, and cystic degeneration and sinus formation, with resulting skin necrosis (3). Liquid silicone injections into the breasts caused similar complications and like paraffin, masked the development of other breast pathology (3).

Also to be condemned is the recent wave of enthusiasm for augmentation by injection of fat harvested from the abdomen or buttocks by suction-assisted lipectomy. The fat does not remain viable, and when it disappears, often leaves large cystic cavities. It may also form microscopic calcifications that confuse the mammographer. In spite of this, fat injection remains a means of breast augmentation available in our society, although significant health risks may result from its use.

Over the years, reports have circulated of other foreign bodies injected into breasts for enlargement. The complications of all of these injections are inflammation, nodules, masses, cysts, and pain. Future examination of breasts so treated is made difficult, and these patients may require subcutaneous or total mastectomies for relief (4–6).

In the 1950s, Ivalon sponges made of polyvinyl were used for breast augmentation, but fibrous tissue growth into and around these open-cell sponges caused hardness, asymmetry, and irregularity in the breast and a high incidence of infection with sinus formation (7, 8).

The modern era of breast augmentation began in 1964 with a presentation by Cronin and Gerow (9) on their experience with a gel-filled silicone bag. All subsequent refinements in breast augmentation have been attempts to control and resolve the difficulties with capsular contracture around this prosthesis.

The silicone implants now used are made from a heat-stable, inert rubber compound, dimethylsiloxane (9). For 25 years, this medical-grade silicone has been used for breast procedures. Numerous refinements in shape and quality of the implants have increased the safety of this procedure and improved aesthetic results, but the problem with capsule contracture remains unsolved.

Implant Types

The *gel-filled implant*, originally described in 1962, is a thin-walled, gell-filled sac with a teardrop shape, held in position by a fixation patch on the posterior wall (9, 10). The purpose of the fixation patch was to permit tissue ingrowth to secure the implant on the chest wall, but its elimination resulted in a lower incidence of capsule contraction. The thin outer shell allowed microscopic leakage of gel into the surrounding tissue, known as "gel bleed." The thicker-walled implant, now popular, allows a significantly lower amount of "gel bleed" and is available in multiple sizes and shapes, depending on the correction desired. The most popular shapes are the low-profile, teardrop or contour implant, and the round implant. Each is measured in centimeters of projection and cubic centimeters of fill and is designed to provide varying amounts of anterior projection and volume.

The *saline inflatable implant* was introduced in 1965 and was very popular in the 1970s because the incidence of capsular contracture was less when compared with its gel-filled counterpart (11). However, this implant tends to "go flat" from spontaneous deflation, with resorption of the saline. The single-lumen, saline-filled, inflatable implant has now evolved into our current, temporary, tissue expander. It is used when it is necessary to enlarge the "pocket" that has been dissected beneath the breast so that it can accommodate a permanent prosthesis of appropriate size (12).

The double-lumen, *adjustable implant* evolved as an attempt to combine the desirable qualities of the gel-filled and saline implants (13). Originally it was felt that the outer saline layer would help prevent the problem of capsular contracture, but this concept has not stood the test of time. However, the adjustable implant remains very popular because size discrepancies can be easily accommodated, and the outer saline lumen permits the injection of steroids or antibiotics.

The *polyurethane-covered implant* was introduced in the early 1970s (14–17). It is a silicone-gel prosthesis covered by a fine layer of polyurethane to prevent capsular contractures (18). Recently, favorable results from its use have been reported, but the potential long-term effect of polyurethane on the host remains unknown (19).

The choice of a prosthetic device depends largely on the surgeon's preference, and most surgeons use a variety of different implants based on the patient's anatomy and preference.

Indications for Surgery

The primary indications for breast augmentation are loss of breast volume postpartum and micromastia. Patients with micromastia are deficient in both skin and underlying breast tissue. This may be partial or total, bilateral or unilateral. When unilateral agenesis is present, augmentation is not considered cosmetic surgery.

Preoperative considerations are very important before undertaking breast augmentation, including a history of other breast problems, a family history of breast cancer, and a careful breast examination. Most women's breasts are not perfectly symmetric, the left usually being the larger, and any asymmetry, no matter how minor, must be demonstrated to the patient. Differences in nipple height, diameter, and projection, or abnormal muscular or breast protrusion not noted preoperatively will definitely be criticized postoperatively.

As with other surgical procedures, patients taking aspirin or antiinflammatory compounds should be cautioned about the increased potential for bleeding and hematoma formation associated with these drugs and the long-term increased likelihood of capsular contracture.

Incisions

Preoperative discussion with the patient of the incisions available is essential. The axillary incision is cosmetically appealing because it leaves no scars on the breast, and lay people do not associate an incision in the axilla with breast augmentation. This is a "blind" procedure, since the exposure necessary for dissection of the pocket is difficult to obtain. It may cause underarm numbness as a result of cutting superficial nerves. If there are complications, such as bleeding or capsular contracture, an incision in a different location may be required to correct the problem.

The circumareolar incision is popular because it is hidden, being well disguised when placed at the inferior junction of the areola and skin. It is associated with an increased risk of nipple numbness, and it may leave a scar within the breast that may confuse a later examiner. Surgical exposure is difficult, especially when the implant is placed subpectorally.

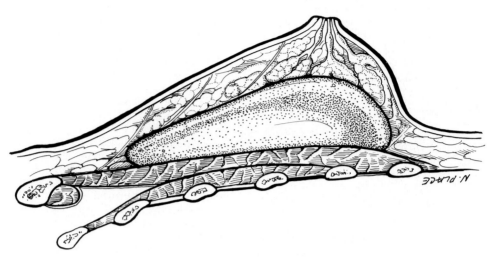

Figure 17.1.   Breast implant in the subglandular position.

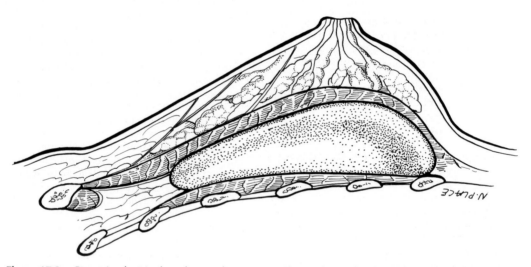

Figure 17.2.   Breast implant in the submuscular position. The implant is separated from the glandular structure of the breast by the pectoralis muscle.

The inframammary crease incision is the most popular and also the safest incision. Exposure is best, and any later complication may be approached through the same incision. However, it is likely to leave a prominent scar beneath the breast, which might be cosmetically objectionable.

Implant Position

Silicone breast prostheses for breast augmentation are placed either above or beneath the pectoralis major muscle (20–24) (Figs. 17.1 and 17.2). Placement beneath the muscle has become more generally used as a result of experience gained from post mastectomy recon-

struction. Most observers feel that the incidence of capsular contracture is less when the implant is in a subpectoral position. The patient's anatomy and the amount of augmentation required are deciding factors in the preoperative consideration of whether the implant is to be placed above or beneath the muscle. Patients with moderate ptosis are not good candidates for subpectoral augmentation unless a large implant is used because a small implant in such a patient will produce a breast mound with excess skin and the nipple draped over it (Figs. 17.3 and 17.4).

Subpectoral breast augmentation is usually painful, since the fibers of the pectoralis major muscle must be incised and elevated, but the

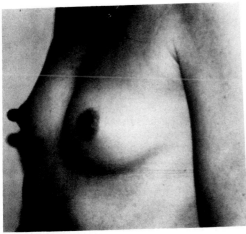

Figure 17.3. Typical patient requesting a breast augmentation. She is 30 years old and has had two children.

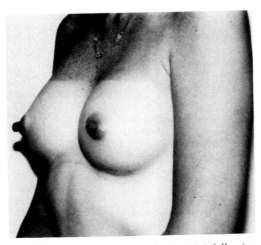

Figure 17.4. Same patient as in Fig. 17.3 following a submuscular breast augmentation.

aesthetic effect is as good as when the prosthesis is placed above the muscle. Palpation is more accurate, and mammograms are easier to interpret when a patient has had a subpectoral augmentation (Figs. 17.5 and 17.6).

When capsular contracture develops after subpectoral augmentation, it is difficult to correct permanently with capsulotomy by external pressure, and an open procedure to sever the constricting scar may be necessary.

Complications of Breast Augmentation

The most common early postoperative complication of breast augmentation is hematoma formation. Since the operation necessitates blind dissection of a submuscular or sub-

glandular "pocket" large enough for the implant, many perforating vessels are stripped and broken and must be ligated or coagulated. The use of small drains is beneficial in reducing the problem of hematoma formation. Currently the risk is less than 1% (16, 18).

Hematomas cause pain, swelling, and discoloration of the skin. They must be evacuated and irrigated, and the bleeding controlled before the implant can be replaced. Failure to evacuate even a small hematoma increases the likelihood of capsular contracture (25).

Infection occurs in less than 1% of cases but is a serious complication, since it may require removal of the implant (26). A swollen, tender, erythematous breast may develop a few days or many weeks after the procedure. Treatment involves removal of the implant, drainage, and antibiotic therapy before the implant can be replaced 6 months later. If the infection occurs on only one side, as is usually the case, most patients prefer to leave the uninfected implant in place even though for 6 months she will be asymmetric. Polyurethane implants are difficult to remove because the porous nature of the external covering permits the ingrowth of connective tissue. Infection may result in prolonged drainage, making it impossible to do a secondary implant.

Any of the three incisions may result in loss of skin or nipple sensation, which may be temporary or permanent, as a result of stretching of skin, muscles, and nerves. Such numbness is not uncommon immediately following surgery. If sensation does not return within a year, it probably will not, and approximately 15% of patients will have permanent loss of sensation (27). Extensive pocket dissection in the area of the fourth intercostal nerve is probably the principal cause for this, but wide dissection may be necessary for proper placement of the implant.

Pain after breast augmentation is similar to that of breast engorgement following pregnancy and usually subsides within 24 to 48 hours. Late pain is often a manifestation of capsular contracture. It is an intermittent burning discomfort, which radiates to the scapula because elevation of a portion of the serratus anterior is necessary to form a suitable pocket. Patients who develop this type of late pain frequently need open capsulotomy to correct the problem.

The scars formed by incisions for breast augmentation are usually acceptable. The axillary scar is hidden by the curve of the thorax, the arm, and the pectoral fold. It gradually fades as it undergoes repeated "dermabrasion" when axillary hair is shaved. The scar resulting from a circumareolar incision is well camou-

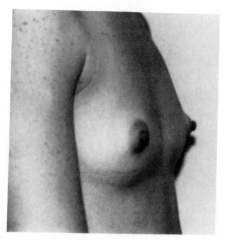

Figure 17.5. A nulliparous 20-year-old desirous of a breast augmentation.

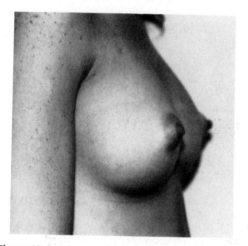

Figure 17.6. Same patient as in Fig. 17.5 following a transaxillary submuscular breast augmentation.

flaged by the areolar pigmentation. There will be a very fine white line in this area in patients who have a deeply pigmented nipple. The scar from the inframammary incision is hidden by a well-developed inframammary fold. Keloid scars can develop in any incision but are amenable to intralesional steroid injections or scar revisions.

An unfortunate occurrence in patients with breast asymmetry is continued asymmetry after augmentation. It is difficult to achieve perfect symmetry even under the best circumstances, but the double-lumen, expandable implant allows size adjustment the day after surgery. This is accomplished through a pediatric feeding tube passed into the adjustable valve percutaneously and brought out through the inframammary crease.

Malpositioning of the implant also occurs, but the risk can be lowered by careful preoperative marking of the patient's skin in the sitting position, identifying the meridian and the ideal inframammary crease. When the implant is placed in a subpectoral position, dissection and release of the pectoralis fascia must be performed below the inframammary crease. The pocket cannot be dissected too far medially because of the attachments of the pectoralis major to the sternum. Lateral dissection is limited by the anterior axillary line. However, inferior displacement of the implant can occur if the pocket is dissected downward too vigorously, or, during submuscular placement, if the insertion of the pectoralis major is not freed sufficiently to prevent downward compression. Postoperative malposition may necessitate a corrective operation.

Breakage or disruption of the implant can occur from trauma or for no known reason. It may occur from vigorous, closed capsulotomy (28). Implant replacement is required. Silicone or gel migration may initiate a granulomatous reaction in the breast.

The capsular membrane that forms around implants consists of a thin layer of fibroblasts surrounded by acellular collagen fibers. It may be soft and not palpable or hard and resistant, for reasons that are not clear. There are two main theories as to why capsules develop: One possibility is that myofibroblasts tend to contract and form scars in reaction to silicone droplets escaping from the implant (29, 30). The second possibility is that contracture is related to low-grade, subclinical infection around the implant, possibly due to *Staphylococcus epidermitis* normally present on the skin (9, 26). This can be cultured from nipple secretions in some cases. In any event, the problem with capsule contracture remains unsolved. It is now generally agreed among plastic surgeons that prevention of capsular contraction mandates the creation of a large "pocket," either above or below the muscle, and that subpectoral implants are less likely to cause the problem, theoretically because when the arm is used the muscle massages the implant. Exercises are prescribed for this purpose, and the patient is advised to move the arm, while massaging the area around the implant for 15 minutes three times a day for the first 6 months following operation. For best results, exercises must be started as soon as they can be tolerated.

Attempts have been made to reduce the incidence of capsular contracture by injecting corticosteroids into the pocket, but the results are controversial (16, 31). High-dose steroids can cause delayed wound healing, thinning of skin flaps, and erosion of subcutaneous tissue, with exposure of the implant. Low-dose steroids may be ineffective.

Oral ingestion of vitamin E has been suggested to decrease capsulization, but its benefits remain unproved (32, 33). At least it has few undesirable side effects. The use of prophylactic antibiotics has had no demonstrable effect on the development of capsulization (16, 26, 34,).

The postsurgical follow-up should be the same as for a woman who has not had breast augmentation. The guidelines presented by the American Cancer Society should be followed, and periodic breast examinations and mammograms should be done. The implant should not alter the ability to do an accurate physical examination, and the patient should be instructed that the implant will provide a smooth surface upon which she can do her own examination.

Extreme caution must be exercised in aspirating a lump or cyst after augmentation, lest puncture of the prosthesis occur. Mammograms can be safely performed, but it is important for the radiologist to view the mammograms as they are being filmed to see that all areas of the breast are evaluated.

When capsule formation does occur, the first attempt to overcome it should be a closed capsulotomy in the plastic surgeon's office, where the surgeon manually compresses the implant, thus disrupting the capsule and increasing the size of the pocket. This procedure is less successful in a patient with a submuscular prosthesis, but when it is above the muscle it is usually an effective mechanism for cure. Complications such as bleeding or rupture of the implant may occur (25, 28, 35, 36).

When external pressure is unsuccessful, open capsulotomy is necessary. This consists either of incisions through, or complete excision of, the capsule depending on the degree of deformity. The contracture tends to recur in approximately 30% of patients (36).

SUMMARY

Patient satisfaction with this procedure remains extremely high, and the complication rate, low. Manufacturing companies are attempting to improve prostheses by changing their characteristics from smooth silicone to an irregular surface to prevent the development of a capsule. The medical-grade silicone used in state-of-the-art implants is tough, inert, and resistant to degradation and trauma. The technique for their manufacture is heat curing and results in complete vulcanization of the gel (16, 29).

The material used in breast implants neither increases nor decreases a woman's risk for developing cancer. Breast cancer is as likely to develop in women who have had breast augmentations as in those who have not, but detection of breast pathology requires some modification in that the shape, consistency, and mobility of the breast must be relearned.

Not all physicians are proficient in examining such a breast. The prosthesis itself can undergo changes, with the development of small projections that can lead to erroneous diagnosis.

Mammographic diagnosis may be difficult because silicone is not opaque to x-rays. The implant compresses breast tissue, and the degree of compression varies depending on the type of implant, whether it is above or behind the muscle, and the individual's anatomy. Tangential views tailored to each patient increase accuracy.

REFERENCES

1. Shipley RH, O'Donnell JM, Bader, KF. Personality characteristics of women seeking breast augmentation. Comparison to small-busted and average-busted controls. Plast Reconstr Surg 1977;60:369.
2. Czerny V. Plastic replacement of the breast with a lipoma. Chir Kong Verhandl 1895;2:216.
3. Chaplin CH. Loss of both breasts from injection of silicone (with additive). Plast Reconstr Surg 1969;44:447.
4. Boo-Bhai K. The complications of augmentation mammaplasty by silicone injection. Br J Plast Surg 1969;22:281.
5. Kopf EH, Vinnik CA, Bongiovi JJ, Dombrowski. Plast Reconstr Surg 1976;73:77.
6. Parson RW, Thering HR. Management of the silicone-injected breast. Plast Reconstr Surg 1977;60:534.
7. Pangman WJ, II. Comments on breast plasty. South Gen Pract Med Surg 1953;115:256.
8. Pickrell K. An evaluation of Etheron as an augmentation material in plastic and reconstructive surgery. A long-term clinical and experimental study. Presented at the Annual Meeting of the American Society of Plastic and Reconstructive Surgery, Hawaii, October 1962.
9. Cronin TD, Gerow FJ. Augmentation mammaplasty: a new "natural feel" prosthesis. In: Transactions of the Third International Congress of Plastic and Reconstructive Surgery. Amsterdam, Excerpta Medica, 1964.
10. Cronin TD, Greenberg RL. Our experiences with the silastic gel breast prosthesis. Plast Reconstr Surg 1970;46:1.
11. Rees TD, Guy CL, Coburn RJ. The use of inflatable breast implants. Plast Reconstr Surg 1973;52:609.

12. McKinney P, Tresley G. Long-term comparison of patients with gel and saline mammary implants. Plast Reconstr Surg 1983;72:27.
13. Hartley JH Jr. Specific applications of the double-lumen prosthesis. Clin Plast Surg 1976;3:247.
14. Brody GS. Discussion of "the Meme implant" by S Herman and "Reconstruction of the breast using polyurethane-coated prostheses" by JE Eyssen, AJ von Werssowetz, and GD Middleton. Plast Reconstr Surg 1984;73:420.
15. Herman S. The Meme implant. Plast Reconstr Srug 1984;73:411.
16. McGrath MH, Burkhardt BR. The safety and efficacy of breast implants for augmentation mammaplasty. Plast Reconstr Surg 1984;74:550.
17. Pollock H. Polyurethane-covered breast implant. Plast Reconstr Surg 1984;74:729.
18. Slade CL, Peterson HD. Disappearance of the polyurethane cover of the Ashley Natural-Y prosthesis. Plast Reconstr Surg 1982;70:379.
19. Hester TR, Jr, Bostwick KKJ, Cukic J. A 5-year experience with polyurethane-covered mammary prostheses for treatment of capsular contracture, primary augmentation mammoplasty, and breast reconstruction. Clin Plast Surg 1988;15:569–584.
20. Biggs TM, Cukier J, Worthing LF. Augmentation mammaplasty: a review of 18 years. Plast Reconstr Surg 1982;69:445.
21. Gruber RP, Friedman GD. Periareolar subpectoral augmentation mammaplasty. Plast Reconstr Surg 1981;67:453.
22. Maxwell GP. Discussion of "Transaxillary subpectoral augmentation mammaplasty: Long-term follow-up and refinements" by JB Tebbetts. Plast Reconstr Surg 1984;74:648.
23. Pickrell KL, Puckett CL, Given KS. Subpectoral augmentation mammoplasty. Plast Reconstr Surg 1977;60:325.
24. Tebbets JB. Transaxillary subpectoral augmentation mammaplasty: Long-term follow-up and refinements. Plast Reconstr Surg 1984;74:636.
25. Williams C, Aston S, Rees TD. The effect of hematoma on the thickness of pseudosheaths around silicone implants. Plast Reconstr Surg 1975;56:194.
26. Courtiss EH, Goldwyn RM, Anastasi GW. The fate of breast implants with infections around them. Plast Reconstr Surg 1979;63:812.
27. Courtiss EH, Goldwyn RM. Breast sensation before and after plastic surgery. Plast Reconstr Surg 1976;58:1.
28. Williams JE. Invited Comment—"Review of closed capsulotomy complications" by RP Gruber and HW Jones. Ann Plast Surg 1981;6:275.
29. Barker DE, Retzky MI, Schultz S. "Bleeding" of silicone from gel bag breast implants, and its clinical relation to fibrous capsule reaction. Plast Reconstr Surg 1978;61:836.
30. Rudolph R, Guber S, Vecchione, T, et al. Myofibroblasts and free silicone around breast implants. Plast Reconstr Surg 1978;62:185.
31. Carrico TJ, Cohen IK. Capsular contracture and steroid-related complications after augmentation mammaplasty. Plast Reconstr Surg 1979;64:377.
32. Baker JL Jr. The effectiveness of alpha-tocopherol (vitamin E) in reducing the incidence of spherical contracture around breast implants. Plast Reconstr Surg 1981;68:696.
33. Peters CR, Shaw TE, Raju DR. The influence of vitamin E on capsule formation and contracture around silicone implants. Ann Plast Surg 1980;5:347.
34. Truppman ES, Ellenby JD. A 13-year evaluation of subpectoral augmentation mammoplasty. In: Owsley JA Jr, Peterson RA, eds. Symposium on aesthetic surgery of the breast. St. Louis, Mosby,1978:341–343.
35. Baker JL, Bartels RJ, Douglas WM. Closed compression technique for rupturing a contracted capsule around a breast implant. Plast Reconstr Surg 1976;58:137.
36. Little G, Baker JL Jr. Results of closed compression capsulotomy for treatment of contracted breast implant capsules. Plast Reconstr Surg 1980;65:30.

SUGGESTED READINGS

Ad-Hoc Committee on New Procedures, American Society of Plastic and Reconstructive Surgery. Report on autologous fat transplantation. 1987:1–5. Chicago, Ill.

Cronin TD. The voice of polite dissent—"Augmentation mammaplasty by the transaxillary approach" by JH Wright and AG Bevin. Plast Reconstr Surg 1976;58:621.

Fredricks S. Skeletal and postural relations in augmentation mammaplasty. Ann Plast Surg 1978;1:44.

Gerow JF. Augmentation mammaplasty: variation on a theme. In: Owsley JQ, Peterson RA, eds. Symposium on aesthetic surgery of the breast. St. Louis, Mosby, 1978, vol 18.

Hetter GP. Satisfactions and dissatisfactions of patients with augmentation mammaplasty. Plast Reconstr Surg 1979;64:151.

Jobe RP. Progress toward the definition of a proper prosthesis for reconstructive mamoplasties. In: Proceedings of the Symposium of the Educational Foundation of the American Society of Plastic and Reconstructive Surgeons, Scottsdale, Arizona, November 23–26, 1975. St. Louis, Mosby, 1978:230–240.

Mahler D, Hauben DJ. Retromammary versus retropectoral breast augmentation—a comparative study. Ann Plast Surg 1982;8:370.

McKinney P, Shedbalker AR. Augmentation mammaplasty using a noninflatable prosthesis through a circumareolar incision. Br J Plast Surg 1974;27:35.

Vistnes LM, Ksander GA, Kosek J. Study of encapsulation of silicone rubber implants in animals. A foreign-body reaction. Plast Reconstr Surg 1978;62:580.

B. BREAST REDUCTION

Breast reduction is designed to reduce the weight of the breast while improving its shape and configuration. It is the most successful operation performed by plastic surgeons, and patient satisfaction with it is extremely high. Many women can benefit from this procedure. Breast reduction allows a patient more comfortable physical activity and relieves weightbearing pain in the neck, shoulders, and back. It may improve a woman's psyche as well as her overall appearance and health. Women with breasts of excessive size should be counseled regarding the benefits of surgery.

HISTORY

Breast reductions have been performed for hundreds of years; the original procedures were amputations (1). In 1923, the German surgeon Kraske (2) was the first to report a breast reduction that removed the lower half of the breast and elevated the nipple-areola complex to a new position. In 1931, Thorek (3) reported on free nipple-areola grafts with a reduction, and Biesenberger (4), whose name is associated with the operation, reported wide lateral undermining and excision of skin. This procedure caused many serious complications related to decreased vascularity of the skin flaps and nipple (4a). In 1949, Aufrict (5) emphasized the importance of reconstructing the "skin brassiere."

The modern era of breast reduction surgery can be attributed to Robert Wise (6), who introduced the "keyhole" pattern in 1956, which emphasized the importance of preoperative marking. This permitted adequate resection of breast tissue, with an improved contour. The Wise keyhole pattern is the basic design of all breast reduction procedures today (6, 6a, 6b).

INDICATIONS

Although the indications for breast reduction are well known, many physicians may be reluctant to recommend the operation because of a lack of understanding of the discomfort suffered by women with breast hypertrophy. These patients frequently complain of neck, back, and shoulder pain and some have postural defects, such as kyphosis, in attempting to mask breast size. There may be deep ridges in both shoulders from brassiere straps.

Heavy breasts also may compress the medial cord of the brachial plexus, beneath the coracoid process and the pectoralis minor muscle, by pulling the shoulder forward, thus depressing the coracoid process and shortening the pectoralis muscle. The resulting pressure on the nerve trunk can cause paresthesias in its ulnar distribution. Reduction mammoplasty is curative (7).

Patients with heavy breasts may have pulmonary difficulties, especially those with asthma or chronic obstructive pulmonary disease. Breast reduction frequently improves their pulmonary function (8).

Also well-accepted is the fact that patients with heavy breasts have psychological problems related to body image. It is usually apparent that they have been quite sensitive about their appearance for many years. They perceive that the attention of others is focused on their large breasts and that other anatomic features are disregarded. Following breast reduction, patients are extremely grateful and happy. Their clothes fit better, and they are more comfortable with their personal appearance. Symptoms are improved, and sense of well-being enhanced (9; see Chapter 5).

Breast reduction is considered essential reconstructive surgery when performed to relieve specific symptomatology that can be shown to be related to the excessive size and weight of the breasts. The amount of breast tissue removed should not be the only criterion used to determine whether the procedure is truly reconstructive or simply cosmetic. Since only the former is usually covered by insurance, it is the surgeon's responsibility to document carefully the clinical indications for the procedure. Photographs are helpful to document size, deep ridges, or intertrigial excoriations.

TYPES OF PROCEDURES

Free Nipple Grafts

The nipple is removed and replaced as a free graft after resection of superfluous breast tissue and redundant skin. Breast reduction utilizing a free nipple graft is a safe rapid procedure that will not only reduce breast size but also provide a good cosmetic result. Utilization of the free nipple graft should be considered in elderly and poor-risk patients because of reduced anesthesia time and lower morbidity. It should also be considered in patients undergoing a resection of 2000 g or more of tissue.

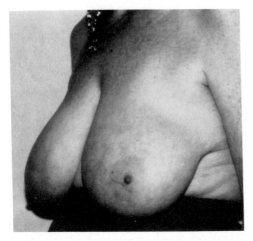

Figure 17.7. An elderly patient desirous of a breast reduction for neck pain, back pain, shoulder pain.

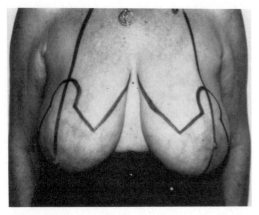

Figure 17.8. Preoperative markings on same patient as in Fig. 17.7. The breast tissue beneath the blue marks will be removed.

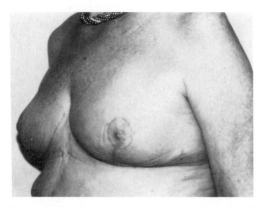

Figure 17.9. Same patient as in Figs. 17.7 and 17.8 following a breast reduction. The nipples were transferred as free nipple grafts.

Detractors of free nipple grafts comment on the loss of nipple sensation, but sensation is diminished after most other breast reductions also (10). The degree of loss is proportional to the volume of tissue removed. Many women with large breasts do not have "normal" nipple sensation to begin with, and quantitative analysis of loss of sensation is very subjective. Another criticism of this type of graft is that there may be some loss of color from the nipple, especially the deeply pigmented nipple. Since the lactiferous ducts must be separated from the nipple, none of the women who have this operation will be able to nurse (3) (Figs. 17.7–17.9).

Dermal Pedicles

All other reduction techniques involve the retention of the nipple-areola complex on the subcutaneous tissue, fat, and breast parynchema in the form of a pedicle graft. The pedicle techniques have evolved from the keyhole pattern described by Wise, and surgeons' names are attached to many modifications of the basic principle.

The *horizontal* technique was described by Strombeck (11) and utilizes preincisional marking of the keyhole pattern around the areola. It is a good operation when the nipple does not have to be elevated significantly. However, technical problems with late nipple retraction, and the fact that the nipple may be difficult to elevate have limited its usefulness.

The *superior and inferior* technique is a vertical bipedicle flap, first introduced by McKissock (12, 13). As with all breast reductions, preoperative marking of the keyhole pattern is essential. This procedure is used by many surgeons today because the results are so satisfactory and the viability of the nipple-areola circulation is high.

The superior pedicle in the flap is thinned to allow folding of the nipple-areola complex on itself. The length of this pedicle should not exceed 40 cm. It is important that the distance from the bottom of the nipple to the inframammary crease not exceed 5 to 6 cm. If the distance from the bottom of the nipple to the inframammary crease is too long, these patients will have their nipples high on the breast mound, a deformity known as the "star gazer" (14, 15).

The *superior only* technique was first described by Weiner and associates (16) in 1973. The superior pedicle is the only support for the nipple-areola complex, and this works well when nipple elevation is limited to 10 cm or less (17).

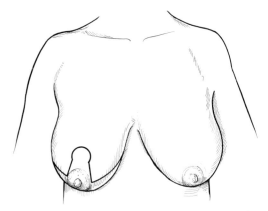

Figure 17.10. *Heavy black line* demonstrates the "keyhole" pattern used frequently for breast reductions and mastopexies.

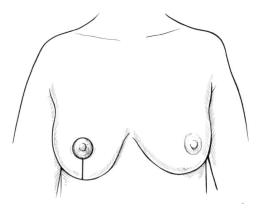

Figure 17.11. *Heavy black line* demonstrates the incision around the nipple along the breast meridian and inframammary crease. These are the locations of incisions for a breast reduction or mastopexy.

The *inferior only* technique evolved in an attempt to maintain normal nipple sensitivity (18, 19). The various modifications of the inferior dermal pedicle have incorporated the fourth and fifth intercostal nerves into the attachments of the breast to the chest wall. It is useful for removing small as well as large amounts of tissue. A critical consideration is the length-to-width ratio of the flap, which should be about 3 to 1. The viability of the inferior flap depends on the parenchymal tissue remaining attached to the pectoralis major. Careful consideration must be given to the distance from the bottom of the nipple to the inframammary crease, which should not exceed 5 to 6 cm.

The techniques listed above will yield good results with careful patient selection. Many modifications have evolved, depending on the individual surgeon's experience and preference (20–22, 30) (Figs. 17.10 and 17.11).

COMPLICATIONS

Hematoma. Since the breast parenchyma is quite vascular, meticulous hemostasis is important, and drains should be used if there is residual oozing. The incidence of hematoma formation is low, but skin ecchymoses are common.

Infections. Infections following breast reduction are rare, but breast ducts harbor bacteria, especially *Staphylococcus aureus*, and resulting infections may compromise the skin flaps or nipple-areola complex.

Hypertrophic scarring. The surgical incisions required for breast reduction may produce thick, wide, hypertrophic scars around the nipple or along the inframammary creases, but they rarely require surgical revision, since scars gradually shrink with time. Patients are usually satisfied with the result even if there is scarring.

Nipple or skin necrosis. Nipple or skin loss is a result of compromised circulation and is the most dreaded complication of breast reduction, since healing is prolonged. The initial treatment is conservative, but if there is total loss, reconstruction must be done in a manner similar to postmastectomy operations (see Part D "Reconstruction").

Fat necrosis. Fat necrosis is common following breast reduction. Nodules and thickening develop deep beneath the incisions, presenting a diagnostic problem if they occur late, since recurrent malignancy must be ruled out. Excision may be necessary.

Loss of nipple sensation. Most breast reductions result in some loss of nipple sensation, but many women have a return of sensation within 2 years. The inferior dermal pedicle was designed in an attempt to help retain nipple sensitivity. Variations in nipple sensitivity cannot be measured, since "normal" nipple sensation is difficult to evaluate. Women with large, hypertrophic breasts frequently have large areolae and minimal nipple sensation. In such patients breast reduction may improve nipple sensation. Sensory changes in the nipple and adjacent skin following breast reduction are directly related to the amount of breast tissue removed; the larger the resection, the greater the loss of sensation (10).

Asymmetry. Postoperative asymmetry is often seen in the years following breast reduction. This complication can be avoided by careful preoperative measuring and marking, with the patient in a standing position. There are usually discrepancies in breast size prior to surgery, and it is almost impossible to produce perfect symmetry in the final result. Patients must be counseled about this preoperatively.

The skin beneath the breast may stretch following breast reduction, resulting in a "bottoming out" of the breast tissue and leaving the nipple-areola complex too high on the breast mound. The nature of the correction required depends on the extent of the deformity. A skin resection below may be all that is required, but a woman who has lost weight may need correction by the placement of a prosthesis.

MAMMOGRAPHY

Changes in the breasts that occur following a reduction can be demonstrated on mammograms. Radiologists are able to differentiate scar from premalignant calcifications or dense parenchymal shadows. In patients at high risk for breast cancer, a preoperative and early postoperative mammogram, should be ordered as a baseline for future comparison. Breast reduction does not reduce the risk of developing breast cancer, and appropriate diagnostic tests should be continued postoperatively.

MASTOPEXY

The degree of breast ptosis is determined by the position of the nipple on the breast mound and is said to be severe when the nipple lies below the submammary fold. When mild, it may best be corrected by breast augmentation with a prosthesis (23).

Mastopexy has evolved along with breast reductions but differs from reduction in that only the skin is removed and the breast tissue remains almost intact. It is designed to elevate sagging breasts that are not oversized and reduce the diameter of the nipple-areola complex, if it is too large. Less than 300 g of parenchyma are usually removed, but shortening the supporting skin serves to raise the breast and realign the nipple-areola complex. The scars following mastopexy may stretch because of the downward pull and become very large. Since these patients are more interested in the cosmetic result than relief of symptoms, circumspection is required in patient selection (24, 25).

SUMMARY

Breast reduction is designed to reduce disproportionately large, sagging breasts and can also reduce the size of the areola. The degree of reduction depends on the patient's needs and the desirability of a good cosmetic result. Patient satisfaction with the procedure is high because it relieves symptoms of neck, back, and shoulder pain as well as intertrigial excoriations. The psychological improvement is often remarkable.

REFERENCES

1. Guinard M. Comment on "Rapport de l'ablation esthetique des tumeurs du sein," par M.H. Morestin. Bull Mem Soc Chir (Paris) 1903;29:568.
2. Kraske H. Die Operationen der atrophischen und hypertrophischen Hangebrust. Munchen Med Wchnschr 1923;70:672.
3. Thorek M. Histological verification of efficacy of free transplantation of nipple. Med J Rec 1931;134:474.
4. Biesenberger H. Deformitaten und kismetische Operationen der weiblichen Brust. Vienna, W Maudrich, 1931.
4a. Maliniac JW. Arterial blood supply of the breast. Arch Surg 1943;47:329.
5. Aufricht G. Mammaplasty for pendulous breasts. Empiric and geometric planning. Plast Reconstr Surg 1949;4:13.
5a. Courtiss E, Goldwyn RM. Reduction mammaplasty by the inferior pedicle technique. Plast Reconstr Surg 1977;59:500.
6. Wise RJ, Gannon JP, Hill JR. Further experience with reduction mammaplasty. Plast Reconstr Surg 1963;32:12.
6a. Penn J. Breast reduction. Br J Plast Surg 1955;7:357.
6b. Wise RJ. A preliminary report on a method of planning the mammaplasty. Plast Reconstr Surg 1956;17:367.
7. Letterman G, Schurter M. The effects of mammary hypertrophy on the skeletal system. Ann Plast Surg 1980;5:425.
8. Goldwyn RM. Pulmonary function and bilateral reduction mammaplasty. Plast Reconstr Surg 1974;53:84.
9. Goin MK, Goin JM, Gianini MH. The psychic consequences of a reduction mammaplasty. Plast Reconstr Surg 1977;59:530.
10. Courtiss EH, Goldwyn RM. Breast sensation before and after plastic surgery. Plast Reconstr Surg 1976;58:1.
11. Strombeck JO. Mammaplasty: report of a new technique based on the two pedicle procedure. Br J Plast Surg 1960;13:79.
12. McKissock PK. Reduction mammaplasty with a vertical dermal flap. Plast Reconstr Surg 1972;49:245.
13. McKissock PK. Reduction mammaplasty by the vertical bipedicle flap technique. Clin Plast Surg 1976;3:309.
14. Dinner MI, Chait LA. Preventing the high-riding nipple after McKissock breast reduction. Plast Reconstr Surg 1977;59:330.
15. Millard DR Jr, Mullin WR, Lesavoy MA. Secondary correction of the too-high areola and nipple after a mammaplasty. Plast Reconstr Surg 1976;58:568.
16. Weiner DL, et al. A single dermal pedicle for nipple transposition in subcutaneous mastectomy, reduction mammaplasty, or mastopexy. Plast Reconstr Surg 1973;51:115.

17. Hugo NE, McClellan RM. Reduction mammaplasty with a single superiorly-based pedicle. Plast Reconstr Surg 1979; 63:230.

18. Ariyan S. Reduction mammaplasty with the nipple-areola carried on a single, narrow inferior pedicle. Ann Plast Surg 1980;5:167.

19. Georgiade NG, Seratin D, Morris R, et al. Reduction mammaplasty utilizing an inferior pedicle nipple-areolar flap. Ann Plast Surg 1979;3:211.

20. Hoopes JE, Maxwell GP. Reduction mammaplasty: a technique to achieve the conical breast. Ann Plast Surg 1979;3:106.

21. Rees TD, Aston SJ. The tuberous breast. Clin Plast Surg 1976;3:339.

22. Mathes SJ, Nahai F, Hester TR. Avoiding the flat breast in reduction mammaplasty. Plast Reconstr Surg 1980;66:63.

23. Owsley JQ Jr. Simultaneous mastopexy and augmentation for correction of the small, ptotic breast. Ann Plast Surg 1979;2:195.

24. Erol OO, Spira M. A mastopexy technique for mild to moderate ptosis. Plast Reconstr Surg 1980;65:603.

25. Gruber RP, Jones HW Jr. The "donut" mastopexy: indications and complications. Past Reconstr Surg 1980;65:34.

26. Woods JE et al. Experience with and comparison of methods of reduction mammaplasty. Mayo Clin Proc 1978;53:487.

C. PROPHYLACTIC MASTECTOMY

A prophylactic mastectomy is a total subcutaneous removal of nearly all breast tissue and may be recommended to prevent breast cancer in certain individuals at risk for the disease. Much controversy surrounds the indications for the operation. Freeman (1), in 1962, first suggested subcutaneous mastectomy. Refinements have evolved with the development of better implants, the knowledge of where they should be placed, and the use of tissue expanders; but even after more than 25 years of evolution, with improvement in results, the operation can be recommended only on an individualized basis.

INDICATIONS

Breast cancer continues to be the most common malignancy in women and the second leading cause of cancer deaths in that sex. It may occur at a relatively young age, when its treatment causes greater emotional trauma. Although breast cancer cannot be totally prevented, subcutaneous mastectomy reduces the risk by removing 90% of the breast parenchyma.

The risk factors for the development of breast cancer are now better understood (see Chapter 18) These include age, with breast cancer increasing in incidence as long as a woman lives. The risk of developing breast cancer is increased fourfold in women with a family history of premenopausal breast cancer in mother or sister, and an even higher risk if bilateral breast cancer was present. There is a 1.5 times greater risk in the daughters of women who had postmenopausal breast cancer. A history of prior breast cancer is most significant; the chance of a second primary in the opposite breast is 8 to 14 times higher than in the general population. An increased risk in women with a history of benign breast disease that shows, on biopsy, the changes of ductal or lobular atypical hyperplasia (see Chapter 6). Lobular or ductal carcinoma in situ, with the probability of multifocal origin, is an even more serious harbinger of future invasive disease. The majority of women with benign breast disease are not at an increased risk of breast cancer, however, and should not be treated by prophylactic mastectomies.

A less known risk factor is a prior history of radiation exposure. This has been documented following the atomic bombings of Hiroshima and Nagasaki and in women who have undergone irradiation treatment for tuberculosis, and benign diseases such as thymus enlargement and acne (2). Radiation of one breast does not appear to increase the risk of breast cancer in the remaining breast (2). Although these and many other risk factors must be taken into account, 75% of the women who develop breast cancer had no positive risk factors at the time of diagnosis.

There are now generally accepted objective indications for recommending a prophylactic mastectomy. Any patient who thinks of undergoing this operation should have a recommendation from two physicians. Plastic surgeons are reluctant to recommend prophylactic mastectomy, since they believe that the recommendation should come from the physicians who know the patient and her care best. The patient's gynecologist, general surgeon, or oncologist is in the best position to do this, and the plastic surgeon may be considered as the final opinion. The procedure is technically feasible, with acceptable cosmetic results, but it does involve removing a normal organ, or one with preinvasive changes, to prevent a disease that may never occur. It is a highly sensitive and emotional issue that requires the most careful consideration. The patient's level of anxiety in this difficult situation must also be taken into account.

The objective indications for recommending prophylactic mastectomy include women with biopsy-proven lobular or ductal carcinoma in situ, proliferative hyperplasia with atypia, proliferative hyperplasia in those over age 45, and ductal epithelial hyperplasia in the premenopausal years (see Chapters 6 and 7)

Lobular carcinoma in situ presents a controversial management problem (3). It is frequently an incidental finding at biopsy, not associated with a palpable mass. It is multicentric and frequently bilateral, and unilateral mastectomy will not prevent cancer in the contralateral breast. It may take 20 years, or a lifetime, before invasive cancer becomes apparent following this diagnosis, and women may elect frequent physical examinations and mammography rather than surgery. Bilateral mastectomies with reconstruction, however, offer the best certainty of remaining free of disease.

Patients with a breast biopsy demonstrating a premalignant lesion are statistically at an increased risk for developing breast cancer. Different series provide different risk statistics; however, it can be stated that women with extensive papillomatosis, large ductal hyperplasia, or the atypias are more likely to develop carcinoma of the breast. It has been reported that the risk is at least 13 to 15 times the normal incidence (2, 4, 5).

The patient with repeated breast biopsies and progressive fibrocystic "disease" is also a candidate for prophylactic mastectomy, although she may not be at greater risk for developing cancer, because of her dread of the many biopsies and the stress associated with recurring breast masses. The term fibrocystic disease is a misnomer since it describes, for the most part, normal hormone-dependent physiologic changes in breast tissue (5). Other categories of benign disease not currently thought to be precancerous include sclerosing adenosis, duct ectasia, fibrosis, mastitis, squamous metaplasia, and both microcysts and macrocysts. The critical determinant is the biopsy and its interpretation, but, unfortunately, the negative sampling of one area cannot provide a guarantee that the rest of the breast is also disease free.

A history of prior mastectomy for breast cancer is an important consideration in recom-

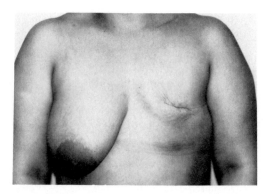

Figure 17.12. A 30-year-old patient following a modified radical mastectomy for carcinoma of the breast.

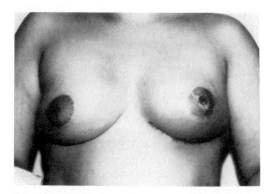

Figure 17.13. Same patient as in Fig. 7.12 following a left breast reconstruction utilizing tissue expansion techniques. The right breast underwent a reduction and subcutaneous mastectomy with reconstruction utilizing a submuscular breast implant. The left nipple was reconstructed sharing the right nipple.

mending prophylactic mastectomy because of the increased likelihood of a new cancer in the contralateral breast, especially when a precancerous mastopathy is known to be present (6–9) (Figs. 17.12 and 17.13).

Women who have had a mastectomy on one side may elect to have a prophylactic mastectomy at the time of the reconstruction. This is most likely to occur in women who have undergone chemotherapy (author's observation).

Some benign tumors of the breast may require prophylactic mastectomy. These include cystosarcoma phylloides, siliconomas, recurrent desmoid tumors, and severe hypertrophy; in general, afflictions that affect most of the breast and cannot be satisfactorily treated with conservative operations.

There are some subjective indications for prophylactic mastectomy, when the patient's psyche is the important factor. Their breasts may be difficult to examine or to follow radiologically, because of density and multiple nodularities, and they become impatient with the suspense and conflicting medical advice, or depressed about the possibility of future malignancy.

Women with constant severe mastodynia may request prophylactic mastectomies. The symptoms may be incapacitating, and such patients are often difficult to examine because of pain and tenderness. However, treatment modalities other than surgery should be used on patients with mastodynia. Mastectomy may not relieve the local pain, or pain may appear in other organs. Counseling is indicated along with medical treatment.

Patients who have had silicone injections in their breasts are still seen today. Liquid silicone forms multiple discrete nodularities, which prevents adequate evaluation of the breast. In these patients, prophylactic mastectomies may be the only treatment.

TYPES OF PROCEDURES

Two basic types of procedures are used for prophylactic mastectomies: total mastectomy or a subcutaneous mastectomy. A total mastectomy is essentially a simple mastectomy in which the nipple is removed and all ductal structures are excised and then replaced as a full-thickness graft. An ellipse of skin may also be removed to reduce the size. The incisions may be either transverse or diagonal. A diagonal incision is a preferable incision for reconstruction as it does not show underneath a brassiere or clothes.

Subcutaneous mastectomy differs from total mastectomy in the placement of the incision and the fact that the nipple remains attached to the skin envelope. The incision must be generous to allow for adequate exposure. In the subcutaneous mastectomy 90% or more of the breast parenchyma is removed, but most of the skin, the nipple-areola complex, and the lymphatic drainage are preserved.

A total mastectomy may be used when patients undergoing prophylactic mastectomies require skin reduction. These may be performed with a "keyhole" pattern as in reduction procedures, or with a transverse incision.

Careful counseling concerning either type of preventive mastectomy is important, since patients must understand that the result will not be a normal breast. The spouse should be included in such conversations. The breast tissue removed is replaced with an inert foreign body made of silicone, with no inherent healing capacity. Skin and nipple sensation is impaired,

and the breast does not feel the same. Capsular contracture, distortion, and asymmetry may occur. Patients undergoing subcutaneous mastectomy frequently require an additional surgical procedure to correct a technical problem within a year or two.

If properly selected and carefully counseled, patients accept the procedure as beneficial. Most feel that the cosmetic results are satisfactory and the risk of cancer is significantly reduced.

The reconstructive techniques used by individual surgeons vary. The implants may be placed in a subpectoralis position. Tissue expanders are the prostheses of choice in most instances. Gradual expansion allows for the healing of skin flaps and nipple-areola complex, but a second procedure is required for removal of the expanders. The end results are usually superior to those of the definitive implant that is placed primarily. The removal of the tissue expander during the secondary procedure allows the surgeon to adjust defects in size, shape, and symmetry.

COMPLICATIONS

The complications of prophylactic mastectomy are the same as those that occur with breast augmentation or reduction and include bleeding, infection, skin or nipple necrosis, capsular contracture, implant disruption, asymmetry, and loss of sensation. Additional surgery may be needed. Patients may have some return of sensation because of reinnervation from the underlying pectoralis muscles and surrounding skin.

Prophylactic mastectomies do not completely prevent breast cancer, but the risk is significantly reduced (10–12). Masses may develop in the residual subcutaneous tissue, which all necessitate biopsy. Patients must be informed about the potential for the future development of such lumps and, possibly, cancer.

SUMMARY

Prophylactic mastectomy is designed to reduce the incidence of breast cancer in women at high risk for the development of malignancy. When careful patient selection is utilized, satisfaction is high. The procedure is not a simple "shelling out of breast tissue" but a formidable operation that should be viewed as a double mastectomy and double reconstruction.

Recommendation for the procedure should come from the general surgeon, oncologist, or gynecologist who knows the patient and her physical condition well. Specific risk factors should be carefully evaluated prior to recommending this procedure.

This procedure should be undertaken only by physicians well-trained in reconstructive breast surgery. The surgeon should be familiar with the various types of implants available and well-versed in tissue expansion and reconstuctive procedures utilizing myocutaneous flaps.

Prophylactic mastectomy is not a cosmetic procedure and should never be undertaken with the idea that the breast will look or feel more natural. It should be performed only when the surgeon and patient feel that the potential complications are less than the risk of developing breast cancer. Aside from prophylaxis, the goal of the operation, from the viewpoint of both the patient and the plastic surgeon is for the woman to appear normal, dressed or undressed.

REFERENCES

1. Freeman, BS. Subcutaneous mastectomy for benign breast lesions with immediate or delayed prosthetic replacement. J Plast Reconstr Surg 1962;30:676.
2. Brown GR, Askew RE, Gallager HS, Hartobagyi GN, Montague ED, et al. Breast cancer. Tex Med September 1987;83:81.
3. Rosen PO, Braun DW, Lynghold B, Urban JA, Kinne DW. Lobular carcinoma in situ of breasts. Cancer 1981;47:813.
4. Calle R, Pilleron JP, Vilcoq JR, et al. Breast carcinoma: experience of the Curie Institute. In: Ames FR, Blumenschein GR, Montague ED, eds. Breast cancer. Austin: University of Texas Press, 1984:121–134.
5. Cancer Committee of the American Pathologists. Is fibrocystic disease of the breast precancerous? Arch Pathol Lab Med 1986;110:171.
6. Zafrani B, Fourquet A, Vilcoq JR, et al. Conservative management of intraductal breast carcinoma with tumorectomy and radiation therapy. Cancer 1986;57:1299.
7. Urban JA, Papchristori D, Taylor J. Bilateral breast cancer. Cancer 1977;40:1968.
8. Keys HM, Bakemeier RF, Saviov E. Breast cancer. In: Rubin P, ed. Clinical oncology: a multidisciplinary approach. Rochester, NY: American Cancer Society, 1983:120–140.
9. Pressman PI. Bilateral breast cancer: the contralateral breast biopsy. Breast 1979;5:29.
10. Jarrett JR, Cutler RG, Teal DF, et al. Aesthetic refinements in prophylactic subcutaneous submuscular reconstruction. Plast Reconstr Surg 1982;69:624.
11. Silverstein MJ, Rosser RJ, Gamagami P, et al. Intraductal breast carcinoma: what constitutes adequate treatment? Cancer 1987;59:1819.
12. Unzeitig GW, Frankl G, Ackerman M, et al. Analysis of the prognosis of minimal and occult breast cancers. Arch Surg 1983;118:1403.

SUGGESTED READINGS

American Joint Committee on Cancer. Breast: manual for Staging of cancer. 3rd ed. Beahrs OH, Henson DE, Hutter RVP, Myers MH, eds. Philadelphia, Lippincott, 1988.

Anderson DE. Genetics and etiology of breast cancer. Breast Dis 1977;31:37.

Bader K, Pellettiere E, Curtin JW. Definitive surgical therapy for the premalignant or equivocal breast lesion. Plast Reconst Surg 1970;46:120.

Baker LH. Breast cancer detection demonstration project: five-year summary report. Cancer 1982;32:4,194.

Bostwick J III, ed. Aesthetic and reconstructive breast surgery. St. Louis, Mosby, 1983.

Deapen MD, Pike MC, Casagrande JT, et al. The relationship between breast cancer and augmentation mammoplasty: an epidemiologic study. Plast Reconstr Surg 1986;77:361.

Egan RL. Role of mammography in the early detection of breast cancer. Cancer 1986;18:279.

Egan RL. Role of mammography in the early detection of breast cancer. Cancer 1969;24:1197.

Fisher B, Redmond C, Fisher ER, et al. Ten-year results of a randomized clinical trial comparing radical mastectomy and total mastectomy with or without radiation. N Engl J Med 1975;312(11):674.

Fisher B. Reappraisal of breast biopsy prompted by the use of lumpectomy: surgical strategy. JAMA 1985;253(4):3585.

Georgiade NG, ed. Reconstructive breast surgery. St. Louis: Mosby, 1976.

Harris JR, Canellos GP, Hellman S, et al. Cancer of the breast—staging. In: DeVita VT, Hellman S, Rosenbert SA, eds. Cancer—principles and practice of oncology. Philadelphia, Lippincott, 1985:1127–1129.

Hoopes JE, Edgerton MT, Shelley W. Organic synthetics for augmentation mammoplasty: their relation to breast cancer. Plast Reconstr Surg 1967;39:262.

Leis HP, Hallager HS, Leis HP, Synderman RD, Urban JA, The breast. eds. St. Louis: Mosby, 1978:490.

Lilla JA, Vistnes LM. Long-term study of reactions to various silicone breast implants in rabbits. Plast Reconstr Surg 1976;57:637.

McGrath MH, Burkhardt BR. The safety and efficacy of breast implants for augmentation mammoplasty. Plast Reconstr Surg 1984;74:440.

Morgernstern L, Gleischman SH, Michel SL, et al. Relation of free silicone to human breast cancer. Arch Surg 1985;120:573.

Schwartz AW, Erich JB. Experimental study of polyvinyl-formal (Ivalon) sponge as a substitute tissue. Plast Reconstr Surg 1960;25:1.

D. RECONSTRUCTION

Because female breasts are symbolic of sexuality in our society, women who have had a mastectomy feel that they have been defeminized, and breast reconstruction improves their self-confidence and self-esteem. The missing breast can never be perfectly duplicated, but a reconstructed breast may feel soft, and a reconstructed nipple may have a nearly normal appearance so that a woman can look normal in clothes. The result must be compared with absence of the breast rather than the appearance before surgery, and the patient is freed from the discomfort and embarrassment of an external prosthesis, with its tendency to be dislodged.

The psychologic enhancement that results from breast reconstruction is important. Women who have had mastectomies experience feelings of guilt, depression, and loss. Following reconstruction, they are less reminded of the negative aspects of the mastectomy and view reconstruction as a positive event that encourages their hope for cure.

The physician caring for patients with breast cancer must be cognizant of the various options available for reconstruction after surgery. Preoperative counseling must inform the patient of the precise goals, likelihood of success, and complications of the operation.

HISTORY

The modern era of breast reconstruction has evolved during the last 20 years as myocutaneous flaps have been developed (1). In the 1950s, breast reconstructions were laborious, staged procedures, utilizing tubed pedicles from the abdomen and taking up to 2 years to complete (2–8) The final results were not aesthetically pleasing. The omentum was tunneled to the chest and covered by a skin graft in an attempt to duplicate a breast, but this was usually unsatisfactory. Currently, myocutaneous flaps and free flaps are used frequently (9). It is due to these refinements that reconstruction is an integral part of the treatment of breast cancer.

INDICATIONS

Although a woman undergoing mastectomy is a candidate for breast reconstruction, not everyone is a good candidate. Consideration of the stage and type of breast cancer is important, but even women with positive axillary nodes, requiring chemotherapy or radiation therapy, are candidates for reconstruction. The decision regarding reconstruction in the patient with a less favorable prognosis depends on good communication among patient, reconstructive surgeon, and oncologist. Regardless of prognosis, the best patients are intelligent, well-motivated women who have a good self-image. Predictably, elderly patients, smokers, and those afflicted with diabetes, obesity, and debilitating diseases have the worst results and the highest rates of complications.

When a woman is diagnosed as having breast cancer, the treatment may be either lumpectomy and radiation therapy or modified radical mastectomy (10, 11). If the latter, consideration of reconstruction, and whether the timing should be immediate or delayed, is mandatory.

Immediate reconstruction is gaining favor (12). It is considered safe, does not result in an increased risk of local recurrence, and is not a contraindication to adjuvant chemotherapy or radiation. The ideal patient is a healthy woman with small breasts and localized disease. Those having immediate reconstruction tolerate mastectomy better emotionally but are less likely to be satisfied with the end result.

The difficulties encountered with immediate reconstruction are usually psychologic rather than technical. The patient may feel that decisions are being forced upon her without her having a true understanding of what is going to happen. It is therefore imperative that the patient understand that reconstruction does not immediately return the breast to a perfect contour but that there will probably be a series of procedures, of which the formation of the primary breast mound at the time of mastectomy is only the first.

A second problem is scheduling. There is a sense of urgency about a breast malignancy, and the general and plastic surgeons must coordinate their schedules to accommodate the needs of the patient.

Delayed reconstructions can be done from several weeks to months following mastectomy, allowing the patient to evaluate her feelings about further surgery. These patients tend to be better satisfied with the result because they have lived with no breast at all. They must understand from the outset that more than one procedure is almost always necessary; these are usually not complicated and can often be done on an outpatient basis.

With modern breast reconstruction, the final result is usually satisfactory. The breast shape resembles that of a normal breast, its consistency is soft, and it is appropriately mobile. The final step is the addition of a well-positioned, symmetric nipple-areola complex. The reconstructive procedure selected depends on the amount and type of remaining skin and whether tissue must be replaced. The shape, size, and texture of the opposite breast are also taken into consideration. The breast is a paired structure, and the two must be matched as closely as possible.

The silicone implant may be used for reconstruction in approximately 25% of the patients, preferably when the other breast is not large and the remaining skin is loose and fairly thick. Many early reconstructions were performed with only a silicone implant beneath the skin. This is a very simple method that can be accomplished through a small incision, but following mastectomy the skin is usually thin and scarred, which results in contracture and erosion around the implant. This early method is no longer considered acceptable (2, 4, 13).

SILICONE IMPLANT RECONSTRUCTION

The first choice in reconstructive procedures is the placement of a silicone implant beneath the pectoralis muscle. The pectoralis is rarely removed during a modern mastectomy. The potential for capsular contracture or implant exposure is reduced, as is the case with simple augmentation procedures, since the pectoralis provides a healthy, protective layer (14).

Unfortunately, the aesthetic result of this procedure may not be ideal because it is often impossible to insert a prosthesis large enough to match the opposite breast. If the mastectomy has been performed through a transverse incision, the conical shape of the breast will be lost. These patients may have to add cotton to their bras to make their breasts symmetrical. Another technical problem with this operation is that failure to detach the distal pectoralis fascia sufficiently may cause the prosthesis to move too high on the chest wall.

The nipple-areola complex is usually reconstructed as a second procedure. Six to 8 weeks are allowed for healing around the implant. Final symmetry is thus improved, as the nipple can be more accurately localized on the breast mound after the edema has subsided.

TISSUE EXPANSION TECHNIQUES

When the mastectomy has caused a deficiency of anterior chest wall skin, tissue expansion should be utilized. The results from this technique are excellent, and it is a less complicated procedure than skin replacement utiliz-

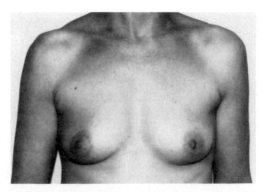

Figure 17.14. Preoperative photograph of a 30-year-old patient who has a breast mass. This mass has not been biopsied, however mammographic findings were suggestive of cancer.

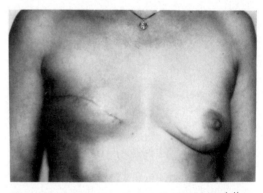

Figure 17.15. Same patient as in Fig. 17.14 following a breast biopsy, modified radical mastectomy and immediate placement of a tissue expander.

ing myocutaneous flaps. It may require months to complete. The tissue expander is a temporary device that stretches the anterior chest wall skin and muscle over a period of weeks. It is placed in a subpectoralis-subserratus position and inflated with saline through a subcutaneous valve. This technique is frequently used with immediate reconstructions because it is quick and safe and allows the submuscular placement of the implant to be done at the time of the mastectomy, before scarring has occurred. It is also effective as a delayed procedure (12, 15, 16).

The small valve through which a fine-gauge needle can be passed to increase gradually the volume of fluid in the expander is placed in a subcutaneous position. The goal is to overstretch the anterior chest wall skin and muscle to a size approximately 30% larger than finally desired. Tissue expansion works best in women who have small breasts and have not received radiation therapy, which causes thickened fibrotic skin. Patients who have been irra-

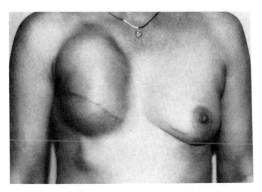

Figure 17.16.   Same patient as in Figs. 17.15 and 17.16 following inflation of the tissue expander.

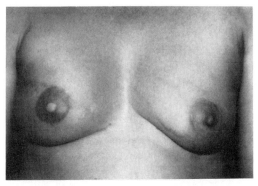

Figure 17.17.   Same patient as in Figs. 17.15–17.17 following removal of the tissue expander, nipple reconstruction, and placement of the permanent implant.

diated often require myocutaneous flaps that provide skin and muscle replacement. After the skin is overstretched, the expander is removed and the permanent implant placed. The skin is allowed to conform to the permanent implant prior to formation of the nipple-areola complex. The inframammary fold can also be remodeled by internally suturing the expander pocket to the periosteum of the sixth or seventh ribs, or by de-epithelializing and apposing adjacent skin surfaces to restore the inframammary fold (Figs. 17.14–17.17).

Immediate reconstruction utilizing the tissue expansion technique has gained wide acceptance because it allows an uncompromised cancer operation without loss of time or greater risk of an inferior result. The psychologic advantage for the patient is significant. Any additional procedures can be done on an ambulatory basis. There is a slight increase in the incidence of infection with this technique; if this occurs, the expander must be removed and other options considered. Risk factors are the same as those described for other plastic

procedures using a prosthesis. Immediate reconstruction does not increase the risk of cancer recurrence, nor does it affect the decision to prescribe adjuvant therapy.

The placement of the mastectomy incision is an important consideration when reconstruction is planned. Horizontal incisions remove the conical shape of the breast. A low diagonal incision facilitates reconstruction and is unlikely to show in a bathing suit or brassiere. Women should be told of the importance of incision placement before undergoing mastectomy.

THE LATISSIMUS DORSI MYOCUTANEOUS FLAP BREAST RECONSTRUCTION

The ability to transfer skin and muscle on their vascular pedicle from the back or abdomen to the anterior chest evolved in the mid-1970s (4, 17–20). The procedure affords soft tissue coverage of the prosthesis with better reconstruction of the normal shape of the breast. The patient is placed in a modified Sims position and an oval island of skin overlying the inferior portion of the latissimus dorsi just behind the posterior axillary line is marked, incised, and elevated along with the underlying muscle (Figs. 17.18 and 17.19).

The myocutaneous flap must be carefully tailored to the size desired. It is dissected free down to the thoracodorsal vessels, and the donor site is closed primarily, after undercutting the edges. The patient is then repositioned to permit frontal exposure, and the mobilized flap is passed under the axillary skin to the mastectomy site, still attached to its vascular pedicle, and fastened in the appropriate place. Beneath this island of skin and muscle a silicone implant is fixed. There is rarely a problem with healing, and the transplanted muscle makes it possible to form initially a large breast. The cosmetic result is excellent. The latissimus dorsi myocutaneous flap can also be combined with a tissue expander when a larger breast is required (Figs. 17.20 and 17.21).

Its chief disadvantage is the additional scar on the patient's back. Patients rarely experience any weakness of the arm or shoulder except in the power stroke associated with swimming. The problem of capsule contracture may occur because of the implant. This procedure requires a general anesthetic and hospitalization for 3 to 5 days. As with all reconstructive breast procedures, the nipple-areola complex is restored at a later time to allow for the new breast mound to stabilize.

The latissimus dorsi myocutaneous flap breast reconstruction may be performed either

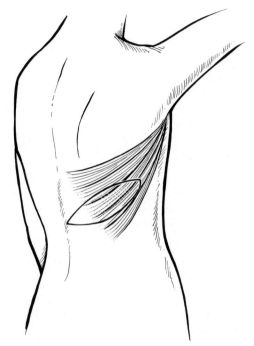

Figure 17.18. The skin-island transposed on the latissimus dorsi myocutaneous flap for breast reconstruction.

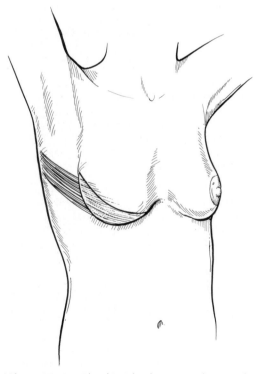

Figure 17.19. The skin-island transposed anteriorly for skin replacement with the latissimus dorsi myocutaneous flap.

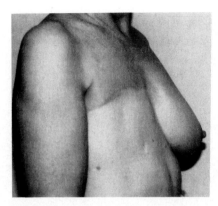

Figure 17.20. A 50-year-old patient following a modified radical mastectomy. She has a large left breast and is deficient in skin on the mastectomy side.

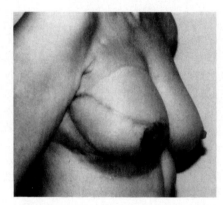

Figure 17.21. Same patient as in Fig. 17.20 following a breast reconstruction utilizing a latissimus dorsi myocutaneous flap. Notice that the original mastectomy scar has faded. The breasts match well for size, shape, and contour.

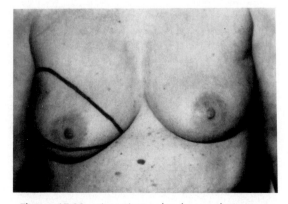

Figure 17.22. A patient who has undergone a breast biopsy. She has infiltrating ductal carcinoma of the breast.

cle, which is provided with arterial perforating vessels from the superior epigastric artery for nourishment. The large volume of tissue thus transplanted obviates the necessity for a prosthesis. Since the superior epigastric artery is a continuation of the internal mammary artery, prior disruption of the internal mammary artery precludes the use of the flap (21, 22).

Either the ipsilateral or contralateral rectus muscle can be used as the carrier. The large transverse oval of skin from one anterior iliac spine to the other, with underlying subcutaneous tissue, fascia, and one entire rectus muscle is transplanted by rotating the mass superiorly to the chest. The abdominal fascia is then closed primarily or reinforced with a synthetic mesh, if there is a tissue deficiency, and the skin is closed by an appropriate plastic maneuver. The breast mound is then formed by tailoring the large flap to the dimensions of an acceptable symmetric breast. A breast prosthesis is seldom needed, and there are no future problems with capsular contraction. The end result is usually excellent from a cosmetic viewpoint (Fig. 17.25).

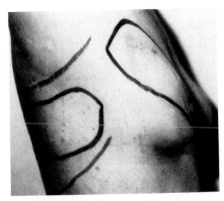

Figure 17.23. Same patient as in Fig. 17.22 marked for an immediate breast reconstruction utilizing latissimus dorsi myocutaneous flap.

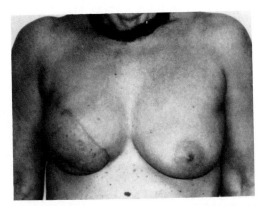

Figure 17.24. Same patient as in Figs. 17.21 and 17.22 following an immediate breast reconstruction utilizing a latissimus dorsi myocutaneous flap. This patient elected not to have the nipple reconstructed.

as an immediate or as a delayed procedure. Usually it is delayed, but the result from immediate reconstruction can be excellent. The primary reason for delay is the magnitude of the procedure when combined with mastectomy and the difficulty of explaining the pros and cons of a secondary operation to a patient whose chief concern is the cure of her cancer. Since transfusions may be necessary, the lack of adequate time for storing autologous blood is also a problem (Figs. 17.22–17.24).

THE RECTUS ABDOMINIS MYOCUTANEOUS FLAP BREAST RECONSTRUCTION

The transverse rectus abdominis myocutaneous (TRAM) flap consists of lower abdominal fat and skin transposed to the breast area on the underlying rectus abdominis mus-

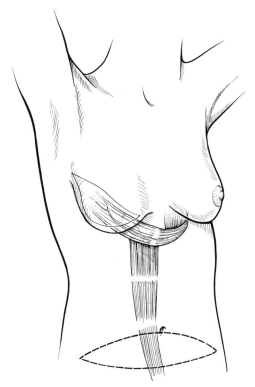

Figure 17.25. Diagramatically represents the lower abdominal skin-island to be elevated on the left rectus muscle. The transverse rectus abdominus myocutaneous flap will provide a large volume of skin and muscle for breast reconstruction.

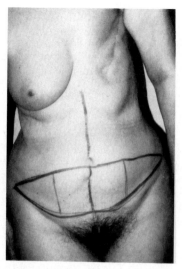

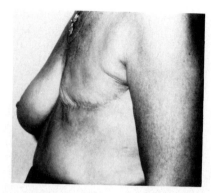

Figure 17.28. An elderly patient following a modified radical mastectomy. She is deficient in skin. Her complaint is that the prosthesis slips when she swims.

Figure 17.26. Demonstrates a patient preoperatively who will undergo a breast reconstruction utilizing the transverse rectus abdominus myocutaneous flap.

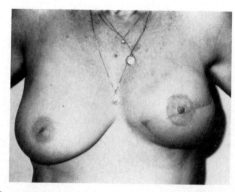

Figure 17.29. Same patient as in Fig. 17.28 following the left breast reconstruction utilizing latissimus dorsi myocutaneous flap. The areola is reconstructed with a groin graft. The nipple is a composite from the right nipple.

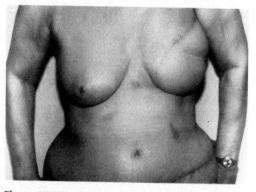

Figure 17.27. Same patient as in Fig. 17.26 following reconstruction using the TRAM flap. A large amount of abdominal skin and muscle has been transposed to reconstruct a large, ptotic breast.

COMPLICATIONS

The major disadvantage is the formidable nature of the operation; it takes 6 to 8 weeks to recover. Problems with skin and fat necrosis may occur, especially among smokers and diabetics. There is also weakness in the abdominal wall following transposition of the muscles. Even when properly reinforced, hernias can develop. Autologous blood transfusions, with their inherent risks, are routine, and hospitalization usually lasts 5 to 7 days. If used for immediate reconstruction, delays in flap healing may retard the initiation of adjuvant chemotherapy or irradiation. For these reasons this is not the primary choice of the available procedures, and it should be reserved for special

cases when less complicated procedures will not suffice (Figs. 17.26 and 17.27).

NIPPLE AREOLAR RECONSTRUCTION

The breast reconstruction is completed with the addition of the nipple-areolar complex. The pigmented areolar skin is reconstructed with a full-thickness graft harvested from the patient's upper-inner thigh. This is normally pigmented skin that contracts when taken as a full-thickness graft. The hair follicles are carefully removed from the posterior aspect of the graft. The graft is then sutured into the de-epithelialized site on the reconstructed or redundant upper eyelid tissue. Tatooing techniques have also been used for areolar reconstruction. Nipple projection is more commonly provided by constructing a localized flap based on a subcutaneous pedicle of tissue elevated on the reconstructed breast mound. Various grafting techniques have been used to help maintain nipple projection. Currently, nipple prostheses are being manufactured to help provide additional nipple projection and to help reconstruct the conical shape of the breast (Figs. 17.28 and 17.29).

REFERENCES

1. Hohler H. Reconstruction of the Female Breast after Radical Mastectomy. In J.M. Converse (ed) Reconstructive Plastic surgery, Vol. 7, 2nd Ed. Philadelphia: Saunders, 1977, p 3661.
2. Alexander JE, Block LL. Breast reconstruction following radical mastectomy. Plast Reconstr Surg 40:175, 1967.
3. Berson MI. Derma-fat-facia transplants used in building up the breasts. surgery 15:451, 1944.
4. Georgiade NG. Reconstruction of the Breasts Following Mastectomy. In N.G. Georgiade (ed) Reconstructive Breast Surgery. St. Louis: Mosby, p. 292, 1976.
5. Goldwyn RM. Vincenz Czerny and the beginnings of breast reconstruction. Plast Reconstr Surg 61:673, 1978.
6. Letterman GS, Schurter M. total mammary gland excision with immediate breast reconstruction. Am Surg 21:835, 1955.
7. Longacre JJ. The use of local pedicle flaps for reconstruction of the breast after subtotal or total extirpation of the mammary gland and for the correction of distortion and atrophy of the breast due to excessive scar. Plast Reconstr Surg 11:380, 1953.
8. Millard DR. Breast reconstruction after a radical mastectomy. Plast Reconstr Surg 58:283, 1976.
9. Shaw WW: Breast reconstruction by superior gluteal microvascular free flaps without silicone implants. Plas. and Reconstr. Surg., Vol. 72, 4:490–501, 1983.
10. Veronesi U, Costa A, Grandi C. Surgical treatment of primary breast cancer. Schweiz. Med. Worschenschr. 107:987, 1977.
11. Westdahl PR. Selection, workup and surgical technique of conservation surgery and axillary dissection. Front Radiat Ther Oncol 17:48, 1983.
12. Noone RB, Murphy JB, Spear SL, et al. A 6-year experience with immediate reconstruction after mastectomy for cancer. Plast Reconstr Surg 76:258, 1985.
13. Freeman BS. Experiences in reconstruction of the breast after mastectomy. Clin Plast Surg 3:277, 1976.
14. Gruber RP, Kahn RA, Lash H, et al. Breast reconstruction following mastectomy: A comparison of submuscular and subcutaneous techniques. Plast Reconstr Surg 67:312, 1981.
15. Radovan C. Reconstruction of the breast after radical mastectomy using temporary expander. ASPRS Plast Surg Forum 1:41, 1978.
16. Radovan C. Breast reconstruction after mastectomy using the temporary expander. Plast Reconstr Surg 69:195, 1982.
17. Baroudi R, Pinotti JA, Keppke EN. A transverse thoraco-abdominal flap for closure after radical mastectomy. Plast Reconstr surg 61:547, 1978.
18. Cooper GG, Webster MHC, Bell G. The results of breast reconstruction following mastectomy. Br J Plast surg 37:369, 1984.
19. Cronin TD, Upton J, McDonough JM. Reconstruction of the breast after mastectomy. Plast Reconstr Surg 59:1, 1977.
20. McCraw J. Late Findings in Latissimus Dorsi Breast Reconstruction. Presented at the American Association of Plastic Surgeons Meeting, Chicago, May 1984.
21. BunkisJ, Walton RL, Mathes SJ, Krizek TJ, Vasconez LO: Experience with the transverse lower rectus abdominis operation for breast reconstruction. Plas. and Reconstr. Surg., Vol.72, 6:819-826, 1983.
22. Hartrampf CR, Scheflan M, Black PW: Breast reconstruction with a transverse abdominal island flap. Plast. Reconstr. Surg. 69: 216, 1982.

SUGGESTED READINGS

Asplund, O. Capsular contracture in silicone gel and saline-filled breast implants after reconstruction. Plast Reconstr Surg 73:270, 1984.
Birnbaum L, Olsen JA. Breast reconstruction following radical mastectomy, using custom designed implants. Plast Reconstr Surg 61 355, 1978.
Bostwick J, III, Vasconez LO, Jurkiewicz MJ. Breast reconstruction after a radical mastectomy. Plast Reconstr Surg 61:682, 1978.
Bosworth JL. Chossein NA. Limited surgery and radiotherapy in the treatment of localized brest cancer: An overview. surg Clin North Am 64:1115, 1984.
Guthrie RH. Breast reconstruction after radical mastectomy. Plast Reconstr Surg 57:14, 1976.
Hartwell SW, Anderson R, Hall MD, Esselstyn C. Reconstruction of the breast after mastectomy for cancer. Plast Reconstr Surg 57:152, 1976.
Hokin JAB. Mastectomy reconstruction without a prosthetic implant. Plast Reconstr Surg 72:810, 1983.
Pearl RM, Wisnicki J. Breast reconstruction following lumpectomy and irradiation. Plast Reconstr Surg 76:83, 1985.
Pontes R. single stage reconstruction of the missing breast. BR J Plast Surg 26:377, 1973.
Scheflan M, Dinner MI. The transver abdominal island flap: I. Indications, contraindications, results and complications. Ann Plast Surg 10:24, 1983.

18

Epidemiology of Breast Cancer

Barrie Anderson
Elaine Smith

Breast cancer kills almost as many U.S. citizens every year as were killed in combat in the entire 8 years of the Vietnam War. In 1988 135,900 cases were diagnosed and 42,300 women died from this disease. Breast cancer is the leading cause of death from cancer in American women between the ages of 15 and 54, and second in women age 55 and older (Fig. 18.1) (1). This record of carnage continues despite several decades of intensive efforts to improve treatment, and the achievement of major technologic advances in diagnosis. To date little has been accomplished in the area of prevention.

The role of epidemiologic research in the prevention of disease is identifying risk factors that can then be eliminated. Epidemiologic studies of breast cancer can yield clinical and statistical associations that may elucidate the process by which a carcinogen stimulates development of clinical cancer.

Identification of risk factors for breast cancer starts with examination of incidence rates in populations. Caution must be used in comparing international rates because of differences in availability of medical care, which can then affect rates of diagnosis (2). Underdeveloped or poor regions may therefore be prone to underreporting bias.

Possible risk factors are then evaluated in retrospective case comparison and correlation studies. Such studies are easily confounded by unrelated variables. Causality may be established when the association is strong, can be replicated, is biologically plausible, precedes the onset of cancer, and shows a dose-response relationship. It is difficult to prove causality in human cancers.

Cohort studies are usually prospective evaluations of groups of individuals exposed to a risk factor. Cohorts are followed over time and compared with similar but unexposed individuals. Because data are less subject to recall bias and confounding variables they are more reliable in identifying true risk factors. However, cohort studies are time consuming and costly.

The advantages and disadvantages of each type of study must be borne in mind when reviewing the results of epidemiologic inquiries into breast cancer causation.

In evaluating risk it is customary to calculate the relative risk ratio. This is a particularly useful measure when the disease under consideration is rare in the population being considered and when the interval after exposure is long. Low levels of risk (≤ 2) can be misleading and should be interpreted with caution. Several highly publicized risk factors for breast cancer have a relative risk ratio of 2 or less (Table 18.1) (3).

Attributable risk describes the proportion of cancers in exposed individuals that can be attributed to exposure to a given factor. Attributable risk is a measure of the possible impact of risk avoidance on prevention of disease.

BREAST CANCER RISK

Cancer is a disease with more than one cause, reflecting interactions of many mechanisms. What further confounds and obscures relationships is the latency between carcinogen exposure and disease development. Finally, susceptibility to a carcinogen may vary with age and physiologic factors.

Only two identified factors confer major risk for breast cancer—sex and age. Cancer of the

218

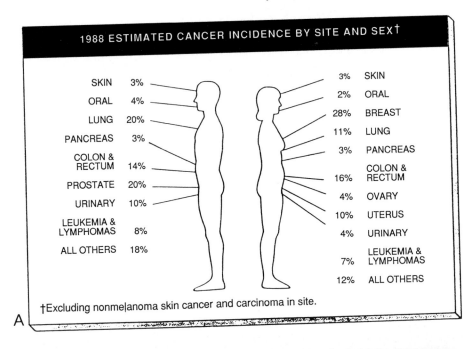

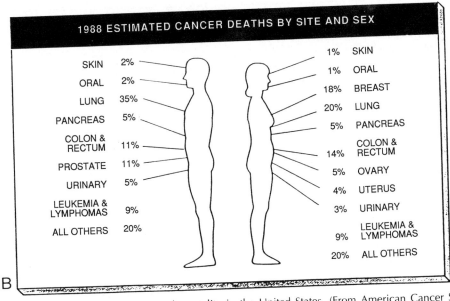

Figure 18.1. **A, B,** Cancer incidence and mortality in the United States. (From American Cancer Society. Cancer statistics 1988. CA 1988;38:5–22.)

breast affects females almost entirely, and it increases in frequency with age (Fig. 18.2).

REPRODUCTIVE AND HORMONAL FACTORS

Many aspects of reproductive and hormonal function have been extensively studied and correlated with the risk for breast cancer in different populations. Most large epidemiologic studies confirm the increased risk associated with early menarche and late menopause and the protective effect of early age at first pregnancy (4–10).

With late menopause, menstrual cycles become longer, and there is greater variability

Table 18.1.   Risk Factors for Breast Cancer in Females[a]

Factor	High Risk	Low Risk	Magnitude of Risk Differential[b]
Age	Old age	Young age	>>>
Country of residence	North America, Northern Europe	Asia, Africa	>>>
Socioeconomic class	Upper	Lower	>>
Marital status	Never married	Ever married	>
Place of residence	Urban	Rural	>
Place of residence	Northern US	Southern US	>
Race	White	Black	>
Age at first birth	Older than 30	Younger than 20	>>
Oophorectomy	No	Yes	>>
Body build	Obese	Thin	>>
Age at menarche	Early	Late	>
Age at menopause	Late	Early	>
Family history of premenopausal bilateral breast cancer	Yes	No	>>>
History of cancer in one breast	Yes	No	>>>
History of fibrocystic disease	Yes	No	>>
Any first-degree relative with breast cancer	Yes	No	>>
History of primary cancer in ovary or endometrium	Yes	No	>>
Radiation to chest	Large doses	Minimal exposure	>>

[a]From Kelsey JL. A review of the epidemiology of human breast cancer. Epidemiol Rev 1979;1:74–109.
[b]>>>, relative risk of greater than 4.
>>, relative risk of 2–4.
>, relative risk of 1.1–1.9.

than with menopause at an earlier age (11). Endometrial biopsy in premenopausal women with breast cancer compared with age-matched controls showed only 17% of the women with cancer had secretory endometrium, as compared with 68% of the control group (12). Thus, anovulatory cycles and unopposed estrogen increase with late menopause.

Early bilateral salpingo-oophorectomy or natural menopause before the age of 45 cuts the risk to less than half of that with menopause at age 55 or greater (10, 13, 14). Removal of only one ovary is less protective, and hysterectomy alone does not change the risk (14, 15). The greatest protective effect is seen when surgical menopause occurs before the age of 35 (14), with less protection persisting up to the age of 50 (10). This difference is eradicated when replacement estrogen therapy is given (9).

The "estrogen window hypothesis" has been proposed as an explanation for this effect; it theorizes that unopposed estrogen stimulation after menarche and before menopause is the most favorable state for tumor induction. This is based on the assumption that anovulatory cycles are more frequent with early menarche and late menopause, and that ovulatory cycles are induced by pregnancy (16).

The importance of unopposed estrogen has been challenged by the observation that risk for development of breast cancer appears to be proportional to the cumulative number of regular ovulatory cycles (17). In addition, early menarche is associated with early establishment of ovulatory cycles (18, 19); young women who begin menses at a later age take a longer time to establish regular cycles (11). Breast cancer patients have a history of earlier initiation of regular cycles than do controls (19). Women who establish regular menses within 1 year after menarche have two times the risk of later development of breast cancer than do those who took 5 or more years to establish regular menses (20). Teenage daughters of breast cancer patients appear to ovulate more frequently than controls matched for age and onset of menarche (21, 22).

Data correlating histologic changes in the breast with menstrual phase are few and in conflict; some show breast mitotic activity to be maximum in the luteal phase (23), and others find more mitoses in the proliferative phase (24). However, tritiated thymidine labeling of in vitro benign breast tissue revealed a cyclic pattern of proliferation of the terminal duct cells. The labeling index was lowest early in the cycle (days 2 to 15) and elevated late (days 16 to

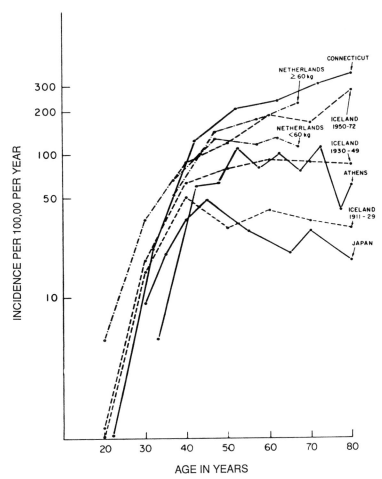

Figure 18.2. Age-specific incidence rates for breast cancer. *Solid line:* Connecticut, USA, 1970–1974; Athens, Greece. 1966–1967; Miyagi Prefecture, Japan, 1959–1960. *Dashed line*: Iceland, 1911–1929, Iceland, 1930–1949, Iceland, 1950–1972. *Broken line*: Rotterdam and The Hague, the Netherlands, 1972–1974, women <60 kg, women ≥60 kg. (From Kelsey JL. A review of the epidemiology of human breast cancer. *Epidemiol Rev* 1979;1:74–109.)

1). There was also a negative correlation with the age of the patient, with a mean turnover time of 22 days at age 20 and 147 days at age 40 (25). Secretions are greatest in the luteal phase.

Prolactin has been implicated in the development of breast cancer. It stimulates growth of mammary epithelial cells, particularly just prior to menarche. The prolactin-stimulating antihypertensive reserpine was initially thought to be associated with breast cancer risk (26, 27) because of its effect on prolactin secretion. However, subsequent studies found no positive association (28), and the suspicion of causality was not supported when cases were further matched by follow-up after the diagnosis of hypertension (27).

The prolactin association is further weakened by the observation that women who have lactated have no increased risk of breast cancer (29). If prolactin increased risk, prolonged prolactin stimulation during lactation would be expected to have that effect, and it does not. In fact, premenopausal women who have lactated may have a decreased risk (30). This protective effect persists after data are controlled for age, parity, age at first pregnancy, age at menarche, and education. There is no protective effect in postmenopausal women.

Another hormonal relationship has been identified through a major prospective study of urinary excretion of androgen and corticosteroid metabolites (31). Androsterone and etiocholanolone excretion measured from age 30 to

55 is subnormal in women who subsequently develop breast cancer and in unaffected sisters of breast cancer patients (32). It is hypothesized that androgens may protect through their inhibition of mammary epithelial cell growth (31).

Risk for development of breast cancer is related to age at first full-term birth (33, 34). The risk for those delaying first full-term delivery until 30 years of age or older is 2.2 times greater than for those delivering before 20 years of age (13). Risk increases over nulliparity with delay of first birth beyond age 35 (8, 35). Incomplete pregnancy has little (36) or no protective effect (35), and interruption of the first pregnancy in the first trimester may possibly increase cancer risk (20). Abortion after completion of the first-term pregnancy conferred no incrased risk. An increasing number of births may give a small additional protective effect (8), especially if they occur at an early age (34). However, there is no additional protective effect of subsequent births when data are controlled for age at first birth (35). This protective effect of the first birth is not due to relative infertility in women who delay birth, since the same effect was found whether childbirth occurred within 2 years of marriage or later (33). Prolactin levels are significantly decreased after pregnancy, but this effect is not confined to women whose pregnancies occurred at an early age (37). Therefore, prolactin is unlikely to be the mediating factor.

The influence of oral contraceptives on breast cancer risk has been extensively studied. Most major reports have concluded that there has been no increased overall risk for breast cancer due to use of oral contraceptives (1, 6, 38–47). However, there may be an increased risk in some subgroups. Use by older women around the time of menopause may increase risk slightly (38), with a 15-fold increased risk for premenopausal users age 51 to 55 (40). Although use of oral contraceptives before the first-term pregnancy may increase the risk of breast cancer (39, 48–50), large well-controlled studies report no increased risk regardless of length of use (42). There have been some reports of increased risk for development of breast cancer with oral contraceptive use in women with a diagnosis of benign breast disease (38, 51), but most studies have concluded that there is no increased risk (38, 42, 44, 51) or that there may be protection against future development of fibrocystic disease but not against the hyperplastic variety that is premalignant (52); see Chapter 6.

There has been concern that oral contraceptives may act as tumor promoters, especially in the older user. Oral contraceptive steroids can stimulate mammary epithelial growth in vitro (53). However, there is no in vitro difference in cell proliferation in human breast ducts between patients exposed to oral contraceptives and those unexposed (25). Some investigators have reported an increased risk with increasing length of use (49), while others have not (42–44). Some have even observed a long-term protective effect (6, 45, 46).

There is no increased risk of oral contraceptive use in women who have first-degree relatives with breast cancer (41, 42). Although a possible risk has been reported with high progestogen formulations, especially in young women with prolonged usage (50), this association has not been confirmed (44, 47).

The influence of estrogen replacement therapy has been studied extensively. There appears to be no significant influence of oral estrogen replacement therapy on breast cancer risk regardless of the dose, duration, or other risk factors (6, 54–57). Although increased risk can be seen with long-term use at high dosage (58–61), these differences have been either small or statistically not significant.

The protective effect of surgical menopause is canceled by the use of estrogen replacement, but risk is not increased above normal (9, 38, 54, 55, 59, 61, 62). Breast cancer risk may be increased in subgroups of women who have used oral estrogen with intact ovaries (60, 62), women who use injectable estrogen (55), women with a family history of breast cancer (58), or women who have received high doses of estrogen in pregnancy (63). Increased risk is also seen with estrogen use in the presence of benign breast disease (60), especially if the benign disease develops after the start of estrogen replacement therapy (59, 60) or if it contains ductal epithelial hyperplasia (9).

RISK FROM OTHER BREAST DISEASE

The influence of benign breast disease on the development of breast cancer is related to the histologic type of benign disease present. Numerous studies have suggested that women who have undergone a breast biopsy or who have a history of fibrocystic disease (5, 64–68) have an increased risk of developing breast cancer. However, women whose breast lesion contains atypical epithelial changes have up to six times the risk of those without such changes (13, 63, 66–72). The incidence of epithelial atypia parallels the incidence of cancer in some high-risk ethnic groups (64). The type of hyperplasia appears to vary with menopausal status, with premenopausal women having papillary proliferation and postmenopausal women having cribriform intraductal proliferation (71). Women with biopsy-only treatment of ductal carcinoma in situ have a 28% chance of developing cancer in the same breast (73). When atypical hyperplasia is accompanied by a family history of breast cancer the risk rises to 11 times that for individuals whose fibrocystic disease has no epithelial atypia and in whom there is no family history (70, 73). This increased risk is similar to that when carcinoma in situ is found (67).

The breast lesion that confers the greatest risk for subsequent development of breast cancer is cancer in the opposite breast (71). Women who had bilateral subcutaneous mastectomies for treatment of cancer were found to have a 13% bilaterality rate for carcinoma in situ, with 30% having severe dysplasia in the opposite breast (74). Postmortem studies confirm this high rate of bilaterality, with invasive disease found in the opposite breast in 25% (75).

INTERNATIONAL DIFFERENCES IN RISK

International statistics reveal widely varying rates of breast cancer among different national groups (Table 18.2). Descriptive studies of breast cancer incidence and mortality abound (1, 2, 76) and are useful in suggesting several lines of inquiry into the causes of these differences.

The first association that is evident in reviewing national and international statistics is that breast cancer incidence is greatest in affluent societies. Economic indicators such as the gross national product are closely correlated with national breast cancer incidence and mortality rates (77). The relationship to socioeconomic class is apparent if the statistics of developed nations are compared with those of developing regions. Breast cancer incidence in the United States and Canada is six times that in Asia or Black Africa. Incidence in Western Europe is four times that in Japan. South America, the Caribbean region, and Eastern Europe have intermediate rates (2).

Although racial groupings might seem at first glance to be strongly influential, a more extensive analysis lessens this impression. Breast cancer incidence in black American women is more closely related to white American women than to black African women. Furthermore, Japanese immigrants to Hawaii and the United States have a risk that is more closely related to American women than to women in Japan.

The Third National Cancer Survey found a positive association of high socioeconomic class, as measured by college education and income, with incidence of cancer of the breast

Table 18.2.   Cancer Around the World 1982–1983: Age-Adjusted Death Rates per 100,000 Population for Selected Sites for 50 Countries[a]

Country	Breast Female
United States	26.7 (16)
Australia	24.9 (20)
Austria	25.2 (19)
Barbados	21.3 (25)
Belgium	32.2 (5)
Bulgaria	16.5 (33)
Canada	28.4 (14)
Chile	15.6 (34)
Costa Rica	12.9 (37)
Cuba	18.2 (29)
Czechoslovakia	24.0 (21)
Denmark	31.6 (8)
Dominican Republic[b]	6.5 (47)
El Salvador	1.7 (50)
England and Wales	34.5 (2)
Finland	19.6 (27)
France	23.8 (22)
Germany, D.R.	20.2 (26)
Germany, F.R.	26.8 (15)
Greece	18.0 (30)
Hungary	25.3 (18)
Iceland	25.5 (17)
Ireland	32.2 (5)
Israel	29.0 (13)
Japan	6.2 (48)
Kuwait	12.7 (38)
Luxembourg	29.1 (12)
Malta and Gozo	34.9 (1)
Martinque[b]	16.9 (32)
Mauritius	7.3 (45)
Mexico[b]	7.2 (46)
Netherlands	32.7 (4)
New Zealand	32.2 (5)
Northern Ireland[c]	29.4 (10)
Norway	21.7 (24)
Panama	9.6 (44)
Paraguay	12.1 (40)
Peru[b]	5.8 (49)
Poland	17.7 (31)
Portugal	18.7 (28)
Puerto Rico	11.5 (41)
Romania	15.2 (36)
Scotland	33.9 (3)
Singapore[c]	12.6 (39)
Surinam[b]	10.6 (42)
Sweden	22.9 (23)
Switzerland	31.6 (8)
Uruguay	29.2 (11)
Venezuela[c]	10.6 (42)
Yugoslavia[b]	15.5 (35)

[a]From American Cancer Society. Cancer statistics 1988. CA 1988;38:5–22.
[b]1982 only.
[c]1983 only
NOTE: Figures in parentheses are order of rank within site and sex group.

(78). In a large study in Los Angeles County (79) age-adjusted breast cancer rates were compared by socioeconomic class as determined by a combination of income and education. The rate for the highest socioeconomic class was 50% greater than that for the lowest. There was no difference among social classes in age at menarche or menopause. The only known breast cancer risk factor associated with social class was age at first birth. Median age at first pregnancy in the highest socioeconomic class was significantly older than that in the lowest class (24.6 years vs. 20.3 years). Even after correction for age at first birth a significant effect of socioeconomic class is seen (8, 35). When socioeconomic status was similar, breast cancer patients did not differ from controls in regard to height, weight, obesity, prior breast disease, hormone use, parity, or nursing (80). In a high-risk society with uniformly high socioeconomic class, there is no significant difference in age at menarche, age at first full-term birth, or age at menopause when breast cancer patients are compared with age-matched controls selected from a population registry (81).

ROLE OF HEREDITY

There is significant heterogeneity for cancer risk among relatives of breast cancer probands (82). In the general population any family history of breast cancer increases risk for the individual two to three times (13, 29, 83–86). However first-degree female relatives of patients with premenopausal bilateral disease have a nine- to 14-fold increase in risk as compared with relatives of patients with unilateral postmenopausal disease (83, 86), and 47 to 51 times the risk in women with no family history (84).

There are some families with a high incidence of breast cancer related to an autosomal dominant allele transmitted by either maternal or paternal lines (87, 88). Disease is characterized by multifocal primaries and early age of onset (83, 89). Women carrying the susceptibility allele have a risk of breast cancer that is 12% by age 35, 50% by age 50, and 87% by age 80. This allele appears in the same chromosomal region as glutamate pyruvic transaminase (GPT). However, since GPT has no physiologic relationship to breast cancer, it is not useful as a marker. In families with genetic susceptibility to breast cancer there may also be other associated cancers such as cancer of the ovary, endometrium, and other sites (87, 88).

Cultured skin fibroblasts in women with high-risk hereditary breast cancer have been found to have increased hyperdiploidy (90). Numerous hormonal differences have been identified in daughters of women who developed breast cancer at an early age. These women have significantly higher levels of estrogen, progesterone, and prolactin measured in the luteal phase of the menstrual cycle (22, 91). Low levels of plasma androgens have been found in sisters of breast cancer patients (35). Mammograms in both breast cancer patients and their daughters and younger sisters show characteristic patterns of extensive ductal prominence (P2) or sheets of increased density (DY) (92, 93).

Attempts to distinguish the high-risk familial breast cancer patient from other breast cancer patients may be useful in identifying those individuals at high risk for early development of breast cancer.

DIET

To this point the risk factors described are either intrinsic or difficult to change. As a factor that may possibly be subject to control, diet has received a great deal of attention and study. Some have concluded that differences in breast cancer risk are explained by excessive fat and meat consumption (77, 94, 95). However, one of these reports (77) also concluded that economic indicators, such as gross national product, are as closely correlated with breast cancer incidence and mortality as are dietary fat and meat consumption. In another (94), most of the increased risk associated with meat eating was seen in women in the highest social class. It has been suggested that these data may also reflect a significant effect of economic factors on the quality of cancer incidence data (77).

No association of dietary fat (96) or serum cholesterol, β-lipoprotein or total lipids (97) with increased breast cancer risk has been found. Lack of association of dietary meat with breast cancer risk is confirmed in studies of meat-abstaining nuns, most of whom joined their religious order as adults (98) and lactoovovegetarian Seventh Day Adventists, 60% of whom were adult converts and 40% of whom were born into the religion (99). In none of these groups was there any decrease in breast cancer risk. A major prospective cohort study concluded that a moderate decrease in adult fat intake would be unlikely to result in a substantial decrease in the incidence of breast cancer (100).

It has also been suggested that protective mechanisms might be found in diet. However, vegetarians and nonvegetarians differ little in breast cancer rates (99) and no protective factors associated with diet have been found in the U.S. population (101).

It may be that caloric intake has its influence through alteration of total body weight, which has a pronounced effect on breast cancer risk. The influence of body weight on breast cancer risk varies in relationship to menopause. Although some studies have concluded that there is a statistically significant association of increased body weight with risk in both premenopausal and postmenopausal women (6, 13, 102), most have reported no association in the premenopausal woman but statistically significant increased risks in the postmenopausal group (4, 6, 94, 103–106).

Another dietary factor that has been the subject of scrutiny is alcohol intake. Some case-control studies have indicated that there is increased risk with moderate drinking (78, 107, 108). However, one major well-controlled study identified factors influencing alcohol consumption as age, religion, education, occupation, marital status, body mass, and smoking and found no dose relationship with increasing alcohol consumption and no increased risk when patients were controlled for age at first pregnancy and parity (109). It is probable that moderate alcohol consumption is associated more closely with other identified risk factors such as socioeconomic status, which influence the true risk factors of age at first pregnancy and body mass.

LOCAL CARCINOGENS IN BREAST SECRETIONS

A field of research that has received scant attention is the physiology of the breast and passage of known environmental carcinogens into breast fluid. Transport of drugs, pesticides, and almost any other compound from plasma to milk across the mammary membrane in women has been documented to occur at levels that may equal or even exceed those found in the maternal serum (110). Data on transfer of carcinogenic agents is almost nonexistent. In animals N-nitrosodiethylamines have been found to be transmitted into the milk of nursing hamsters (111, 112) and rats (113), with subsequent development of tracheal cancers in the offspring (111). Transmission has not been as easily documented in humans (114). Aflatoxins, identified hepatocellular carcinogens, have been found in human breast milk (115) but have no known relationship to breast cancer. Alcohol has been documented to reach breast tissues (116).

There are few published studies analyzing lobular secretions or duct contents in the nonlactating breast. A study measuring blood and breast secretions in four nonlactating women after a high nitrite-nitrate meal detected no volatile nitrosamines in breast fluid but also found no change in blood levels (117).

The possibility of differences in metabolism and excretion of carcinogens exists but has not been studied.

RADIATION

Ionizing radiation is the only known risk factor for breast cancer that most probably acts by causing DNA damage. Exposure to radiation with low linear energy transfer (LET) increases the risk of breast cancer (118, 119). Individuals exposed to atomic bomb radiation at Hiroshima and Nagasaki (120, 121), radiated for postpartum mastitis (122) or various benign breast diseases (123), or subjected to multiple fluoroscopies for documentation of pneumothorax in treatment of tuberculosis (124, 125) have all had increased risk for the development of breast cancer (119). It appears that sensitivity to radiation induction of breast cancer varies by age at exposure and may be strongest in childhood (118–120), falling off with age after the teens and 20s and becoming negligible with exposure over age 40 to 50 (121, 123). Scatter radiation from mantle treatment of Hodgkin's disease does not appear to increase risk for breast cancer (126).

There is little or no synergism between radiation and other risk factors, including family history, ovarian hormone factors, or age at first childbirth. Women whose breasts were irradiated at the time of first childbirth but not subsequent births and those who subsequently developed cystic breast disease seemed to be at greater-than-expected risk (127).

Although risk is linear with no level at which exposure to ionizing radiation is totally safe (119), the relative risk of diagnostic x-rays and mammograms has been judged to be insignificant when compared with the benefits obtained from such x-rays (128).

OTHER FACTORS

Other factors that have been studied and found to have no association with the development of breast cancer include caffeine intake (129), cigarette smoking (78, 130, 131), and use of hair dyes (132). A viral etiology is not supported by the epidemiology of breast cancer and no B-type RNA virus has been found in human milk (29, 133). Prospective studies of psychological factors measured on Minnesota Multiphase Personality Inventory (MMPI) scales of depression, sensitization, and lying found no significant association of any psychological state or predisposing factor to later development of breast cancer (134). The small but consistent predominance of left-sided breast cancer is probably related to the fact that 55%

of women have a larger left breast, thus placing unequal volumes of tissue at risk (135).

THEORY OF CARCINOGENESIS

Moolgavkar and associates (136) have proposed a two-stage model for carcinogenesis in which clinical cancer is the end result of two discrete permanent events at the cellular level. The first event is a mutation that transforms a stem cell to an intermediate cell. A subsequent event then transforms the susceptible intermediate cell into a malignant cell. Anything that decreases the number of stem cells, generally by promoting differentiation, will lead to a decreased number of susceptible intermediate cells and thus to a decrease in cancer risk. Increased transformation of stem cells leads to more cells in the susceptible intermediate population. Increased cells at risk or increased exposure to agents provoking the second event then promotes malignant transformation (137).

Applied to breast cancer, this theory predicts the shape of the age-incidence curve and the effect of known risk factors. Breast cell growth is stimulated by hormones at puberty and becomes less active with decreased hormones at menopause. The first birth leads to permanent cell differentiation with removal of cells from the susceptible pool. The length of time from menarche to first birth determines the number of intermediate cells that will later be influenced by exposure to hormones and other agents. Early age at first birth thus protects the individual from normal risks.

Radiation increases risk by increasing the number of first cellular events transforming normal cells to susceptible intermediate cells. The effect of radiation is greater when cells are dividing rapidly, such as at puberty, and less at times when they are not. The longer intermediate cells are present before involution at menopause, the greater the time for exposure to the agents causing the second cellular event. Thus the radiation-induced risk for breast cancer is greatest in the teenage years and less with increasing age at exposure.

After the first transforming event, hormonal and other as yet unidentified influences act to promote transformation of intermediate cells to malignant cells throughout the individual's lifetime. As the number of intermediate cells varies, so also will the cancer risk induced by exposure to the cancer-promoting factor (35, 100). Risk factors for breast cancer are complex and probably interactive (138). Socioeconomic factors may affect reproductive patterns and then act through nutrition to affect body mass and composition, thereby influencing endo-

crine and metabolic process. Environmental contaminants and carcinogens may act directly on mammary cells to promote neoplasia (138).

NONATTRIBUTABLE RISK

While many hormonal, genetic, and environmental factors have been associated with the development of breast cancer, identified risk factors account for only 21% of breast cancer risk in women from age 30 to 54 and 29% from age 55 to 84 (139). Combinations of specific factors may lead to greater risk in a relatively small number of women, particularly those in the hereditary group. However, the great majority of risk owned by American women is nonattributable (80, 139). Because the interrelationship of identified risk factors and the ultimate causes of breast cancer remain unclear (138), it is not yet possible to identify changes in life-style or hormone status that could decrease mortality from breast cancer. All women must be considered at high risk for the development of breast cancer.

SUMMARY

Breast cancer is the most common cancer in American women, and second only to lung cancer as a cause of cancer death. Numerous reproductive and hormonal factors have been associated with its development. A small percentage of cases belong to a hereditary cancer syndrome. Epidemiologic characteristics of breast cancer are explained by the theory of carcinogenesis, which posits two irreversible events at the cellular level: In the first event, stem cells are transformed to intermediate cells, which are then susceptible to carcinogenic transformation. The second event completes the transformation process and leads to the development of clinical cancer.

Although identification of the individual with the hereditary form of breast cancer can lead to the use of detection and prevention measures to promote early diagnosis and treatment, this is a relatively small group of women and there will be no significant impact on the incidence of breast cancer in the general population. Since most risk is currently nonattributable and therefore not modifiable, all women must be considered at nearly equally high risk for the development of breast cancer. Any measures taken to promote earlier detection and treatment must therefore be directed at the entire female population. If the death toll from breast cancer is to be decreased significantly it must be through promotion of screening and application of effective treatment.

REFERENCES

1. American Cancer Society. Cancer statistics. 1988; CA 1988;38:5–22.
2. Waterhouse J, Muir C, Correa P, Shanmugaratnam K, Powell J. Cancer incidence in five continents. IARC Sci Publ No. 15 1976.
3. Kelsey JL. A review of the epidemiology of human breast cancer. Epidemiol Rev 1979;1:74–109.
4. Choi NW, Howe GR, Miller AB, et al. An epidemiologic study of breast cancer. Am Journal Epidemiol 1978;107:510–521.
5. Helmrich SP, Shapiro S, Rosenberg L, et al. Risk factors for breast cancer. Am J Epidemiol 1983;117:35–45.
6. Kelsey JL, Fischer DB, Holford TR, et al. Exogenous estrogens and other factors in the epidemiology of breast cancer. J Natl Cancer Inst 1981;67:327–333.
7. Lubin JH, Burns PE, Blot WJ, et al. Risk factors for breast cancer in women in northern Alberta, Canada, as related to age at diagnosis. J Natl Cancer Inst 1982;68:211–217.
8. Thein-Hlaing, Thein-Maung-Myint. Risk factors of breast cancer in Burma. Int J Cancer 1978;21:432–437.
9. Thomas DB, Persing JP, Hutchinson WB. Exogenous estrogens and other risk factors for breast cancer in women with benign breast diseases. J Natl Cancer Inst 1982;69:1017–1025.
10. Trichopoulos D, MacMahon B, Cole P. Menopause and breast cancer risk. J Natl Cancer Inst 1972;48:605–613.
11. Wallace RB, Sherman BM, Bean JA, Leeper JP, Treloar AE. Menstrual cycle patterns and breast cancer risk factors. Cancer Res 1978;38:4021–4024.
12. Grattarola R. The premenstrual endometrial pattern of women with breast cancer. Cancer 1964;17:1119–1122.
13. Brinton LA, Hoover R, Fraumeni JF. Epidemiology of minimal breast cancer. JAMA 1983;249:483–487.
14. Feinleib M. Breast cancer and artificial menopause: a cohort study. J Natl Cancer Inst 1968;41:315–329.
15. Hirayama T, Wynder EL. A study of the epidemiology of cancer of the breast: II. The influence of hysterectomy. Cancer 1962;15:28–38.
16. Korenman SG. The endocrinology of breast cancer. Cancer (suppl) 1980;46:874–878.
17. Henderson BE, Ross RK, Judd HL, Krailo MD, Pike MC. Do regular ovulatory cycles increase breast cancer risks? Cancer 1985;56:1206–1208.
18. Apter D, Vihko R. Early menarche, a risk factor for breast cancer, indicates early onset of ovulatory cycles. J Clin Endocrinol Metab 1983;57:82–86.
19. Henderson BE, Pike MC, Casagrande JT. Breast cancer and the estrogen window hypothesis. Lancet 1981;2:363–364.
20. Pike MC, Henderson BE, Casagrande JT, Rosario I, Gray GE. Oral contraceptive use and early abortion as risk factors for breast cancer in young women. Br J Cancer 1981;43:72–76.
21. Henderson BE, Ross RK, Pike MC, Casagrande JT. Endogenous hormones as a major factor in human cancer. Cancer Res 1982;42:3232–3239.
22. Trichopoulos D, Brown JB, Garas J, Papaioannou A, MacMahon B. Elevated urine estrogen and pregnanediol levels in daughters of breast cancer patients. J Natl Cancer Inst 1981;67:603–606.
23. Ferguson DJP, Anderson TJ. Morphological evaluation of cell turnover in relation to the menstrual cycle in the "resting" human breast. Br J Cancer 1981;44:177–181.
24. Vogel PM, Georgiade NG, Fetter BF, Vogel S, McCarty KS. The correlation of histologic changes in the human breast with the menstrual cycle. Am J Pathol 1981;104:23–34.
25. Meyer JS. Cell proliferation in normal human breast ducts, fibroadenomas and other ductal hyperplasias measured by nuclear labeling with tritiated thymidine: Effects of menstrual phase, age, and oral contraceptive hormones. Hum Pathol 1977;8:67–81.
26. Boston Collaborative Drug Surveillance Program. Reserpine and breast cancer. Lancet 1974;2:669–671.
27. Kodlin D, McCarthy N. Reserpine and breast cancer. Cancer 1978;41:761–768.
28. Laska EM, Siegel C, Meisner M, Fischer S, Wanderling J. Matched-pairs study of reserpine use and breast cancer. Lancet 1975;2:296–300.
29. Henderson BE, Powell D, Rosario I, et al. An epidemiologic study of breast cancer. J Natl Cancer Inst 1974;53:609–614.
30. Byers T, Graham S, Rzepka T, Marshall J. Lactation and breast cancer: evidence for a negative association in premenopausal women. Am J Epidemiol 1985;121:664–674.
31. Bulbrook RD, Hayward JL, Spicer CC. Relation between urinary androgen and corticoid excretion and subsequent breast cancer. Lancet 1971;2:395–398.
32. Wang DY, Bulbrook RD, Hayward JL. Urinary and plasma androgens and their relation to familial risk of breast cancer. Eur J Cancer 1975;11:873–877.
33. Lilienfeld AM, Coombs J, Bross IDJ, Chamberlain A. Marital and reproductive experience in a community wide epidemiological study of breast cancer. Johns Hopkins Med J 1975;136:157–162.
34. MacMahon B, Purde M, Cramer D, Hint E. Association of breast cancer risk with age at first and subsequent births: A study in the population of the Estonian Republic. J Natl Cancer Inst 1982;69:1035–1038.
35. MacMahon B, Cole P, Lin TM, et al. Age at first birth and beast cancer risk. A summary of an international study. Bull WHO 1970;43:209–221.
36. Vessey MP, McPherson K, Yeates D, Doll R. Oral contraceptive use and abortion before first term pregnancy in relation to breast cancer risk. Br J Cancer 1982;45:327–331.
37. Musey VC, Collins DC, Musey PI, Martino-Saltzman D, Preedy JRK. Long-term effect of a first pregnancy on the secretion of prolactin. N Engl J Med 1987;316:229–234.
38. Brinton LA, Hoover R, Szklo M, Fraumeni JF. Oral contraceptives and breast cancer. Int J Epidemiol 1982;11:316–322.

39. Harris NV, Weiss NS, Francis AM, Polissar L. Breast cancer in relation to patterns of oral contraceptive use. Am J Epidemiol 1982;116:643–651.

40. Jick H, Walker AM, Watkins RN, et al. Oral contraceptives and breast cancer. Am J Epidemiol 1980;112:577–585.

41. Lipnick RJ, Buring JE, Hennekins CH, et al. Oral contraceptives and breast cancer. A prospective cohort study. JAMA 1986;255:58–61.

42. Miller DR, Rosenberg L, Kaufman DW, Schottenfeld D, Stolley PD, Shapiro S. Breast cancer risk in relation to early oral contraceptive use. Obstet Gynecol 1986;68:863–868.

43. Royal College of General Practitioners. Breast cancer and oral contraceptives: findings of the Royal College of General Practitioners' study. Br Med J 1981;282:2089–2093.

44. Sattin RW, Rubin GL, Wingo PA, Webster LA, Ory HW. Oral contraceptive use and the risk of breast cancer. Steroid Hormone Study of the Centers for Disease Control and the National Institute of Child Health and Human Development. N Engl J Med 1986;315:405–411.

45. Schlesselman JJ, Stadel BV, Murray P, et al. Breast cancer in relation to early use of oral contraceptives. No evidence of a latent effect. JAMA 1988;259:1828–1833.

46. Trapido EJ. A prospective cohort study of oral contraceptives and breast cancer. J Natl Cancer Inst 1981;67:1011–1015.

47. Vessey M, Baron J, Doll R, McPherson K. Yeates D. Oral contraceptives and breast cancer: final report of an epidemiological study. Br J Cancer 1983;47:455–462.

48. McPherson K, Neil A, Vessey MP, Doll R. Oral contraceptives and breast cancer. Lancet 1983;1:1414–1415.

49. Meirik O, Lund E, Adami H-O, Bergstrom R, Christoffersen T, Bergsjo P. Oral contraceptive use and breast cancer in young women: a joint national case-control study in Sweden and Norway. Lancet 1986;2:650–654.

50. Pike MC, Henderson BE, Krailo MD, Duke A, Roy S. Breast cancer in young women and use of oral contraceptives. Possible modifying effect of formulation and age at use. Lancet 1983;2:926–930.

51. Fasal E. Paffenbarger RS. Oral contraceptives as related to cancer and benign lesions of the breast. J Natl Cancer Inst 1975;55:767–773.

52. LiVolsi VA, Stadel BV, Kelsey JL, Holford TR, White C. Fibrocystic breast disease in oral contraceptive users. A histopathological evaluation of epithelial atypia. N Engl J Med 1978;299:381–385.

53. Longman SM, Buehring GC. Oral contraceptives and breast cancer. In vitro effect of contraceptive steroids on human mammary cell growth. Cancer 1987;59:281–287.

54. Hiatt RA, Bawol R, Friedman GD, Hoover R. Exogenous estrogen and breast cancer after bilateral oophorectomy. Lancet 1984;54:139–144.

55. Hulka BS, Chambless LE, Deubner DC, Wilkinson WE. Breast cancer and estrogen replacement therapy. Am J Obstet Gynecol 1982;143:638–644.

56. Kaufman DW, Miller DR, Rosenberg L, et al. Noncontraceptive estrogen use and the risk of breast cancer. JAMA 1984;252:63–67.

57. Wingo PA, Layde PM, Lee NC, Rubin G, Ory HW. The risk of breast cancer in postmenopausal women who have used estrogen replacement therapy. JAMA 1987;257:209–215.

58. Hoover R, Glass A, Finkle WD, Azevedo D, Milne K. Conjugated estrogens and breast cancer risk in women. J Natl Cancer Inst 1981;67:815–820.

59. Hoover R, Gray LA, Coles P, MacMahon B. Menopausal estrogens and breast cancer. N Engl J Med 1976;295:401–405.

60. Ross RK, Paganini-Hill A, Gerkins VR, et al. A case-control study of menopausal estrogen therapy and breast cancer. JAMA 1980;243:1635–1639.

61. Brinton LA, Hoover RN, Szklo M, Fraumeni JF. Menopausal estrogen use and risk of breast cancer. Cancer 1981;47:2517–2522.

62. Jick H, Walker AM, Watkins RN, et al. Replacement estrogens and breast cancer. Am J Epidemiol 1980;112:586–594.

63. Beral V, Colwell L. Randomized trial of high doses of stilboestrol and ethisterane in pregnancy: long-term followup of mothers. Br Med J 1980;281:1098–1101.

64. Bartow SA, Pathok DR, Black WC, Key CR, Teaf SR. Prevalence of benign, atypical and malignant breast lesions in populations at different risk for breast cancer. A forensic autopsy study. Cancer 1987;60:2751–2760.

65. Donnelly PK, Baker KW, Carney JA, O'Fallon WM. Benign breast lesions and subsequent breast carcinoma in Rochester, Minnesota. Mayo Clinic Proc 1975;50:650–656.

66. Hutchinson WB, Thomas DB, Hamlin WD, Roth GJ, Peterson AV, Williams B. Risk of breast cancer in women with benign breast disease. J Natl Cancer Inst 1980;65:13–20.

67. Kodlin D, Winger EE, Morgenstern NL, Chen U. Chronic mastopathy and breast cancer: a followup study. Cancer 1977;39:2603–2607.

68. Page DL, Vander Zwaag R, Rogers LW, Williams LT, Walker WE, Hartmann WH. Relation between component parts of fibrocystic disease complex and breast cancer. J Natl Cancer Inst 1978;61:1055–1063.

69. Black MM, Barclay THC, Cutler SS, Hankey SJ, Hankey BF, Asire AJ. Association of atypical characteristics of benign breast lesions with subsequent risk of breast cancer. Cancer 1972;29:338–343.

70. Dupont WD, Page DL. Risk factors for breast cancer in women with proliferative breast disease. N Engl J Med 1985;312:146–151.

71. McCarty KS Jr, Kesterson GHD, Wilkinson WE, Georgiade N. Histopathologic study of subcutaneous mastectomy specimens from patients with carcinoma of the contralateral breast. Surg Gynecol Obstet 1978;147:682–688.

72. Ohuchi N, Abe R, Kasai M. Possible cancerous change of intraductal papillomas of the breast. Cancer 1984;54:605–611.

73. Page DL, Dupont WD, Rogers LW, Landenberger M. Intraductal carcinoma of the breast; followup after biopsy only. Cancer 1982;49:751–758.

74. Beller FK, Nienhaus H, Neidner W, Holzgreve W. Bilateral breast cancer. The frequency of undiagnosed cancer. Am J Obstet Gynecol 1986;155:247–255.

75. Nielsen M, Jensen J. Andersen J. Precancerous and cancerous breast lesions during lifetime and at autopsy. A study of 83 women. Cancer 1984;54:612–615.

76. Parkin DM, Stjernsward J, Muir CS. Estimates of the workwide frequency of twelve major cancers. Bull WHO 1984;62:163–182.

77. Armstrong B, Doll R. Environmental factors and cancer incidence and mortality in different countries with special reference to dietary practices. Int J Cancer 1975;15:617–631.

78. Williams RR, Horm JW. Association of cancer sites with tobacco and alcohol consumption and socioeconomic status of patients: interview study from the Third National Cancer Survey. J Natl Cancer Inst 1977;58:525–547.

79. Henderson BE, Pike MC, Ross RK. Epidemiology and risk factors. In: Bonadonna G, ed. Breast cancer: diagnosis and management. New York: John Wiley & Sons, 1984:3:15–33.

80. Wynder EL, MacCornack FA, Stellman SD. The epidemiology of breast cancer in 785 United States caucasian women. Cancer 1978;41:2341–2354.

81. Adami H-O, Rimsten A, Stenkvist B, Vegelius J. Reproductive history and risk of breast cancer. A case-control study in an unselected Swedish population. Cancer 1978;41:747–757.

82. Lynch HT, Fain PR, Golgar D, Albano WA, Maikiard JA, McKenna P. Familial breast cancer and its recognition in an oncology clinic. Cancer 1981;47:2730–2739.

83. Anderson DE. A genetic study of human breast cancer, J Natl Cancer Inst 1972;48:1029–1034.

84. Anderson DE. Genetic study of breast cancer: identification of a high-risk group. Cancer 1974;34:1090–1097.

85. Bain C, Speizer FE, Rosner B, Belanger C, Hennekens CH. Family history of breast cancer as a risk indicator for the disease. Am J Epidemiol 1980;111:301–308.

86. Sattin RW, Rubin GL, Webster LA, et al. Family history and the risk of breast cancer. JAMA 1985;253:1908–1913.

87. King M-C, Bishop DT, Preliminary analysis for linkage of glutamate-pryruvate transaminase and breast cancer susceptibility in a Morman kindred. In: Cains J, Lyon JL, Skolnick M, eds. Banbury Report 4. Cancer incidence in defined populations. New York: Cold Spring Harbor Laboratory, 1980:379–384.

88. King M-C, Go RCP, Elston RC, Lynch HT, Petrakis NL. Allele increasing susceptibility to human breast cancer may be linked to the glutamate-pyruvate transaminase locus. Science 1980;208:406–408.

89. Albano WA, Recabaren JA, Lynch HT, et al. Natural history of hereditary cancer of the breast and colon. CA 1982;50:360–363.

90. Lynch HT, Albano WA, Danes BS, et al. Genetic predisposition to breast cancer. Cancer 1984;53:612–622.

91. Henderson BE, Gerkins V, Rosario I, Casagrande JT, Pike MC. Elevated serum levels of estrogen and prolactin in daughters of patients with breast cancer. N Engl J Med 1975;293:790–795.

92. Wolfe JN, Albert S, Belle S, Salane M. Familial influences on breast parenchymal patterns. Cancer 1980;46:2433–2437.

93. Wolfe JN, Albert S, Belle S, Salane M. Breast parenchymal patterns: analysis of 332 incident breast carcinomas. Am J Roentgenol 1982;138:113–118.

94. Hirayama T. Epidemiology of breast cancer with special reference to the role of diet. Prev Med 1978;7:173–195.

95. Miller AB, Kelly A, Choi NW, et al. A study of diet and breast cancer. Am J Epidemiol 1978;107:499–509.

96. Katsouyanni K, Willett W, Trichopoulos D, et al. Risk of breast cancer among Greek women in relation to nutrient intake. Cancer 1988;61:181–185.

97. Hiatt RA, Friedman GD, Bawol RD, Ury HK. Breast cancer and serum cholesterol. J Natl Cancer Inst 1982;68:885–889.

98. Kinlen LJ. Mortality in relation to abstinence from meat in certain orders of religious sisters in Britain. In: Cains J, Lyon JL, Skolnick M, eds. Banbury Report 4. Cancer incidence in defined populations. New York: Cold Spring Harbor Laboratory, 1980:135–139.

99. Phillips RL, Kuzma JW, Lotz TM. Cancer mortality among comparable members versus nonmembers of the Seventh-Day Adventist church. In: Cains J, Lyon JL, Skolnick M, eds. Banbury Report 4. Cancer incidence in defined populations. New York, Cold Spring Harbor Laboratory, 1980:93–102.

100. Willett WC, Stampfer MJ, Colditz GA, Rosner BA, Hennekens CH, Speizer FE. Dietary fat and the risk of breast cancer. N Engl J Med 1987;316:22–28.

101. Mettlin C. Diet and the epidemiology of human breast cancer. Cancer 1984;53:605–611.

102. DeWaard F, Baanders-von Halewijn EA. A prospective study in general practice on breast cancer risk in postmenopausal women. Int J Cancer 1974;14:153–160.

103. DeWaard F. Breast cancer incidence and nutritional status with particular reference to body weight and height. Cancer Res 1975;35:3351–3356.

104. DeWaard F, Cornelis JP, Aoki K, Yoshida M. Breast cancer incidence according to weight and height in two cities of the Netherlands and in Aichi Prefecture, Japan. Cancer 1977;40:1269–1275.

105. Lin TM, Chen KP, MacMahon B. Epidemiologic characteristics of cancer of the breast in Taiwan. Cancer 1971;2:1497–1504.

106. Mirra AP, Cole P, MacMahon B. Breast cancer in an area of high parity: Sao Paulo, Brazil. Cancer Res 1971;31:77–83.

107. Schatzkin A, Jones DY, Hoover RN, et al. Alcohol consumption and breast cancer in the epidemiologic followup study of the first national

health and nutrition examination survey. N Engl J Med 1987;316:1169–1173.

108. Willett WC, Stampfer MJ, Colditz GA, Rosner BA, Hennekens CH, Speizer FE. Moderate alcohol consumption and the risk of breast cancer. N Engl J Med 1987;316:1174–1180.

109. Harris RE, Wynder EL. Breast cancer and alcohol consumption. A study in weak associations. JAMA 1988;259:2867–2871.

110. Knowles JA. Excretion of drugs in milk—a review. J Pediatr 1965;66:1068–1982.

111. Mohr U, Althoff J. Carcinogenic activity of aliphatic nitrosamines via the mothers milk in offspring of Syrian golden hamsters. Proc Soc Biol Med 1971;136:1007–1009.

112. Spielhoff R, Bresch H, Honig M, Mohr U. Milk as a transport agent for diethyl nitrosamine in Syrian golden hamsters. J Natl Cancer Inst 1974;53:281–282.

113. Schoental R, Gough TA, Webb KS. Carcinogens in rat milk. Transfer of injested diethylnitrosamine into the milk of lactating rats. Br J Cancer 1974;30:238–240.

114. Lakritz L, Pensabene JW. Survey of human milk for volatile N-nitrosamines and the influence of diet on their formation. Food Chem Toxicol 1984;22:721–724.

115. Wild CP, Pionneau FA, Montesano R, Mutiro CF, Chetsanga CJ. Aflatoxin detected in human breast milk by immunoassay. Int J Cancer 1987;40:328–333.

116. Lawton ME. Alcohol in breast milk. Aust NZ J Obstet Gynaecol 1985;25:71–73.

117. Melikan AA, LaVoie EJ, Hoffmann D, Wynder EL. Volatile nitrosamines: analysis in breast fluid and blood of non-lactating women. Food Cosmet Toxicol 1981;19:757–759.

118. Boice JD Jr, Land CE, Shore RE, Norman JE, Tokunaga M. Risk of breast cancer following low-dose radiation exposure. Radiology 1979;131:589–597.

119. Land CE, Boice JD Jr, Shore RE, Norman JE, Tokunaga M. Breast cancer risk from low-dose exposure to ionizing radiation. Results of parallel analysis of three exposed populations of women. J Natl Cancer Inst 1980;65:353–376.

120. McGregor DH, Land CE, Choi K, et al. Breast cancer among atom bomb survivors, Hiroshima and Nagasaki 1950–1969. J Natl Cancer Inst 1977;59:798–811.

121. Tokunaga M, Land CE, Yamamoto T, et al. Breast cancer among atomic bomb survivors. In: Boice JD Jr., Fraumen JF Jr, eds. Radiation carcinogenesis: epidemiology and biological significance. New York: Raven Press, 1984:45–56.

122. Shore RE, Hempelmann LH, Kowaluk E, et al. Breast neoplasms in women treated with x-rays for acute postpartum mastitis. J Natl Cancer Inst 1977;59:813–822.

123. Baral E, Larsson L-E, Mattsson B. Breast cancer following radiation of the breast. Cancer 1977;40:2905–2910.

124. MacKenzie I. Breast cancer following multiple fluoroscopies. Br J Cancer 1965;19:1–8.

125. Myrden JA, Hiltz JE. Breast cancer following multiple fluoroscopies during artificial pneumothorax of pulmonary tuberculosis. Canad Med Assoc J 1969;100:1032–1034.

126. Janjan NA, Wilson F, Gillin M, et al. Mammary carcinoma developing after radiotherapy and chemotherapy for Hodgkin's disease. Cancer 1988;61:252–254.

127. Shore RE, Woodard ED, Hempelmann LH, Pasternack BS. Synergism between radiation and other risk factors for beast cancer. Prev Med 1980;9:815–822.

128. Adelstein SJ, Uncertainty and relative risks of radiation exposure. JAMA 1987;258:655–657.

129. Phelps HM, Phelps CE. Caffeine ingestion and breast cancer. A negative correlation. Cancer 1988;61:1051–1054.

130. Rosenberg L, Schwingl PJ, Kaufman DW, et al. Breast cancer and cigarette smoking. N Engl J Med 1984;310:92–94.

131. Stockwell HG, Lyman GH. Cigarette smoking and the risk of female reproductive cancer. Am J Obstet Gynecol 1987;157:35–40.

132. Hennekins CH, Speizer FE, Rosner B, Bain CJ, Belanger C, Peto R. Use of permanent hair dyes and cancer among registered nurses. Lancet 1979;1:1390–1393.

133. Henderson BE. Type B virus and human breast cancer. Cancer 1974;34:1386–1389.

134. Hahn RC, Petitti DB. Minnesota Multiphasic Personality Inventory–rated depression and the incidence of breast cancer. Cancer 1988;61:845–848.

135. Senie RT, Rosen PP, Lesser ML, Snyder RE, Schottenfeld D, Duthie K. Epidemiology of breast carcinoma. II: factors related to the predominance of left-side disease. Cancer 1980;46:1705–1713.

136. Moolgavkar SH, Day NE, Stevens RG. Two-stage model for carcinogenesis: epidemiology of breast cancer in females. J Natl Cancer Inst 1980;65:559–569.

137. Moolgavkar SH, Knudson AG Jr. Mutation and cancer. A model for human carcinogenesis. J Natl Cancer Inst 1981;66:1037–1052.

138. Petrakis NL. Genetic factors in the etiology of breast cancer. Cancer 1977;39:2709-2715.

139. Seidman H, Stellman SD, Mushinski MH. A different perspective on breast cancer risk factors: some implications of the nonattributable risks. CA 1982;32:301–313.

19

Surgery for Breast Cancer

Douglas Marchant

Untreated breast cancer has a surprisingly predictable 5-year survival, and controversy concerning optimal management has existed since the earliest descriptions by Celsus and Galen in the first and second centuries AD (1). Contemporary treatment must therefore reflect an understanding of the natural history of breast cancer and the necessity for long-term follow-up.

HISTORY

Surgical removal of the breast was described in the first and second centuries AD. The lesions observed were far advanced and the treatment, unsuccessful. Later refinements in surgical technique resulted in lower operative mortality, but cures were infrequent. In 1867 C.H. Moore (2) suggested that the entire breast be removed with a wide margin of skin. Halsted's mastectomy was first mentioned in 1891, and by 1894 he had performed 50 "complete mastectomies (3)." This radical mastectomy, as the operation came to be known, was enthusiastically adopted in this country and abroad. Because the lesions for which the Halsted procedure was designed were far advanced, the operation was not associated with an increase in cure, although there was a dramatic reduction in chest wall recurrences. During the next several decades, the results of the radical mastectomy improved, principally due to earlier diagnosis and more selective use of the operation.

Because the radical mastectomy did not include resection of the internal mammary lymph nodes, it was suggested that the classic operation be extended to include a resection of the internal mammary nodes and the chest wall. In 1951, Urban (4) described an extended radical mastectomy that included an en bloc dissection of the chest wall.

It is now widely accepted that cancer of the breast is a systemic disease and that the majority of patients will not be cured even with the most extensive local treatments. This has resulted in a more conservative approach and participation of the patient in treatment planning. These less severe surgical procedures have largely replaced the classic Halsted radical mastectomy.

ROLE OF THE PRIMARY CARE PHYSICIAN

Most patients with breast cancer are referred to surgeons for appropriate additional evaluation and treatment. However, the primary care physician, who should participate in these consultations, has these three responsibilities:

1. wise counsel concerning risk factors;
2. the performance of a satisfactory breast examination; and
3. an understanding of diagnostic studies, including screening of asymptomatic patients.

Although this information is presented in other chapters it is important to emphasize the significance of screening and the evaluation and treatment of the occult lesion. Mammography is the only screening method that can provide a geographic representation of an abnormal finding. Recent consensus meetings have resulted in a uniform set of guidelines for screening. However, only 11% of the population are being screened according to these guidelines. As more patients are screened, an increasing number of occult lesions will be discovered. These include asymmetric densities and the geographic cluster of microcalcifications. In either case, a decision must be made to repeat the films to clarify the diagnosis, to repeat the films in several months to assess stability, or to recommend "localization" and biopsy.

231

If localization is recommended, the patient should be referred to a surgeon and a radiologist experienced in this technique. Most of these lesions are benign; however, approximately 15 to 20% represent carcinoma, either in situ or invasive. Biopsy often becomes part of the definitive treatment.

If localization is recommended the patient is taken to the radiology suite, where under local anesthesia a small needle is placed in the vicinity of the occult lesion. Since the majority of these biopsies are performed under local anesthesia, it is essential that the needle be placed as close to the lesion as possible. The patient is taken to the operating suite and a biopsy is performed. The incision must be chosen carefully since the biopsy may represent the definitive treatment. The area in question is removed and submitted for specimen radiography. If the lesion is present, the wound is closed. The pathologist must obtain tissue for receptor analysis and mark the margins with ink to determine the completeness of the incision when the permanent microscopic sections are reviewed (see Chapter 16).

It should be obvious that treatment planning requires a multidisciplinary approach including the primary care physician, the radiologist, surgeon, medical oncologist, and radiation oncologist. It is the responsibility of the primary care physician to be aware of these "centers of excellence."

THE DOMINANT MASS

The discovery of a mass is a judgement call. It must be emphasized that once a lesion has been described as a mass, measured, or drawn on a diagram, it must be resolved. The single exception is the young teenager for whom elective excision is appropriate. Physical examination will be discussed in other chapters, however, it is important to emphasize that the physician must look for subtle changes. The appearance of a large mass, skin thickening, or dimpling imply late disease, for which any treatment usually is ineffective.

Once it has been decided that a mass is present, several pretreatment evaluations are required. The first is the mammogram. This is performed not only to confirm the presence of the mass but to determine whether there are other nonpalpable lesions in the same or in the contralateral breast. It must be emphasized that a negative mammogram in the presence of a three-dimensional mass does not preclude referral for open biopsy (see Chapter 16).

The physician should describe the history in detail and the findings, preferably using a diagram. If cancer is discovered, a staging procedure is utilized. This refers to the grouping of patients according to the extent of their disease. This is useful in determining the correct surgical procedure and estimating prognosis. Breast cancer initially is staged on a clinical basis, i.e., the physical examination and laboratory or radiologic evaluations. The most widely used staging system is the one adopted by the International Union Against Cancer (UICC) and the American Joint Committee on Cancer (AJCC), which is based on the findings prior to surgery and is known as the TNM system (i.e., tumor, nodes, metastases); see Chapter 16. Additional surgical staging includes the histology, nodal status, and receptor analysis.

SURGICAL OPTIONS FOR LOCAL TREATMENT

Several factors influence the definitive surgical treatment for breast cancer. Important considerations include the size and histology of the lesion and the skill and experience of the multidisciplinary team and the wishes of the patient. Treatments discussed include

1. radical mastectomy;
2. modified radical mastectomy;
3. simple mastectomy;
4. subcutaneous mastectomy;
5. quadrantectomy, including axillary dissection; and
6. wide local excision, with or without axillary dissection.

There is no doubt that the conservative approach appeals to many patients; however, statistics clearly indicate that most patients are treated with the modified radical mastectomy. This operation has replaced the Halsted radical mastectomy. The patient care and research committee of the American College of Surgeons' Commission on Cancer reported in a 1982 audit that 55% of patients treated had undergone a modified radical mastectomy and 28% had a Halsted radical operation. Comparable figures from the 1978 audit revealed that nearly 50% of the women treated had a Halsted mastectomy and only 28%, a modified radical mastectomy. It is estimated that at least 80% of all patients undergoing surgical treatment for breast cancer have the modified radical procedure (5).

RADICAL MASTECTOMY

There are few indications today for the classic radical mastectomy. This operation assumed that cancer spread locally, involving the deeper structures of the breast and the pectoral

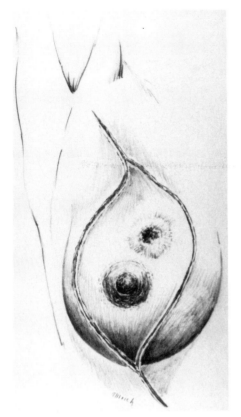

Figure 19.1. Vertical incision for radical mastectomy, encompassing lesion with a skin margin of at least 4 cm and extending toward axilla.

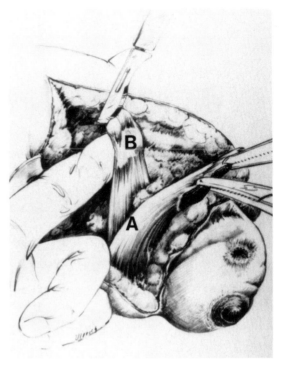

Figure 19.2. Radical mastectomy. Insertion of the pectoralis major (A) has been cut and the muscle reflected medially. The insertion of the pectoralis minor (B) is being severed to expose the axillary contents.

muscles, and then, in a predictable manner, the regional nodes. The operation requires a vertical incision with excision of sufficient skin to include the primary tumor and the nipple-areolar complex (Fig. 19.1). Relatively thin skin flaps are developed medially and laterally or if the incision is more oblique or even transverse, superiorly and inferiorly. The pectoralis major muscle is identified and removed, leaving the clavicular head. It is divided at its humoral and sternal attachments. At this point, the dissection is carried laterally toward the latissimus dorsi muscle until the pectoralis minor is encountered. This is divided at the corocoid process and axillary dissection is performed (Figs. 19.2 and 19.3).

This operation is a more standardized procedure than are the operations described as modified mastectomy. It is essentially the same procedure that was performed by Halsted almost 100 years ago and, as previously noted, is largely replaced today by the modified operation. Large lesions are probably best treated with external radiation and then removed; lesions that involve the pectoral fascia can be ex-

cised with a portion of the muscle and the area then treated with postoperative radiation.

There are four complications associated with the radical mastectomy: infection, necrosis of the skin, seroma, and edema.

Infection is rare and occurs in less than 10% of cases. It is more common in older patients, and treatment with prolonged catheter drainage and appropriate antibiotics will resolve the problem.

Skin necrosis is unusual since very thin skin flaps are the exception rather than the rule. Some patients have "very thin skin," making it difficult to obtain a safe plane for dissection, and discrete areas may as a result be poorly vascularized. It is rare for these areas to require additional treatment, and healing usually takes place by secondary intention.

A seroma may develop if the drains are removed prematurely. This complication requires continued aspiration, which may result in infection. This complication can be avoided by providing continued drainage until the skin flaps are securely attached to the chest wall (Fig. 19.4).

Lymphedema is unusual in the early postoperative period, but the later development of this complication is a distressing problem for

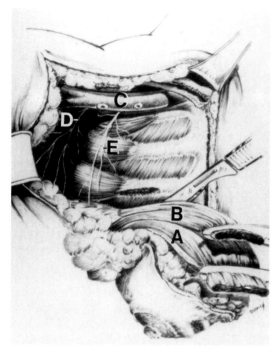

Figure 19.3. Radical mastectomy. The fat, connective tissue and lymphatics still attached to the breast and pectoral muscles (A, B) have been swept away from the undersurface of the axillary vein (C). The thoracodorsal nerve (D) and the long thoracic nerve (E) have been preserved. The latter lies on the serratus anterior muscle.

the patient. It usually results from a low-grade infection in the hand or arm, with ascending lymphangitis. The patient must be instructed to avoid trauma to the hand or arm; if infection does occur, appropriate antibiotics must be administered promptly.

MODIFIED RADICAL MASTECTOMY

This is, in essence, a total mastectomy and axillary node dissection with preservation of the pectoral muscles. There are a number of modifications including the removal of the pectoralis minor muscle. Most contemporary surgeons agree, however, that the operation today is best performed with preservation of both the pectoralis major and the pectoralis minor muscles. The axillary dissection is more difficult than in the true radical mastectomy, but with appropriate relaxation of the muscles a satisfactory dissection can be performed.

A modified mastectomy is the procedure of choice for patients with large operable lesions, for patients with smaller lesions and relatively small breasts, and for patients who refuse conservative treatment. It is also the procedure of

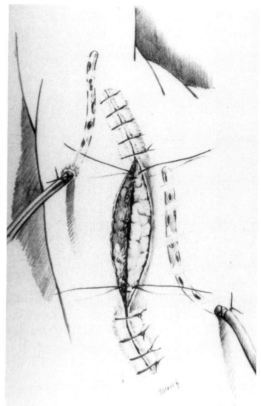

Figure 19.4. Radical mastectomy. The incision is being closed in two layers, leaving one suction drain in the axilla and one on the chest wall.

choice for large lesions demonstrated by mammography and proven by biopsy. In some cases the incision chosen for open biopsy precludes conservative treatment and mastectomy must then be performed. For example, if a circumareolar incision is chosen and the lesion is at some distance from the nipple, too much breast tissue must be removed to achieve a cosmetic closure.

The arm is placed on an arm board at right angles to the patient or elevated on a cross bar to relax the pectoralis muscles and permit a more complete axillary dissection (Fig. 19.5). A transverse incision is utilized for the majority of lesions (Fig. 19.6). Some patients will request immediate or delayed reconstruction which can be performed more cosmetically with this incision. Following the axillary dissection, the arm should be returned to the patient's side. This is helpful in planning the closure. Skin flaps are developed superiorly and inferiorly, and the dissection is carried down to the chest wall medially. The breast is then removed together with the pectoralis major fascia. The dissection is continued until the hu-

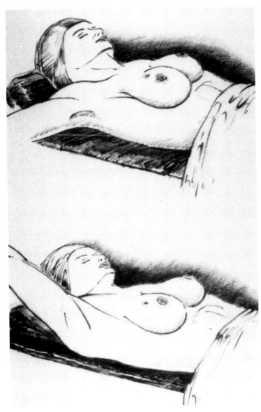

Figure 19.5. Modified radical mastectomy. The patient's position for the operation; above, arm at right angles to the trunk; below, arm extended upward (Paté).

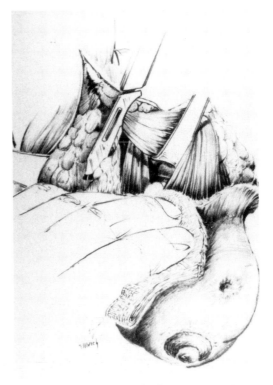

Figure 19.6. Modified radical mastectomy. Breast has been mobilized and is ready for removal above the muscles. Insertion of pectoralis major is being retracted to allow dissection of axillary lymphatics at levels I & II.

moral head of the pectoralis major muscle is identified together with the costocoracoid fascia. When this fascia is entered, the axillary fat is immediately apparent, and axillary dissection is performed (Fig. 19.7). The nodes lateral to the pectoralis major muscle and immediately beneath the pectoralis minor muscle are removed. With proper exposure and sharp dissection, a minimum of 12 to 15 axillary nodes should be recovered. The number of nodes actually removed depends on the thoroughness of the surgeon and the diligence of the pathologist at the surgical desk. Repeated recovery of one or two nodes suggests either that the surgeon is not performing a true modified radical mastectomy or that the pathologist is careless in locating the lymph nodes in the specimen. Drainage is provided by suction catheters placed under the medial flap and in the axilla. These exit through separate stab wounds and, as noted previously, are removed when all drainage has ceased. The wound is closed in layers, being careful to obtain a cosmetic closure. A simple nonpressure dressing is all that is required. The scar resulting from this operation is usually not unsightly.

TOTAL (SIMPLE) MASTECTOMY

This operation is described as a simple or total mastectomy, but it is a radical procedure as far as the patient is concerned. It implies that the entire breast including the nipple areolar complex and the fascia of the pectoralis major muscle is removed. The modified radical mastectomy previously described is in essence a simple mastectomy with an axillary dissection. Thus, the operative procedure for the simple mastectomy is identical to that of the initial stages of the modified radical mastectomy. The location of the incision is carefully chosen and the skin flaps meticulously developed.

The indications for this procedure are:

1. in situ carcinoma—ductal or lobular (DCIS and LCIS);
2. recurrences after partial mastectomy with axillary dissection, or axillary irradiation with or without breast irradiation;

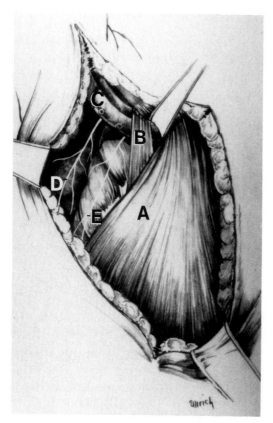

Figure 19.7. Modifed radical mastectomy. Breast has been removed, leaving pectoral muscles (A, B), axillary vein (C), and thoracodorsal and long thoracic nerves (D, E) intact.

3. bulky or ulcerated lesions or distant metastases when local control will improve the quality of life;
4. elderly patients or those who are poor operative risks and in whom there is no axillary adenopathy and no evidence of distant disease; or
5. selected cases when prophylactic removal of the opposite breast is recommended.

There is considerable debate concerning the best treatment for patients with documented in situ ductal carcinoma (6–8). The standard treatment continues to be total mastectomy. However, there are selected cases for whom conservative surgery (i.e., quadrantectomy or wide local excision) may be considered. Newer protocols include the addition of postoperative radiation therapy.

Local recurrence following appropriate treatment is unusual, occurring in less than 10% of cases. Recurrences following conservative treatment are managed by removal of the breast, and the prognosis appears to be equal to that following initial modified radical mastectomy.

The use of total mastectomy in elderly and debilitated patients requires some explanation. These lesions usually are discovered by physical examination. The diagnosis can be confirmed by open biopsy using local anesthesia or by fine-needle aspiration. Because adjuvant chemotherapy is not an option for these patients, total removal of the breast without axillary dissection is appropriate, and, depending on estrogen receptor status, tamoxifen can be routinely administered without significant side effects. The operation can be quickly performed, with minimal blood loss and a decreased hospital stay.

Finally, for selected patients who request or who are candidates for prophylactic mastectomy, a total mastectomy is the operation of choice. It is the only operation that completely removes all the breast tissue. A subcutaneous mastectomy is inadequate. Studies have indicated that even with the most carefully performed subcutaneous mastectomy, breast tissue remains under the areola and is found in other locations in 80% of the cases. It is not a prophylactic procedure, although there are no studies indicating whether removal of 80% of the breast tissue would yield an equivalent reduction in risk. In addition, the subcutaneous mastectomy may result in a less-than-satisfactory cosmetic result. Some complications are associated with this operation, including immediate hematoma and subsequent scarring and fibrosis.

BREAST PRESERVATION PROCEDURES

Several consensus development conferences have dealt with the treatment of primary breast cancer to determine treatment recommendations that provide the best chance for disease-free survival. These conferences have considered whether conservative treatment including dissection of the axillary lymph nodes followed by irradiation to the breast is as effective as the modified or radical mastectomy (9–14).

While the concept of conservative treatment has gained favor, there has been continued controversy concerning the technical details of the surgery and the radiation therapy. Several definitions dealing with these issues were proposed at a consensus conference in New York in 1985 (15):

Conservative surgery implies wide local excision and resection of the tumor with 1 or 2 cm of adjacent breast tissue designed to provide clear margins.

Quadrantectomy implies the resection of the tumor with the involved quadrant of the breast including the overlying skin. The terms lumpectomy and segmental mastectomy are imprecise.

Axillary dissection implies the removal of the axillary contents from the tail of the breast to the latissimus dorsi, the axillary vein superiorly, and the lateral border of the pectoralis minor medially. The use of the term axillary sampling is discouraged because it is not a precise definition concerning the extent of the surgical procedure performed.

The use of breast conservation procedures involves four important criteria: (*a*) patient selection; (*b*) surgery of the primary tumor; (*c*) radiotherapy of the primary tumor; and (*d*) surgery of the axilla.

The principal advantage of conservative treatment is cosmetic. There are no data to indicate that the conservative approach provides improved survival when compared with the radical or modified radical mastectomy. Thus, the surgeon must select patients for whom an adequate resection results in acceptable cosmesis. Patients who are poor candidates include those with widely separated tumors in the same breast, those whose mammograms reveal diffuse disease in many quadrants, and those with large tumors and relatively small breasts. Patients with central lesions involving the nipple-areolar complex can be treated by resection of the nipple, with careful attention to the final cosmetic result. Reconstruction of the nipple has been accomplished following appropriate radiation therapy. Age does not seem to be a consideration. Patients in their middle 70s often request conservative treatment for cosmetic reasons, and younger patients may request not only total mastectomy but prophylactic mastectomy in order to avoid further concerns about the recurrence of cancer in the treated breast and the development of new cancer in the opposite breast.

Adequate surgical resection implies grossly clear margins. The surgeon at the time of the operation marks the specimen for orientation by the pathologist. The pathologist then "inks" the margins to assist in the examination of the permanent sections. In all cases the pathologist must also mark the specimen to indicate the deep margin. Tissue is submitted for estrogen and progesterone receptor analysis without disturbing the resected margins. If the margins are "positive" following wide local excision, additional tissue must be removed. Close margins (1 to 2 mm) require either "boost" radiotherapy or reexcision. Additional, or boost, radiation therapy interferes with the cosmetic result, and often the best procedure is to reexcise the area and proceed with standard radiotherapy.

The timing of reexcision is important. If the margins can be adequately evaluated during the wide local excision, no further surgery will be required. This is not often the case, and reoperation, either under local anesthesia or general anesthesia, will be required. When reexcision is performed several weeks after the initial biopsy, significant induration and ecchymosis at the operative site make it difficult, if not impossible, to define the extent of the dissection and provide a satisfactory cosmetic result and clear margins.

It is generally agreed that adequate breast preservation procedures result in a survival rate equal to that obtained with the modified radical mastectomy. The major advantage of the conservative treatment is the final cosmetic result, and this requires considerable surgical skill. The incision must be chosen to provide adequate removal of tissue and acceptable cosmesis, realizing that the entire breast will be treated with radiation therapy. The axillary incision should be marked with the patient in sitting position along a skin fold. The author prefers to perform the axillary dissection first with a separate set of instruments. The previously marked incision is made and the pectoralis major muscle, identified. The costocorocoid fascia is incised and the axillary contents cleared by sharp dissection. Hemostasis is achieved with fine silk sutures, and if the wound is dry, no drain is employed. Only a few subcutaneous sutures are needed, and the skin is closed with fine sutures to provide a satisfactory cosmetic closure (Fig. 19.8).

With a separate set of instruments the wide local excision is carried out (Fig. 19.9). This requires removal of the previous incision and careful orientation of the specimen for the pathologist. Once the tissue has been removed and carefully oriented, the breast is reconstructed with a minimum of sutures and careful hemostasis. The skin is closed and a pressure dressing is applied. Intermittent suction often results in a defect that is very obvious, especially if the patient is sitting or standing. The author has found that with adequate hemostasis, a large pressure dressing held in place with a 6-inch Ace bandage provides a very satisfactory cosmetic result with little or no induration or ecchymosis. Most of the patients can be discharged within 48 hours, and they immediately begin active arm motion. This is important because of the fibrosis that may be associated with the subsequent radiotherapy.

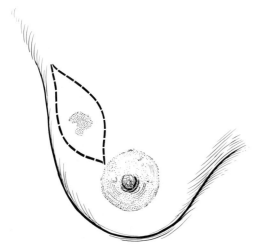

Figure 19.8. Radial incision for wide local resection. (Incision can also be parallel to areolar margin.)

The entire breast should be treated with 180 to 200 rads/day for a total of 4500 to 5000 rads. Doses in excess of 5000 rads result in fibrosis and retraction and an unacceptable cosmetic result. This is particularly true of patients who require boost therapy. The author prefers to reexcise the area and avoid this cosmetic complication. There is controversy concerning the technique for boost or supplemental radiation. However, whichever technique is employed, it should not diminish the cosmetic result.

It is especially important for the primary physician to realize that the choice of the surgical procedure is a joint decision discussed with the patient and her family and reconfirmed by the multidisciplinary team after review of a

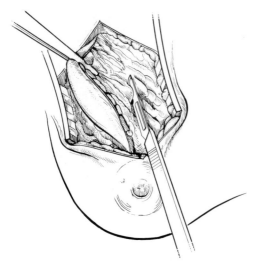

Figure 19.9. Wide local excision of skin, and subcutaneous and lobular tissue around breast cancer.

number of factors including the stage of the lesion, location of the primary tumor, the histology, mammographic findings, and the compliance of the patient.

There are advantages and disadvantages associated with the conservative and radical approaches. Obviously, the main advantage of the conservative approach is the preservation of the breast. However, the price to be paid is the extended radiation treatments and the real concern of some patients that future symptomatology in the retained breast is associated with recurrent tumor. In the more radical approach, treatment is accomplished in a few days, and obviously cancer cannot recur in the removed breast.

The complications associated with the radical and modified radical mastectomy have been discussed. With breast preservation procedures, there is less lymphedema and less restriction of arm motion. Complications can be kept to a minimum with meticulous surgical technique.

ADJUVANT THERAPY

The role of adjuvant therapy is discussed in detail elsewhere (see Chapter 21); however, the timing of this therapy must be integrated with the radiotherapy schedule. Patients with positive nodes are candidates for adjuvant therapy, and recently it has been recommended that node negative patients receive some form of adjuvant therapy as well. There is no agreement either concerning the concomitant use of chemotherapy and radiotherapy or a sequential treatment program. The author's practice is to initiate three cycles of chemotherapy, complete the radiotherapy, and add three additional cycles of chemotherapy to complete the adjuvant program. For post menopausal patients, tamoxifen is the adjuvant program of choice. There are recent data to suggest that radiation therapy is more effective when not combined with tamoxifen (R. Schmidt-Ulrich, personal communications). The author therefore has delayed the tamoxifen administration until completion of the radiation therapy cycle.

RECONSTRUCTIVE SURGERY

Many patients elect reconstructive procedures. If mastectomy is the procedure of choice, the author's practice is to request consultation with the plastic surgeon prior to the scheduled surgical procedure. There are several operative procedures available for reconstruction, and the indications vary depending on the size of the breast, previous treatment, and the anticipated result relative to the opposite breast. In some cases following mastectomy and reconstruction, it is necessary to perform a reduction mammoplasty on the opposite side. This is a lengthly procedure, and many surgeons prefer to perform this as a second operation. There are certain situations that in the author's opinion require careful evaluation of the operative specimen before any reconstructive procedure is performed. If mammographic evidence suggests multifocal disease and the biopsy confirms extensive involvement, postoperative adjuvant radiation treatment may be required, seriously compromising the cosmetic result. This type of surgery is a team effort and requires consultation with the plastic surgeon and the multidisciplinary team performing the local treatment.

FOLLOW-UP

Patients are seen in the immediate postoperative period by the reach to recovery team. They are matched depending on the surgical procedure performed. The patients also are seen by the physiotherapist and may or may not return to voluntary counseling or other similar support groups. The patients should continue to be followed by the multidisciplinary team for the first year every 3 months and for the second and third year every 4 months. A yearly mammogram is obtained and if indicated, a repeat bone scan and other studies to detect metastatic disease. Quality of life is important, and patients are urged to discuss reconstructive procedures and psychosexual concerns. While the team approach is important to determine the best surgical procedure to be performed and to carry out the combined surgical or adjuvant treatment programs, each patient should have her own physician, preferably the surgeon responsible for the initial operative procedure. Triage to oncology or radiation oncology can be arranged as required. Consultation with the primary care physician responsible for referral is encouraged. The informed primary care physician can provide additional support and continuity that would otherwise be lacking.

BREAST CANCER AND PREGNANCY

Breast cancer is infrequent during pregnancy. Numerous studies have indicated that the major problem is delay in diagnosis. If age and stage are comparable, pregnancy, per se, has little influence on prognosis (16–18). Therefore, pregnancy should neither delay prompt diagnosis nor definitive treatment. The issues to be resolved are surgical curability; appropri-

ate therapeutic action; and dangers inherent in a subsequent pregnancy.

Breast examination should be part of every prenatal visit; if any abnormality is noted, appropriate diagnostic tests should be performed. Fine-needle aspiration is as effective during pregnancy as in the nonpregnant patient, and open biopsy can be performed under local anesthesia without adverse sequelae. This is true during lactation as well. The breasts can be emptied prior to biopsy, and the biopsy performed under local anesthesia with careful attention to meticulous surgical technique and hemostasis. In the author's experience, there are no adverse effects with this approach. It is absolutely essential that any mass be resolved during pregnancy or lactation.

During the first trimester once the diagnosis of cancer has been established, prompt treatment including mastectomy and axillary dissection should be performed. Patients presenting during the last trimester, depending on the maturity of the fetus, may be observed until the delivery of a mature fetus is achieved and prompt therapy is then carried out. When the diagnosis is established during the middle trimester, the patient must be treated without delay and observation to reach maturity is unjustified.

If regional involvement is discovered a decision must be made concerning adjuvant therapy. Some studies have indicated that chemotherapy administered during the second and third trimesters has no adverse effect upon the fetus (19). It is wise to discuss these options with the patient, particularly if she wishes to keep the pregnancy. There are no long-term results available regarding the effect of chemotherapy on the newborn.

Breast preservation procedures are contraindicated during pregnancy because of the potential effect of radiation on the fetus. Given this option, few patients have requested termination of the pregnancy in favor of the breast (see Chapter 22).

SUMMARY

It is unlikely that there will be major changes in the technique of excisional surgery for breast cancer within the next few years. On the other hand, it is clear that less surgery will be performed. The majority of patients with diagnosed breast cancer undergo modified radical mastectomy. With increased screening, smaller lesions are discovered and breast preservation procedures will become an ever increasing option.

Regardless of the type of surgery, the best survival rate is for women with small primary tumors and negative lymph nodes. For T1 N0 lesions the cure rate should approach 90% at 5 years and 75% at 10 years. When the lymph nodes contain tumor cells, the cure rate drops to between 25 to 63%, depending on the number of lymph nodes involved and the size of the primary tumor (20).

The role of the primary care physician is critical. He or she should be aware of the guidelines for screening, and promptly refer for appropriate diagnostic studies and treatment. Contemporary management requires a multidisciplinary team including the surgeon, radiation oncologist, and medical oncologist with appropriate support from pathology and diagnostic radiology. The media provides a relentless flow of information concerning the treatment of breast cancer and patients deserve immediate access to the very best treatment including the increasing option of breast preservation procedures.

REFERENCES

1. Bloom HJG, Richardson WW, Harris EJ. Natural history of treated breast cancer (1805–1933). Comparison of untreated cases according to a histological grade of malignancy. Br Med J 1962;11:213.
2. Moore ZH. On the influence of inadequate operations on the theory of cancer. R Med Chir Soc (Lond) 1867;1:245.
3. Halsted WS. The results of operations for the cure of cancer of the breast performed at the Johns Hopkins Hospital. 1894–1895;4:297.
4. Urban JA, Marjani MA. Significance of internal mammary lymph node metastases in breast cancer. AJR 1971;111:130.
5. Wilson RE. Progress in breast cancer treatment, today and tomorrow. Am Coll Surg Bull 1983;68:2.
6. Lagios MD, Westdahl PR, Margolin FR, et al. Duct carcinoma in situ, relationship of extent of non-invasive disease to the frequency of occult invasion, multicentricity, lymph node metastases, and short term treatment failures. Cancer 1982;50:1309.
7. Fisher ER, Sass R, Fisher B, et al. Pathologic findings from the National Surgical Adjuvant Breast Project (protocol 6).1. Intraductal carcinoma (DCIS). Cancer 1986;57:197.
8. Lagios MD, Margolin FR, Westdahl PR, Rose MR. Mammographically detected duct carcinoma in situ. Frequency of local recurrences following tylectomy and prognostic effects of nuclear grade on local recurrence. CA 1989;63:618–625.
9. Fisher B, Bauer M, Margolese R et al. Five-year results of a randomized clinical trial comparing total mastectomy and segmental mastectomy with or without radiation in the treatment of breast cancer. N Engl J Med 1985;312:665.
10. Harris JR, Hellman S. The results of primary radiation therapy for early breast cancer at the Joint Center for Radiation Therapy. In: Harris JR, Hellman S, Silen W, eds. Conservative management of breast cancer. Philadelphia, Lippincott, 1983:47.
11. Veronesi V, Zucali R, Luini A. Local control and survival in early breast cancer: the Milan trial. Int J Radiat Oncol 1986;12:717.
12. Fisher B, Redmond C, Fisher ER, et al. Ten-year results of a randomized clinical trial comparing radical mastectomy and total mastectomy with or without radiation. N Engl J Med 1985;312:674.
13. Langlands AO, Prescott J, Hamilton T. A clinical trial in the management of operable cancer of the breast. Br J Surg 1980;67:170.
14. Hayward J. The surgeon's role in primary breast cancer. Breast Cancer Res Treat 1981;1:27.
15. Harris JR, Hellman S, Kinne DW. Special report: limited surgery and radiotherapy for early breast cancer treatment. N Engl J Med 1985;313:1365.
16. King RM, Welch JS, Martin JK et al: Carcinoma of the breast associated with pregnancy. Surg Gynecol Obstet 1985;160:228.
17. Nugent P, O'Connell TX. Breast cancer and pregnancy. Arch Surg 1985;120:1221.
18. Harvey JC, Rosen PP, Ashikari R, et al. The effect of pregnancy on the prognosis of carcinoma of the breast following radial mastectomy. Surg Gynecol Obstet 1981;153:723.
19. Murray CL, Reichert JA, Anderson J, Twiggs LB. Multimodal cancer therapy for breast cancer in the first trimester of pregnancy. JAMA 1984;252:2607.
20. Townsend CM. Management of breast cancer—surgery and adjuvant therapy. Clin Symp (Ciba-Geigy) 1987;39:(4)3–32.

20

Role of Radiation Therapy in the Management of Breast Cancer

David H. Hussey
Antonio P. Vigliotti

Radiation therapy has been used to treat breast cancer since the turn of the century, soon after the discovery of x-rays. Since then, it has played a variety of roles in the management of this disease. It has been used as the sole treatment modality or in combination with surgery or chemotherapy. It has been used to treat the breast only, the regional lymph nodes only, and both the breast and the regional lymph nodes. Radiation therapy has also played a major role in the palliation of recurrent disease, locally advanced cancer, and distant metastasis.

Considerable information has been accumulated over the past several decades regarding the natural history of breast cancer and the effectiveness of various treatment modalities. As a result, there have been profound changes in the management of this disease. Twenty years ago, most patients were treated with a radical mastectomy, and radiotherapy was commonly used postoperatively to treat the chest wall and the regional lymphatics (1). Today, most patients are treated with lesser radical surgical procedures, and many receive treatment by simple excision and radiation therapy. Chemotherapy is also used if there is extensive nodal disease.

BASIC PRINCIPLES OF RADIOTHERAPY

Radiosensitivity

Forty years ago, radiosensitivity was assumed to be related to tumor histology (2). It was thought that for each histology there was a specific cancericidal dose that was required for local tumor control. Tumors were classified as radiosensitive or radioresistant on the basis of the clinical responses observed. Squamous carcinomas of the oral cavity and cervix had been successfully treated with interstitial radium and were considered to be relatively radiosensitive, whereas adenocarcinomas of the breast and other sites had been treated with relatively low doses of kilovoltage x-rays with little success and were considered to be radioresistant. For many sites, regional lymph node metastases were considered to be more resistant than the primary tumor. This was because the primary tumor could be effectively treated with implants, and the nodal disease was difficult to control because of the poor skin-sparing properties of the x-ray beams then available. At the time, little consideration was given to the volume of cancer in the selection of a treatment modality.

At present, the size of a tumor is recognized as the principal feature determining the effectiveness of irradiation. All epithelial tumors, including squamous carcinomas of the upper respiratory tract and cervix and adenocarcinomas of the breast, prostate, uterus, and colon, are thought to be equally sensitive (2, 3), and cancers in regional lymph nodes are believed to be no less radiosensitive than cancers at the primary site.

The two biological factors that determine the probability of local control by irradiation are the number of malignant cells and the proportion of malignant cells in a hypoxic state. Radiobiology experiments have shown that

241

Table 20.1.   Probability of Control as a Function of Radiation Dose and Tumor Volume[a]

Dose, cGy	Squamous Cell Carcinoma of the Upper Respiratory and Digestive Tracts	Adenocarcinoma of the Breast
3000–3500[b]		
3000–4000[b]	60–70% subclinical[d]	60–70% subclinical[c]
4000[b]		
	>90% subclinical[d]	80–90% subclinical[c]
5000[b]	60% T_1 lesions of nasopharynx	
	~50% 1- to 3-cm neck nodes	>90% subclinical[c]
6000[b]	80–90% T_1 lesions of pharynx and larynx	
	~50% T_3 + T_4 lesions of tonsillar fossa	
	~90% 1- to 3-cm neck nodes	
	~70% 3- to 5-cm neck nodes	
7000[b]	80–90% T_2 lesions of tonsillar fossa and supraglottic larynx	90% clinically positive nodes 2.5–3 cm[e]
	~80% T_3 + T_4 lesions of tonsillar fossa	
7000–8000 cGy/8–9 wk		65% 2–3 cm primary
8000–9000 cGy/8–10 wk		30% >5 cm primary
8000–10,000 cGy/10–12 wk		56% >5 cm primary
		75% 5–15 cm primary

[a]Adapted from Fletcher GF. Textbook of radiotherapy. 3rd ed. Philadelphia, Lea & Febiger, 1980: 194–196.
[b]1000 cGy in five fractions per week
[c]Calculated from the percentage of appearance of supraclavicular failures as compared with the expected percentage.
[d]Calculated from the percentage of failures appearing in the initially clinically uninvolved area of the neck as compared with the expected percentage.
[e]The control rate is corrected for the percentage of nodes that would be positive histologically had an axillary dissection been performed.

hypoxic cells are significantly more resistant to effects of ionizing radiation than are normally oxygenated cells. The proportion of cells that are hypoxic is directly related to the size of the cancer and its vascular supply. Smaller doses are required to eradicate small aggregates of cancer cells than palpable masses, because small aggregates have fewer cells and smaller hypoxic compartments. As the volume of cancer increases, so does the importance of the hypoxic compartment.

Fletcher (3) has correlated the probability of local tumor control with the size of the neoplasm and the radiation dose delivered (Table 20.1). A dose of 4000 cGy in 4 weeks controls subclinical aggregates in 80 to 90% of patients. A dose of 5000 cGy in 5 weeks controls subclinical aggregates in greater than 90% of patients, and it controls 2- to 3-cm nodal metastases in approximately 50% of patients. A dose of 7000 cGy in 7 weeks controls 1- to 3-cm nodes in about 90% of patients and 3- to 5-cm nodes in about 70%.

Combined Surgery and Radiotherapy

The rationale for combined surgery and radiation therapy is based on modern surgical and radiobiologic principles (2). Surgical failures usually result from residual microscopic disease. On the other hand, radiation therapy

failures usually result from inability to eradicate bulky masses. When combined, the two modalities of treatment are complementary—surgery is used to remove gross masses that are too large to be eradicated by moderate doses of irradiation and radiation therapy is used to eradicate microscopic extensions of tumor that cannot be excised. Partial removal of a tumor achieves little because it does not reduce the number of malignant cells to a microscopic level.

Preoperative Radiotherapy

The arguments in favor of preoperative radiotherapy are that (a) inoperable lesions may be made operable, (b) the extent of the surgical resection may be diminished, (c) radiotherapy treatment portals may be smaller than would be required postoperatively, (d) microscopic disease is more radiosensitive before surgery because it has a better blood supply, and (e) the viability of tumor cells that may be disseminated by surgical manipulation is diminished, thereby reducing the risk of distant metastasis. The arguments against preoperative radiotherapy are that (a) wound healing is more difficult after irradiation, (b) the dose that can be delivered safely preoperatively is less than that which can be given postoperatively, and (c) surgery may be more difficult after preoperative irradiation because it may obscure differentiation of cancer from normal tissues.

Postoperative Radiotherapy

The arguments in favor of postoperative irradiation are that (*a*) the anatomic extent of the tumor is better defined by the surgery, making it easier to determine the areas that need radiotherapy, (*b*) a greater dose of radiation may be given postoperatively, and (*c*) surgical resection is easier and healing is better in unirradiated tissues. The arguments against postoperative irradiation are that (*a*) distant metastasis may result from cells spread by the surgical procedure; (*b*) surgery disrupts the vascularity of the tumor bed, theoretically increasing radioresistance; and (*c*) radiation therapy might have to be postponed if surgical healing is delayed, allowing cancer cells to repopulate in the interval.

PRIMARY TUMOR AND ROUTES OF SPREAD

Radiation therapy is similar to surgery in that it is a localized form of treatment. However, radiation therapy can be used to treat areas that are not easily treated with surgery, e.g., the chest wall, the internal mammary nodes, and the supraclavicular nodes. The decision to treat the breast or chest wall should be based on the risk of local failure in these sites and the probability of controlling the disease with irradiation. The decision to treat the regional lymph nodes should be based on the relative probabilities of regional spread and occult distant metastasis and the likelihood of controlling the regional nodal disease without normal tissue complications. A knowledge of the routes of spread is necessary to plan treatment effectively (Fig. 20.1).

Primary Tumor

Breast cancer usually presents as a painless lump, and the site of origin in the breast is related to the volume of breast tissue. More breast tumors arise in the upper-outer quadrant (39%) or central areas (29%) than in the upper-inner (14%), lower-outer (9%), and lower-inner (5%) quadrants (4). The decision to use adjuvant radiotherapy is based partly on the location of the primary tumor in the breast.

As breast cancer enlarges, it infiltrates locally into the breast parenchyma, extending along the mammary ducts or through the breast lymphatics. It may also extend to overlying skin or the deep pectoral fascia. There may be tumor extension well beyond the palpable mass.

Breast cancers are frequently multifocal in origin, and thus there is a need to treat the entire breast, either with surgery or radiotherapy. Qualheim and Gall (5) found independent multifocal lesions in 54% of breast cancers surveyed by whole-organ paraffin sections. In 37% of the specimens, the cancers were detected in quadrants remote from the principal lesion. Multifocal cancers are responsible for some of the local failures seen following treatment with partial mastectomy alone. At the Cleveland Clinic 11% of patients treated with quadrantectomy alone developed recurrent cancer in the area of resection, and an additional 7% developed new tumors in other quadrants (6). In the National Surgical Adjuvant Breast Project (NSABP) B-06 protocol, 28% of patients treated with partial mastectomy without irradiation subsequently developed clinical evidence of recurrent cancer in the breast (7).

Regional Lymph Node Metastasis

The regional lymphatic drainage of the breast is to the axillary, internal mammary, and supraclavicular lymph nodes (Fig. 20.1). The axillary lymph nodes are involved most commonly, followed by the internal mammary, and then the supraclavicular lymph nodes.

Axillary Lymph Nodes

Approximately 55% of patients with operable breast cancers have metastasis in the axillary lymph nodes (8), and this high incidence suggests a need to treat the axilla. The probability of axillary nodal involvement is directly related to the size of the primary tumor and its location. Haagensen (4) found that the incidence of axillary metastasis is 24% for tumors smaller than 2 cm, 40% for those 2 to 4 cm in size, and 57% for those to 5 to 8 cm in size. Approximately 40% of patients with primary tumors in the medial half of the breast have positive axillary nodes, compared with 60% of those with tumors in the central or outer half of the breast.

Physical examination of the axilla is associated with high false-negative and false-positive rates. Approximately 40% of patients with clinically negative axillae have positive nodes at axillary node dissection, and at least one-fourth of patients thought to have positive nodes on physical examination are found to have negative axillae at surgery (NSABP B-04) (8, 9). Axillary nodal status is an important prognostic indicator, and it is commonly used to determine treatment policy.

In recent years, axillary lymph node dissections have been performed routinely for staging purposes. However, the extent of the dissection required for staging has been a

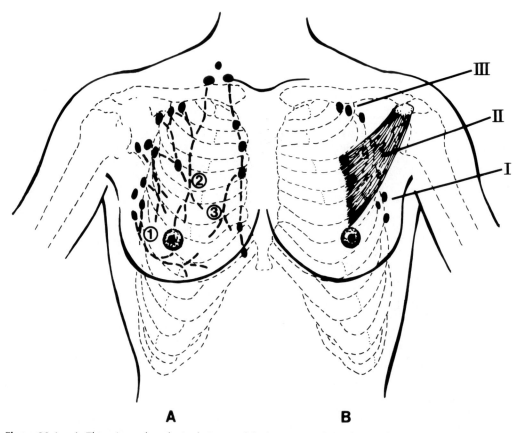

Figure 20.1. **A**, The primary lymphatic drainage of the breast is to the axillary, internal mammary, and supra-clavicular lymph nodes. Three pathways have been described: *1*, The principal pathway drains the medial and lateral portions of the breast, extending to the pectoral group of axillary lymph nodes located between the second and third intercostal spaces. Some of these pass directly to the central or superior axillary lymph nodes. *2*, The transpectoral pathway originates in the periphery of the mammary gland and passes through or around the pectoralis muscle to end in an intrapectoral node (Rotter's node), the high axillary nodes, or, rarely, the supraclavicular nodes. *3*, The internal mammary pathway drains the central and medial portions of the breast. It perforates the intercostal muscles close to the sternum, terminating in the internal mammary nodes. The lymphatics of the skin overlying the breast are arranged radially. The vessels overlying the lateral half of the breast extend to the axilla, and those of the upper portion of the breast terminate in the axillary or supraclavic-ular nodes. The skin from the medial part of the breast is drained by lymphatics extending to the internal mammary nodes or cross midline to join the lymphatics overlying the opposite breast. **B**, The axillary lymph nodes are divided into three levels: level I, the proximal or low axillary nodes lying inferior and lateral to the pectoralis minor muscle; level II, the middle or retropectoral nodes located behind the pectoralis minor mus-cle; and level III, the distal or apical nodes, located superior to the pectoralis minor muscle.

controversial issue. Veronesi and associates (10) have shown that metastasis to the axilla oc-curs in a regular, progressive fashion (Table 20.2). Metastasis to the low axillary lymph nodes almost always develops first, and the middle and upper axillary nodes are involved subsequently. In Veronesi's series, only 1.5% of patients with positive axillary nodes had me-tastasis limited to the middle and/or upper axil-lary nodes without involvement of the lower axilla. Therefore, complete axillary dissections are not needed to correctly assess the status of the axilla. This is important because complete axillary dissections result in greater morbidity, particularly in patients receiving axillary irradiation.

The prognosis of patients with breast cancer depends on the number of histologically posi-tive nodes. Patients with fewer than 4 positive nodes have a lower incidence of internal mam-mary node involvement, a lower incidence of distant metastasis, and better survival than pa-tients with 4 or more positive lymph nodes (4, 8, 11).

Table 20.2. Distribution of Positive Axillary Lymph Nodes By Level of Involvement[a, b]

Sites of Involvement	Incidence, %
Level I	98.5[c]
Level I only	58.3
Level I + level II and/or III	40.3
Level II	39.1
Level II only	1.1
Level II + level I and/or III	38
Level III	18.9
Level III only	0.4
Level III + level I and/or II	18.6

[a]Modified from Veronesi U, Rilke F, Luini A, et al. Distribution of axillary node metastases by level of invasion: an analysis of 539 cases. Cancer 1987;59:682–687.
[b]An analysis of 539 patients undergoing complete axillary dissection. Average number of nodes removed was 20.5 per patient.
[c]Only 1.5% of patients with positive nodes had metastasis to levels II or III without involvement of level I.

Internal Mammary Nodes

Approximately 25% of patients with operable breast cancers have metastasis to the internal mammary lymph nodes (11). The probability of involvement of this site is related to the location of the primary tumor and the status of the axillary lymph nodes. Handley (11) found that 30% of patients with inner-quadrant or central tumors had metastasis to the internal mammary lymph nodes, compared with only 14% of patients with outer-quadrant tumors. He also noted that 35% of those with positive axillary nodes had internal mammary lymph node involvement, compared with only 8% of those with negative axillae. This information is important for planning radiotherapy treatment portals, since it points out the need to treat this area in patients with medially located primary tumors and positive axillary nodes.

Internal mammary node involvement has a negative influence on survival. Valagussa and associates (12), in a randomized study of radical vs. extended radical mastectomy, showed that patients with positive internal mammary nodes had a significantly poorer survival rate than the general study population. The 10-year survival rate for patients with negative axillary nodes and positive internal mammary nodes was only 46%, compared with 82% for the total group with negative axillary nodes. Likewise, the 10-year survival rate for patients with both positive axillary and internal mammary nodes

was 20.5% compared with 40% for the total group with positive axillary nodes.

Supraclavicular Metastasis

Supraclavicular metastasis usually occurs following extensive involvement of the axilla and/or internal mammary lymph nodes. However, it can occur in an isolated fashion if the skin over the upper half of the breast is involved. Dahl-Iversen (13) found that 18% of patients with positive axillary nodes also had spread to the supraclavicular nodes, whereas no supraclavicular metastases were found in patients without axillary lymphadenopathy. Clinically evident supraclavicular metastasis is almost always associated with distant metastatic spread (4).

Distant Metastasis

Hematogenous metastasis occurs early in the natural course of the disease. The most commonly involved sites are bone, lungs, and liver. Bony metastasis may be osteolytic or osteoblastic. Patients with positive axillae have a high risk of distant metastasis, even if the local disease is controlled, and supraclavicular metastasis is almost synonymous with distant spread. The 10-year survival rate for patients without axillary lymph node metastasis is approximately 65%; for those with one to three positive nodes, 40%; and for those with four or more positive nodes, 15% (14). Half of all patients with four or more positive axillary nodes will have clinical evidence of metastatic disease within 18 months. Breast cancer that is locally recurrent after radical mastectomy is associated with distant metastasis in approximately 90% of patients. However, the majority of patients with recurrent tumors following partial mastectomy and radiotherapy can be salvaged by surgery.

THEORIES REGARDING THE SPREAD OF BREAST CANCER

Two theories have dominated thinking regarding the natural history of breast cancer, and each has had a significant influence on the philosophy of treatment (Fig. 20.2). Neither theory is entirely correct. For many years, the recommended treatment for regionally localized breast cancer was radical mastectomy with en bloc resection of the breast and the regional lymphatics. This treatment approach was based on the concept that breast cancer is primarily a local disease and its spread occurs in a stepwise fashion—first to the regional lymph nodes and then to distant sites. If this theory were correct, one would expect to find a signif-

Theories Regarding the Spread of Breast Cancer

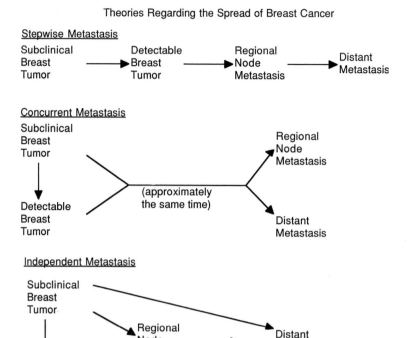

Figure 20.2.   Theories regarding the spread of breast cancer.

icant population of patients with disease confined to the primary site and the regional lymphatics, and treatment of the regional lymph nodes should have a significant impact on ultimate survival.

In recent years, a second theory has emerged. In this theory, breast cancer is thought to spread to the regional lymph nodes and distant sites at approximately the same time. Proponents of this theory believe that regional lymph node metastasis is an indicator of distant spread, and not a precursor. This concept has resulted from the observation that treatment of the regional lymphatics has not improved survival rates significantly. For example, the NSABP B-04 protocol results show similar 5-year relapse-free survival rates for clinically node-negative patients treated with radical mastectomy (60%), simple mastectomy and regional lymphatic irradiation (65%), and simple mastectomy without the regional lymphatic irradiation (56%) (9).

The truth probably lies somewhere between these two opposing points of view (Fig. 20.2). Breast cancer may metastasize through the lymphatics to the regional nodes or hematogenously to distant sites, and hematogenous spread may occur either independently or as metastasis from regional nodal disease. If this theory were correct, patients would fall into three groups: (a) those with disease in only the breast, (b) those with disease in both the breast and the regional lymphatics without distant metastasis, and (c) those with distant metastasis. The first group would be cured if the breast was adequately treated, and the third group would die of their disease regardless of the outcome of locoregional therapy. Thus, neither would benefit from regional lymphatic treatment. It is the second group of patients, those with regional metastasis but without distant spread, who could be salvaged by treatment of the regional lymph nodes.

The reason why clinical studies have failed to demonstrate a significant improvement in survival with regional therapy is that this second patient population is relatively small. Bross and Blumenson (15), using data from early NSABP trials, determined that 63% of patients with operable breast cancers already had occult distant metastasis and that the tumor was confined to the breast in 22% of patients (Table 20.3). Only 15% of patients had regional

Table 20.3. Mathematical Model: Distribution of Patients with and without Occult Axillary Disease or Distant Metastasis (Clinically $T_{1-2}N_0$)[a]

	Systemic Status		
Status of the Axilla	No Distant Metastasis, %	Distant Metastasis, %	Total, %
Negative nodes	22.0	26.0	48.0
Positive nodes	15.3[b]	36.7	52.0
Total	37.3	62.7	100

[a]Adapted from Bross IDJ, Blumenson LE. Predictive design of experiments using deep mathematical models. Cancer 1971; 28:163–1646. (Based on data from NSABP trials).
[b]Theoretically only 15.3% could potentially benefit with regard to cure from treatment of the axilla.

metastasis without distant spread and thus could benefit from regional therapy.

There is clinical evidence to support this view. Rutqvist and Wallgren (16) followed 458 young breast cancer patients for periods of 20 to 51 years. All were treated with radical or modified radical mastectomy, and 97% received postoperative radiotherapy. The actuarial survival rate at 40 years was 53% for patients with negative axillary nodes; more important, 19% of the patients with positive axillary nodes survived 40 years. Thus, a small subset of patients with regional lymph node metastasis was "cured" for an extended period of time. Similar improvements in survival with regional therapy have been detected for selected subsets of patients in a variety of clinical trials (see Adjuvant Radiation Therapy).

The value of treatment of the primary tumor is well-established (17). It is a means of controlling the local cancer, and it clearly improves survival. Bloom and associates (18) plotted the natural history of untreated breast cancer by reviewing the records of 250 patients seen prior to 1933. The survival of this untreated group was compared with that of a later group of patients treated by surgery with or without radiation therapy. The patients who received treatment had a much better survival than those who were left untreated (10-year survival: 34% vs. 3.6%). Further evidence of the value of early treatment comes from mammography screening studies, which have shown a 25 to 30% reduction in breast cancer deaths for the population of women who undergo screening (19).

PATTERNS OF FAILURE

Treatment failures may occur as a result of inability to control the disease in the breast or on the chest wall (local failure), inability to control disease in regional lymph nodes (regional failure), or metastasis to distant sites (distant metastasis). In a review of patients with locoregional recurrences following radical mastectomy or modified radical mastectomy alone,

Bedwinek and associates (20) found that about two-thirds of the patients had failures on the chest wall, one-third in the supraclavicular area, one-sixth in the axilla, and one-ninth in the internal mammary area.

Chest Wall Recurrence

In the early 1940s, Haagensen (4) reviewed his experience with radical mastectomy and found 120 patients with unfavorable clinical features. Half of the patients developed recurrent tumor on the chest wall or in the regional lymphatics, and only one survived 5 years free of disease. This led to the development of Haagensen's criteria of clinical inoperability and the five "grave signs" of breast cancer (Table 20.4). These criteria form the foundation of the Columbia Clinical Staging System. In this staging system, a patient is classified as inoperable if she possesses any one of the signs of clinical inoperability or any two of the grave signs of breast cancer. Haagensen (4) found that 42% of the patients who had two or more grave signs developed locally recurrent cancer and only 2% were alive free of disease at 5 years.

In 1966, Donegan and associates (22) reviewed the records of 704 patients selected for treatment with radical mastectomy alone on the basis of the Haagensen criteria. They found that the incidence of chest wall recurrence correlated well with the size of the primary tumor and the number of axillary nodes involved (Fig. 20.3). Overall, approximately 15 to 25% of patients with operable breast cancers develop chest wall recurrences if the surgery is not followed by postoperative radiation therapy. The incidence increases steadily with the size of the primary tumor and the number of histologically involved axillary lymph nodes (Table 20.5). In Donegan's study, only 6.5% of patients with negative nodes developed chest wall recurrence, whereas 38% of those with heavily infested axillae did.

The clinical criteria for chest wall irradiation are based on results such as those reported by

Table 20.4.   Columbia Criteria of Clinical Inoperability and the Five "Grave Signs" of Breast Cancer[a]

Criteria of Inoperability	Grave Signs
1. Extensive edema of the skin over the breast	1. Edema of the skin involving less than one-third of the breast
2. Satellite nodules of the skin over the breast	
3. "Inflammatory" carcinoma	2. Skin ulceration
4. Distant metastasis	3. Solid fixation of the tumor to the chest wall
5. Parasternal or supraclavicular node metastases	4. Axillary lymph node >2.5 cm
6. Edema of the arm	5. Fixed axillary nodes.

[a]From Haagensen CD, ed. Diseases of the breast. Philadelphia, Saunders, 1971: 622–629.

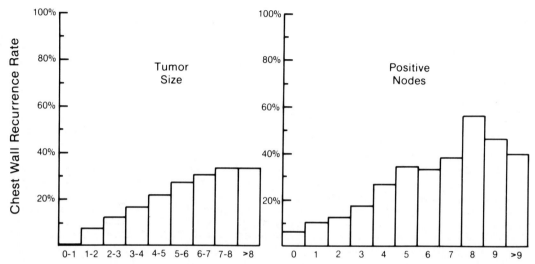

Figure 20.3.   Frequency of chest wall recurrences following treatment with radical mastectomy alone as a function of the size of the primary tumor and the number of positive axillary nodes. (Adapted from Donegan WL, Perez-Mesa CM, Watson FR. A biostatistical study of locally recurrent carcinoma. Surg Gynecol Obstet 1966;122:529–540.)

Haagensen and Donegan. Fletcher has advocated postoperative chest wall irradiation in patients (a) with primary tumors greater than 5 cm in diameter; (b) with any of the five grave signs; (c) with incomplete resection; (d) with pathologic evidence of skin, nipple, perineural, or lymphatic invasion; or (e) with involvement of more than 20% of the axillary lymph nodes. With postoperative radiotherapy, failures on the chest wall are reduced approximately fourfold (2).

Axillary Nodal Recurrence

Axillary recurrence is rare after a classic radical mastectomy (Table 20.5). In the NSABP B-04 study (8, 9), only 2% of the patients with clinically negative axillae treated with radical mastectomy developed axillary recurrences as the first manifestation of treatment failure, although 39% of patients had positive nodes histopathologically. Even in patients receiving no

treatment to the axilla, the axillary recurrence rate is less than would be expected, since only 17.8% of the patients treated with a total mastectomy alone (without treatment to the axilla) developed recurrent tumor in the axilla requiring subsequent axillary dissection.

This observation has been used as evidence to support the theory that host-defense mechanisms are able to control subclinical disease in the axilla. However, this observation may not be entirely valid. First, 35% of the patients randomized to treatment with total mastectomy alone had partial axillary dissections during surgery for the primary tumor, most likely those with lateral tumors having a greater risk of axillary infestation (8). Second, some of the axillary recurrences may not have been counted because they were not amenable to treatment with axillary dissection because of location, fixation, or concurrent distant metastasis. Third, breast cancer can be a slowly evolving tumor, so that some axillary recurrences

Table 20.5. Histopathologic Status and Local Failure Rates By Site for Patients Treated By Radical Mastectomy with or without Adjunctive Radiotherapy

Area	% Histopathologically Positive (Ref.)	% Recurrence in Area (Ref.)	
		Without Radiotherapy	With Radiotherapy
Chest Wall			
Histologically negative axilla		6.5 (22)	2 (23)[a]
1–3 nodes positive		12 (22)	8 (23)[a]
≥4 nodes positive		38 (22)	11 (23)[a]
Axillary Nodes			
Clinically negative	39 (8)	2 (25)	0.4 (23)[b]
Clinically positive	73 (8)	1 (25)	0.6 (23)[b]
Internal Mammary Nodes			
Lateral tumor, histol. neg. axilla	6 (11)	2 (24)	0 (23)
Lateral tumor, histol. pos. axilla	21.5 (11)	2 (24)	0 (23)
Medial tumor, histol. neg. axilla	11 (11)	5 (24)	0 (23)
Medial tumor, histol. pos. axilla	48 (11)	9.5 (24)	0 (23)
Supraclavicular Nodes			
Histol. neg. axilla	0 (13)	7 (26)	0 (23)
Histol. pos. axilla	18 (13)	20 (26)	1 (23)

[a]Patients with Grave signs.
[b]Relative to histologic status of axillary nodes.

may not have become apparent by the date of analysis.

Although the incidence of axillary recurrences is low following treatment with radical mastectomy alone, this failure rate can be reduced further with the addition of irradiation. Treurniet-Donker and associates (27), reported a 4% 5-year axillary recurrence rate following radical mastectomy alone in node-positive patients with low-risk factors, and it was 15% in patients with poorly differentiated tumors, capsular invasion, or apical axillary involvement. With axillary irradiation, the recurrence rate was reduced to less than 1% in both the high- and low-risk groups.

Internal Mammary Node Recurrences

Although approximately one-fourth of patients with early breast cancer have subclinical metastases in the internal mammary nodes, relatively few develop clinical evidence of recurrent tumor in this area (Table 20.5). This is probably because the internal mammary lymph nodes are situated deep to the sternum, and metastases to this region become clinically evident only after they have grown large enough to produce parasternal bulging or abnormalities on chest x-ray. Overall, the incidence of internal mammary failures is less than 5%. However, 8 to 10% of patients with medially located tumors and positive axillary nodes develop recurrent tumor in the internal mammary area after a standard radical mastectomy (25, 28).

Tumor in the internal mammary lymph nodes can be eradicated by irradiation. Gutt-

mann (29) treated 148 patients with biopsy-proven metastases to internal mammary and/or supraclavicular lymph nodes and found a 60% 5-year survival rate. Autopsies in 20 of these patients showed no evidence of residual tumor in the initially involved areas. At M.D. Anderson Hospital none of the patients treated with radiation therapy to the peripheral lymphatics for medially located tumors and/or positive axillary nodes developed recurrent tumor in the internal mammary area (3).

Supraclavicular Nodal Recurrences

Supraclavicular recurrences are usually easily detected, and because of this, the failure rate in the supraclavicular area correlates well with the expected incidence of involvement (Table 20.5). As previously mentioned, Dahl-Iversen (13) reported an 18% incidence of occult supraclavicular metastasis in patients with positive axillary nodes. Jackson (26), in a review of the literature, found that 15 to 17% of patients treated with radical mastectomy alone failed in the supraclavicular lymph nodes.

When the axillary lymph nodes are positive, the incidence of failures in the supraclavicular area is in the range of 20 to 26% with treatment by radical mastectomy alone (30, 31). If postoperative radiation therapy is delivered, this incidence falls to approximately 1 to 1.5% (2, 32). In a retrospective study from Institut Gustave Roussy, Arriagada and associates (33) found a 14% incidence of supraclavicular failures in patients treated by radical mastectomy alone,

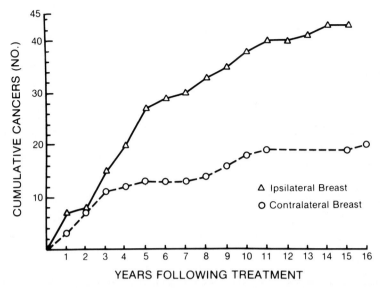

Figure 20.4. Time course of recurrence in the ipsilateral or contralateral breast following treatment with segmental resection and postoperative radiation therapy. A significant proportion of the failures are due to second primary tumors. (Adapted from Kurtz JM, Spitalier JM, Almiric R. Late breast recurrence after lumpectomy and irradiation. Int J Radiat Oncol Biol Phys 1983;9:1191–1194 Pergamon Press.)

compared with less than 1% in those who also received postoperative radiotherapy.

Distant Metastasis

Most failures from breast cancer result from distant metastasis. Approximately 60% of patients with breast cancer have occult distant metastasis at the time of diagnosis (15). Because of this, extensive research has been done to develop adjuvant systemic therapies (chemotherapy or hormone therapy) to be used at the time of initial treatment. Such treatment is given in an effort to destroy occult metastases before they have a chance to become manifest.

Second Primary Breast Tumors

Breast cancers are frequently multicentric and many are associated with large areas of intraductal disease (5). Thus, if the breast is left intact, there is a risk of a new primary tumor developing in the ipsilateral breast. There is also an increased risk of developing a second primary tumor in the contralateral breast. Bilateral synchronous breast cancers are rare, occurring only in 1 to 2% of patients; however, bilateral metachronous cancers have been observed in 7 to 8% of patients (34). The risk of developing a second primary breast cancer is approximately 1% per year (Fig. 20.4). Radiation therapy does not appear to increase the incidence of second primary tumors (36–38).

Time Course of Failure

Locoregional failures following radical mastectomy usually occur within 3 years and rarely after 10 years (38). The prognosis for patients with local recurrence following radical mastectomy is poor and long-term survival is rare, even if effective local therapy is delivered. However, local recurrences after partial mastectomy tend to occur later (Fig. 20.5), and salvage therapy is much more effective. Almost two-thirds of these patients survive 5 years free of disease after salvage mastectomy.

In almost every large series, there are a few patients who die of their disease more than 20 years after treatment. Bloom and associates (18) reviewed the records of 250 patients with untreated breast cancer and found that 18% survived 5 years and 3.6% survived 10 years. The longest survivor lived 18 years and 3 months. Rutqvist and Wallgren (16) followed a series of young patients with operable tumors for 20 to 51 years and found that 6.3% of the cancer deaths occurred after 20 years (Fig. 20.6).

Breast cancers can be very responsive to hormonal manipulation, and it is not infrequent to see patients with advanced disease survive for 10 years following treatment with hormones only. Because of this, bilateral oophorectomy in premenopausal women was one of the earliest forms of systemic therapy for breast cancer. In some of the randomized studies comparing surgery with and without radiation therapy, pa-

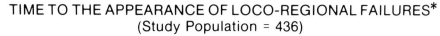

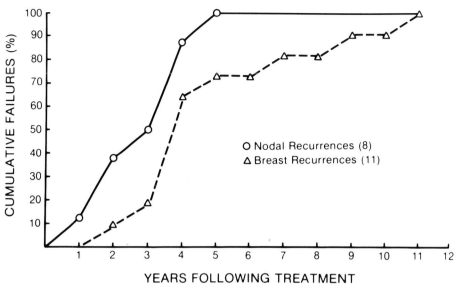

TIME TO THE APPEARANCE OF LOCO-REGIONAL FAILURES*
(Study Population = 436)

O Nodal Recurrences (8)
△ Breast Recurrences (11)

YEARS FOLLOWING TREATMENT

*Adapted from Clarke et al, Int. J. Rad. Oncol. Biol. Phys. 11: 137, 1985

Figure 20.5. Time course of failures in the breast or the regional lymph nodes following treatment with partial mastectomy with and without irradiation in a study population of 436. Whereas, almost all chest wall recurrences and nodal recurrences following radical mastectomy appear within 5 years, a significant percentage of breast recurrences after partial mastectomy appear later. Many of these are second primary breast tumors. (Adapted from Clarke DH, Lê MG, Sarrazin D, et al. Analysis of local-regional relapses in patients with early breast cancer treated by excision and radiotherapy: experience of the Institute Gustave-Roussy. Int J Radiat Oncol Biol Phys 1985;11:137–145, Pergamon Press.)

tients were castrated, making it difficult to evaluate the effectiveness of treatment. Furthermore, once patients develop progressive cancer they are often treated with hormones, making it difficult to evaluate the impact of the initial treatment on overall survival.

A variety of endpoints have been used to evaluate the effectiveness of treatment for breast cancer, and this has made it difficult to compare results between institutions. From the standpoint of cure, 5-year survival rates are meaningless, and even 10-year survival rates have limited usefulness. Some authors have used 5-year relapse-free survival rates, but a significant number of patients develop recurrent tumor between 5 and 10 years. Ten-year relapse-free survival rates or 15-year crude survival rates are appropriate endpoints for the analysis of breast cancer treatment results.

ADJUVANT RADIATION THERAPY

Radiation therapy is often used in combination with a radical, modified radical, or total mastectomy. The rationale for adjuvant radio-

therapy is twofold: (*a*) to decrease the incidence of locoregional failure by controlling subclinical disease on the chest wall or in the regional lymphatics; and (*b*) improve survival by eradicating locoregional disease before it has a chance to disseminate. The effectiveness of adjuvant radiation therapy in the control of locoregional disease is well-established. Its value in improving survival remains a subject of controversy.

Experience with Surgery Alone

The local failure rate following radical mastectomy alone is 5 to 10% if the axillary lymph nodes are negative and 25 to 30% if the axillary nodes are positive (8, 12). As was previously mentioned, failure on the chest wall or in the supraclavicular lymph nodes is relatively common, whereas internal mammary recurrences are unusual (Table 20.5). Recurrences in the axilla are rare following a radical mastectomy.

Some evidence in support of the use of adjuvant radiation therapy comes from clinical trials comparing radical mastectomy with and without internal mammary lymph node dissec-

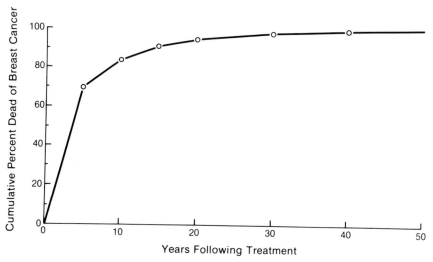

Figure 20.6. Time to death from breast cancer in 458 young breast cancer patients. The actuarial survival rates at 40 years were 53% for those with negative axillary nodes and 19% for those with positive nodes, indicating that a subset of patients with positive nodes was cured of their disease. However, 6.3% of the cancer deaths occurred after 20 years. (Based on data from Rutqvist LE, Wallgren A. Long-term survival of 458 young breast cancer patients. Cancer 1985;55:658–665.)

tion. In the mid 1960s, a large international cooperative trial was performed to compare these two surgical techniques (39). Although there was no significant difference in overall survival between the standard and the extended radical mastectomy groups, a patient subset with medial tumors and positive axillary nodes had significantly better survival with dissection of the internal mammary nodes. A recent update for the patients contributed to this study by the Institut Gustave Roussy showed similar findings at 15 years (Fig. 20.7) (40). These results demonstrate the value of treatment of the internal mammary lymph nodes in patients with a high risk of metastasis to this area.

Radiation Therapy Studies

Indirect evidence for adjuvant radiation therapy comes from a retrospective review from M.D. Anderson Hospital. In general, the patients who received adjuvant radiotherapy at that institution had more advanced tumors than those treated by radical mastectomy alone. For example, only 14% of the patients treated with radical mastectomy alone had positive axillary nodes, compared with 71% of those treated with postoperative radiation therapy and 30% of those treated with preoperative radiation therapy—and the incidence of positive nodes in the latter group was probably reduced by a factor of 2 by the preoperative irradiation. In spite of the differences in tumor extent, the survival rates for all three groups were identical. When analyzed by nodal status,

the 10-year survival rates for the patients who received adjuvant radiotherapy were significantly greater than the survival rate for the group treated with surgery alone (Table 20.6) (41).

In a retrospective study from the Institut Gustave Roussy, Tubiana and associates (42) compared four treatment regiments: (a) standard radical mastectomy alone, (b) radical mastectomy plus postoperative irradiation, (c) extended radical mastectomy alone, and (d) extended radical mastectomy plus postoperative irradiation. The postoperative radiotherapy in this study consisted of 4500 cGy to the chest wall and the regional lymphatics. Again, a marked improvement in locoregional control was seen for the groups that received postoperative radiation therapy, and there was a significant improvement in 5-year survival with internal mammary node treatment for patients with medially located tumors and positive axillary nodes (Fig. 20.7).

The benefits of adjuvant radiotherapy for patients with a high risk of internal mammary lymph involvement has also been demonstrated in several randomized trials. In the late 1960s, a randomized trial of radical mastectomy with or without postoperative radiotherapy was performed at the Norwegian Radium Hospital (43, 44). In the early years of this study, the postoperative therapy was delivered to the chest wall and the regional lymph nodes using low doses of kilovoltage x-rays. In later years, more effective doses were delivered with cobalt-60 gamma rays to the regional nodes only

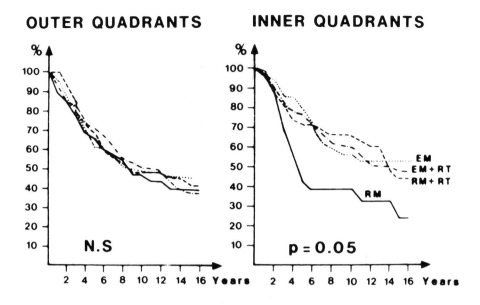

SURVIVAL

Figure 20.7. Institute Gustave Roussy Study: On the left, outer quadrant tumors. No difference among the groups. On the right, 227 patients with medial tumors and positive nodes treated by radical mastectomy or extended radical mastectomy with or without radiotherapy. Survival is significantly lower in the treatment with radical mastectomy alone group than in the three groups in which the internal mammary nodes were either removed or irradiated. Radical mastectomy (RM, *solid line*); extended radical mastectomy (EM, *dotted line*); radical mastectomy plus radiotherapy (RM + RT, *dashed line*); extended radical mastectomy plus radiotherapy (EM + RT, *dot-dash line*). (Adapted from Tubiana M, Arriagada R, Sarrazin D. Human cancer natural history, radiation-induced immunodepression and post-operative radiation therapy. Int J Radiat Oncol Biol Phys 1986;12:477–485, Pergamon Press.)

Table 20.6. M.D. Anderson Hospital study: A comparison of 10-year survival rates for patients treated with radical mastectomy alone, or with preoperative or postoperative radiation therapy[a]

	RM Only	Postoperative RT + RM	Preoperative RT + RM
No. of patients	441	1034	442
With positive axillary nodes, %	14	71	30[b]
10-yr survival, %	54[c]	53[c]	59[c]
Node-negative patients	60	75	70
Node-positive patients	26	44	35

[a]Data from Ref. 41.
[b]Histological status after 4000-cGy preoperative irradiation, which would be expected to sterilize nodes in more than half of the patients.
[c]Overall 10-year survival rates measured from figure.

(no chest wall irradiation). Both radiotherapy techniques reduced the incidence of locoregional recurrences (mastectomy only, 14%; x-rays, 7%; cobalt-60, 4.9%), and the cobalt-60 irradiation resulted in improved survival for patients with medial lesions and positive axillary nodes (Fig. 20.8).

Another randomized trial was performed in the early 1970s at the Radiumhemmet in Stockholm (45). In this study, patients were randomized for treatment with (a) a modified radical mastectomy alone, (b) preoperative radiation therapy followed by a modified radical mastectomy, or (c) a modified radical mastectomy followed by postoperative radiation therapy. Both the preoperative and postoperative radiation therapy groups received 4500 cGy in 5 weeks to the chest wall, the internal mammary, supraclavicular, and axillary lymph nodes. Only 7% of the irradiated patients developed locore-

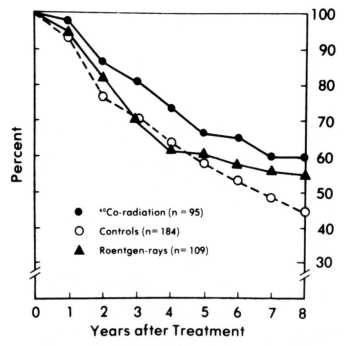

Figure 20.8. Olso study: Comparison of relapse-free survival in patients treated with radical mastectomy alone (controls), radical mastectomy and postoperative Cobalt-60 irradiation, or radical mastectomy and postoperative kilovoltage x-ray irradiation. (From Høst H, Brennhovd IO. The effect of post-operative radiotherapy in breast cancer. Int J Radiat Oncol Biol Phys 1986;12:727–732, Pergamon Press.)

Table 20.7. Stockholm study: A randomized trial of modified radical mastectomy alone or with postoperative radiotherapy or preoperative radiotherapy[a]

	MRM Only	MRM + Preoperative or Postoperative RT
No. of patients	321	639 (316 preop. 323 postop.)
Locoregional failures, %:	26	7
Chest wall recurrences	19.3	5.2
Nodal recurrences	13.1	3.0
Ten-yr survival, % (determinate):		
Node-negative patients	No difference	No difference
Node-positive patients	47	54

[a]Adapted from Wallgren A, Arner O, Bergström J, et al. Radiation therapy in operable breast cancer: results from the Stockholm trial on adjuvant radiotherapy. Int J Radiat Oncol Biol Phys 1986;12:533–537, Pergamon Press.

gional recurrences, compared with 26% of those treated with modified radical mastectomy alone (node-negative patients, 2.5% vs. 20%; node-positive patients, 13% vs. 45%) (Table 20.7). In addition, the 10-year survival rate for node-positive patients was greater for the group receiving adjuvant radiation therapy (54%) than for the group treated with surgery alone (47%) (Fig. 20.9). This is a population that would be expected to have a higher incidence of internal mammary node metastases.

Indications for Adjuvant Radiotherapy

The indications for postoperative irradiation of the peripheral lymphatics are based on the histologic status of the axillary nodes and the location of the primary tumor in the breast. Patients with central or medial quadrant tumors and/or positive axillary nodes have a significant risk of internal mammary node involvement. In the authors' opinion, patients with small (<2 cm) medially located tumors and negative

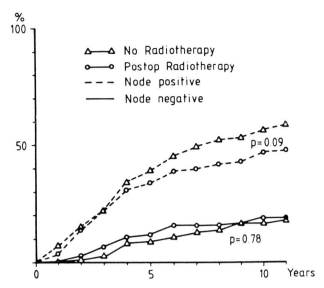

Figure 20.9. Stockholm study: Cumulative incidence of breast cancer deaths in node-negative and node-positive patients treated by modified radical mastectomy alone or by modified radical mastectomy and postoperative radiotherapy. Postoperative radiotherapy improves the survival of patients with positive axillary nodes but does not influence the survival rate for patients with negative axillary nodes. (From Wallgren A, Arner O, Bergström J, et al. Radiation therapy in operable breast cancer: Results from the Stockholm trial on adjuvant radiotherapy. Int J Radiat Oncol Biol Phys 1986;12:533–537, Pergamon Press.)

axillary nodes should receive irradiation to the internal mammary lymph node chain only. Patients with larger tumors in the central or inner quadrants and those with metastasis to the axillary lymph nodes also have significant risk of metastasis to the supraclavicular lymph nodes. In these patients, the lymphatics of the apex of the axilla, the supraclavicular area, and the internal mammary chain should be irradiated. Chest wall recurrences are most likely to occur if the primary tumor has unfavorable characteristics or if there is heavy involvement of the axilla. Consequently, chest wall irradiation is recommended if the tumor in the breast is larger than 5 cm, in the presence of grave signs, or if 20% or more of the axillary lymph nodes are positive.

CONSERVATION SURGERY AND RADIATION THERAPY

In recent years, breast conservation surgery and definitive radiation therapy have gained acceptance as an alternative to radical mastectomy in the management of early breast cancer. Many reports have been published from several centers demonstrating the effectiveness of this treatment regimen (Tables 20.8 and 20.9). A variety of patient selection criteria have been employed for these studies, and a variety of surgical and radiotherapy techniques have been used. In spite of these differences,

there has been remarkable agreement in the results achieved at various centers. Only 5 to 10% of patients have developed recurrent tumor in the treated breast, and the survival rates are at least as good as those achieved with radical mastectomy.

The goal of conservative treatment is preservation of the breast with minimal deformity, without compromising locoregional control or patient survival. Furthermore, by diminishing the sequelae of treatment, women should seek treatment earlier, which should result in improved cure rates for the overall patient population.

Patient Selection Criteria

Careful patient selection is important in the conservative management of breast cancer. The tumor should be in an appropriate location and small enough, in relation to the size of the breast, to ensure a good cosmetic result. In most institutions, patients with subareolar cancers and those with tumors fixed to the skin or chest wall have been excluded. The patient population has usually been limited to those with tumors smaller than 4 cm. However, in some institutions, patients with tumors as large as 7 cm have been successfully treated with definitive radiotherapy (35, 57, 59). Some authors have excluded patients with extensive intraductal carcinomas or widespread micro-

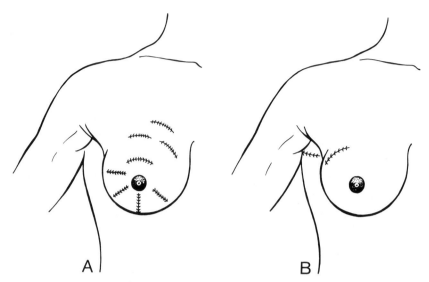

Figure 20.10.   Recommended incisions for breast conservation treatment. **A**, Deformity is minimized with circumferential incisions in the upper half of the breast and radial incisions in the lower half of the breast. **B**, Separate incisions should be employed for the primary tumor and axillary node dissection.

calcification because of the risk of multiple primary tumors (60).

Surgical Techniques

A wide spectrum of surgical techniques has been employed. These have included simple excision, wide excision, segmental mastectomy, quadrantectomy, and partial mastectomy. In some institutions, patients with gross residual tumor have been treated; whereas in others, the tumor bed has been reexcised in patients with a high risk of tumor cut-through. At the National Cancer Institute, patients have been treated by a simple tumor excision, and positive resection margins have been permitted (56). This results in better cosmesis, but could compromise local tumor control. On the other hand, in Milan, a quadrantectomy has been performed with a 3-cm margin (58). This results in considerable deformity, defeating the purpose of conservative treatment. In general, wide local excision with adequate margins is preferable to a segmental mastectomy because cosmesis is the main rationale for conservative treatment. To minimize deformity, surgeons should apply accepted principles of cosmetic surgery (Figs. 20.10 and 20.11).

In the authors' opinion, the tumor bed should be reexcised in high-risk patients. These include patients with uncertain or positive surgical margins and those with microcalcifications on postexcision mammograms. This policy has been employed successfully at M.D. Anderson Hospital and the University of

Pennsylvania (46, 51). Forty-five percent of patients in the University of Pennsylvania series required reexcision (51). However, only 6% developed recurrent tumor in the breast, and the 5-year relapse-free survival rates were 80% for clinical stage I and 69% for clinical stage II. Similar local control and survival rates have been achieved at M.D. Anderson Hospital.

Radiation Therapy Techniques

In most institutions, the whole breast has been treated to a dose of 4500 to 5000 cGy in 4.5 to 5 weeks, and additional treatment has been delivered to the tumor bed with either electrons or an interstitial iridium implant. In general, the total dose has been determined by the tumor burden. If all gross tumor is resected, a dose of 5000 to 6000 cGy in 5 to 6 weeks will control the tumor in more than 90% of patients. However, if the resection margins are positive or gross tumor remains, higher doses are required. No boost was given in the NSABP B-06 protocol, but the surgical margins were always negative. In Creteil and Marseilles, doses of 7000 to 8000 cGy have been given for patients with palpable residual tumor (35, 48, 57).

Treatment of the regional lymphatics has been a controversial issue. In the NSABP B-06 protocol, the nodes were not irradiated regardless of axillary nodal status (7). However, in most institutions, the regional lymph nodes are irradiated in patients with medially located tumors and positive axillary nodes, because of

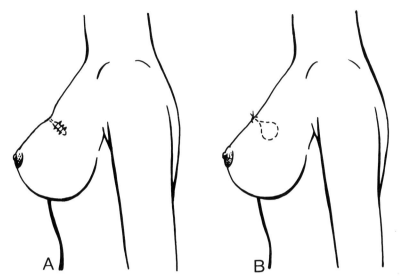

Figure 20.11.   Recommended surgical technique for breast conservation treatment. **A**, Closing the defect at depth can result in skin dimpling. **B**, The incision should be closed at the surface of the skin and allowed to granulate in at depth.

the high risk of subclinical metastasis to these sites (Table 20.5).

Clinical Experience

M.D. Anderson Hospital

Between 1955 and 1980, 291 patients with clinical stage I and II breast cancer were treated with conservation surgery and radiation therapy (46). The breast was treated to a dose of 4500 to 5000 cGy in 5 weeks, followed by a 1000-cGy boost with electrons or a 1500 to 2000-cGy boost with an implant. Regional lymphatic irradiation was used in patients with positive axillary nodes or medially located tumors. Only 5.5% developed recurrent disease in the breast or the regional lymphatics, and the 10-year disease-free survival rates were 78% for stage I and 73% for stage II (Table 20.8). These results compare favorably with those achieved with a radical or modified radical mastectomy at that institution (locoregional failure, 6.7%; 10-year disease-free survival, 80% for stage I and 65% for stage II).

Milan

Between 1973 and 1980, 701 patients with clinical stage T_1N_0 breast cancers were randomized for treatment with (*a*) a classic radical mastectomy alone or (*b*) a quadrantectomy, axillary dissection, and radiation therapy (QUART) (58). A 5000-cGy dose was delivered to the breast through fields that extended 2 cm beyond the midsternal line. This was followed by

a 1000-cGy boost to the tumor bed. A few patients with positive nodes received elective lymph node irradiation, and others received a substantial internal mammary node dose from the tangential breast portals. The overall local control and survival rates were the same for both the radical mastectomy and the QUART groups (Table 20.9). However, in patients with positive axillary nodes, the 5-year relapse-free survival rate was superior for patients treated with a quadrantectomy plus radiation therapy (86.6 vs. 71.6%). This may have been due to eradication of disease in the internal mammary lymph nodes (Fig. 20.12).

Institut Gustave Roussy

A total of 179 patients with stage $T_{1-2}N_{0-1}$ breast cancers were randomized to receive a total mastectomy or local excision plus irradiation (55). Patients in both groups underwent a low axillary dissection, and if the lymph nodes were positive, a complete axillary dissection was performed. The radiation therapy consisted of 4500 cGy to the total breast plus a boost of 1500 cGy to the tumor bed. At 5 years, only 6% of the patients treated with radiotherapy developed a recurrent tumor in the breast, compared with a 10% incidence of chest wall recurrences in the mastectomy group. The 5-year relapse-free survival rate was 84% for patients treated by tumorectomy and irradiation, compared with 72% for those treated by a total mastectomy (Table 20.9).

Table 20.8.   Nonrandomized Studies of Conservation Surgery and Radiotherapy

Study (Ref.)	Clinical Stage	No. Pts.	Technique	Recurrence in Breast	Survival
M.D. Anderson Hospital (46)	I–II	291	Simple excision or segmental resection + RT	5.5% (unlimited follow-up)	State I: 78% 10-yr DFS[a] Stage II: 73% 10-yr DFS[a]
Creteil (47)	I–III (<7 cm)	330	Tumorectomy or biopsy only + RT	13.3%	58% 10-yr NED survival[b]
Institut Curie (48)	I–III (<3 cm)	324	Wide excision + RT	6.5%	90% 5-yr NED survival[b]
Institut Gustave-Roussy (38)	Small T_{1-2} N_{0-1}	436	Simple excision or quadrantectomy + RT	5% at 5 yr	80% 5-yr NED survival[b]
Joint Center for Radiation Therapy (49)	I–II	266	Simple excision biopsy or incomplete resection + RT	Stage I: 3% at 5 yr Stage II: 13% at 5 yr	Stage I: 93% 5-yr survival Stage II: 84% 5-yr survival
Marseilles (50)	I–II	274	Simple excision or wedge resection + RT	12% at 10 yr	74% 10-yr NED survival[b]
University of Pennsylvania (51)	I–II	552	Simple excision + RT	3% at 5 yr (45% had reexcision)	Stage I: 87% 5 yr NED surv.[b] Stage II: 73% 5 yr NED surv.[b]
Yale (52)	I–II	179	Simple excision + RT	6.7% locoregional failures	Stage I: 88% 5 yr RFS[c] Stage II: 66% 5 yr RFS[c]
Princess Margaret Hospital (53)	I–II	1482	Simple excision or segmental resection:		
			No radiation (374 pts.)	24% at 5 yr	71% 10-yr cancer spec. surv.[d]
			Breast RT (662 pts.)	9% at 5 yr	73% 10-yr cancer spec. surv.[d]
			Breast RT + lymphatic RT (446 pts.)	12% at 5 yr	67% 10-yr cancer spec. surv.[d]

[a]DFS, disease-free survival at M.D. Anderson Hospital counts patients dying of intercurrent disease as withdrawn alive.
[b]NED survival, alive with no evidence of disease. However, patients who are salvaged are counted as NED.
[c]RFS, Relapse-free-survival (alive continuously free of tumor).
[d]cancer spec. surv., cancer-specific survival rate at Princess Margaret Hospital, count only cancer-related deaths as failures.

National Surgical Adjuvant Breast Project

The largest randomized trial of conservative therapy was performed by the NSABP B-06 protocol (7). Between 1976 and 1984, 2122 patients with stage I and II breast cancer (<4 cm) were entered into a study comparing (a) total mastectomy, (b) segmental mastectomy only, and (c) segmental mastectomy plus breast irradiation. All patients underwent axillary dissec-tion, and those with positive nodes received melphalan and 5-fluorouracil.

Radiation therapy markedly reduced the failure rate in the breast. Only 7.7% of patients treated with a segmental mastectomy and radiation therapy had recurrent tumor in the breast, compared with 27.9% of those treated with segmental mastectomy alone (Table 20.9). The difference was greatest in the patients with positive nodes (segmental mastectomy plus radiation therapy, 2.1% vs. segmental mastectomy only, 36.2%). Furthermore, the disease-

Table 20.9. Randomized Clinical Trials of Conservation Surgery and Radiotherapy

Study (Ref.)	Clinical Stage	No. Pts.	Technique	Local Recurrence	Survival
Milan (54)	T_1N_0 (≤2 cm)	701	Quadrantectomy + RT	3.4% breast failure	89% 5 yr RFS[a]
			Radical mastectomy	1.4% chest wall failure	86% 5 yr RFS[a]
Institute Gustave-Roussy (55)	T_{1-2} N_{0-1}	179	Simple excision + RT	6% breast failure at 5 yr	84% 5 yr RFS[b]
			Total mastectomy	10% chest wall failure at 5 yr	72% 5 yr RFS[b]
National Surgical Breast Adjuvant Project (7)	I–II ≤4 cm	1843	Segmental mastectomy + RT	7.7% breast failure	Nodes (−): 81% 5-yr DFS[c] Nodes (+): 58% 5-yr DFS[c]
			Segmental mastectomy only	27.9% breast failure	Nodes (−): 68% 5-yr DFS[c] Nodes (+): 55% 5-yr DFS[c]
			Total mastectomy only		Nodes (−): 72% 5-yr DFS[c] Nodes (+): 58% 5-yr DFS[c]
National Cancer Institute (56)	I–II	175	Simple excision (narrow margins)	2% locoregional failure (limited follow-up)	12% disease progression (local &/- or distant failure)
			Total mastectomy	2% locoregional failure (limited follow-up)	14% disease progression (local &/- or distant failure)

[a]RFS, Relapse-free survival (alive continously free of tumor).
[b]RFS, Definition not stated.
[c]DFS, Disease-free survival in NSABP protrocol B-06 refers to patients who are alive continuously free of tumor, although recurrence in the breast is not counted as recurrent tumor if the patient can be salvaged with mastectomy.

free survival rate for the group treated with a segmental mastectomy plus radiation therapy was better than the disease-free survival rates for either of the other groups (Fig. 20.13).

Another finding was that there were fewer local recurrences in the patients with positive nodes who received both postoperative radiation therapy and chemotherapy than in either those with positive nodes who received only chemotherapy postoperatively or those with negative nodes who received only radiation therapy postoperatively. These data suggest that radiation therapy and chemotherapy may be additive or perhaps even synergistic in their action.

LOCALLY ADVANCED BREAST CANCER

The category of locally advanced breast cancer represents a wide spectrum of disease (3, 4). It includes patients with primary tumors larger than 5 cm in diameter, with edema, invasion, or ulceration of the skin, with fixation to underlying structures, with satellite nodules, or with single or multiple axillary nodes measuring more than 2.5 to 3 cm in diameter (Table 20.4). Inflammatory carcinoma is a special category of locally advanced breast cancer that will be discussed in a separate section.

The prognosis for patients with locally advanced breast cancer is poor, both because of a high local failure rate and a high incidence of distant metastasis. Local tumor control is difficult to achieve because of the bulk of the cancer within the breast and the regional lymphatics and because of local extension to critical structures. On the other hand, most of these patients manifest distant metastasis within 2 years, which suggests that occult distant spread was already present when the patient was first seen.

Locally advanced breast cancers can be classified as those that are technically *operable* and those that are technically *inoperable*. Patients with technically operable breast cancer should be treated with a combination of surgery and irradiation—a simple mastectomy if the axilla is clinically negative or an extended simple mastectomy if there are clinically positive, mobile nodes (61–63). A simple mastectomy is pre-

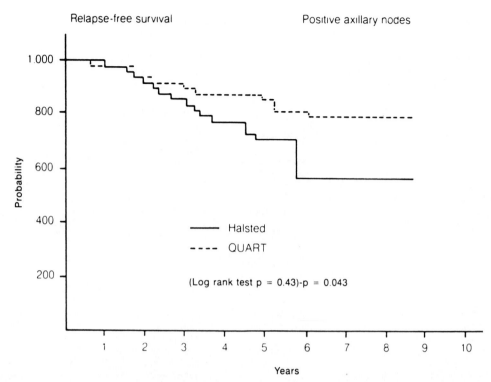

Figure 20.12. Comparison of relapse-free survival in patients with positive axillary nodes treated by quadrantectomy and radiotherapy vs. classic radical mastectomy. (From Veronesi U, et al. Results of quadrantectomy, axillary dissection, and radiotherapy (QUART) in T_1N_0 patients. In: Harris JR, Hellman S, Silen W, eds. Conservative management of breast cancer: new surgical and radiotherapy techniques. Philadelphia: Lippincott, 1983:91–99.)

ferred to a radical mastectomy because there is less surgical manipulation, healthier skin flaps, and more rapid healing, which allows radiation therapy to be instituted earlier. If a patient has a technically inoperable breast cancer, surgery is not feasible and treatment is delivered with radiation therapy and/or chemotherapy.

Toonkel and associates (64), analyzed the results in 470 patients with operable stage III and IV breast cancers. Of these, 381 had all gross tumor removed, and 89 had only a biopsy. Whereas, 79% of those who had the tumor removed had local tumor control with radiotherapy, only 45% of those with a residual mass did. These results were reflected in improved 5-year survival rates—50% for patients who had all gross tumor removed, compared with 14% for those with residual tumor.

In recent years, the trend has been to treat locally advanced breast cancer with chemotherapy initially in order to suppress occult metastases and diminish the tumor burden before local treatment is instituted (63). However, local treatment is needed to eradicate gross tumor that is too large to be controlled with chemotherapy. This treatment policy also allows

oncologists to assess response rates so that the chemotherapeutic regimen can be modified if the tumor is unresponsive.

The selection of the local treatment regimen should be based on the response of the tumor to chemotherapy (63). If the tumor does not respond to chemotherapy, radiation therapy is initiated in an attempt to make the tumor resectable. On the other hand, if the tumor becomes resectable with chemotherapy, surgery generally precedes radiation therapy. If there is a complete clinical response to chemotherapy, radiation therapy may be used to avoid the need for mastectomy. The choice of local treatment is also based on the anatomic extent of the tumor. Patients with tumors that are fixed to the chest wall and those with fixed axillary nodes, supraclavicular metastasis, arm edema, or brachial plexus involvement are usually not candidates for a mastectomy. These patients are more appropriately treated with radiation therapy after chemotherapy.

The best results for patients with technically operable cancers have been achieved with a combination of all three modalities (surgery, radiotherapy, and chemotherapy). Klefstrom

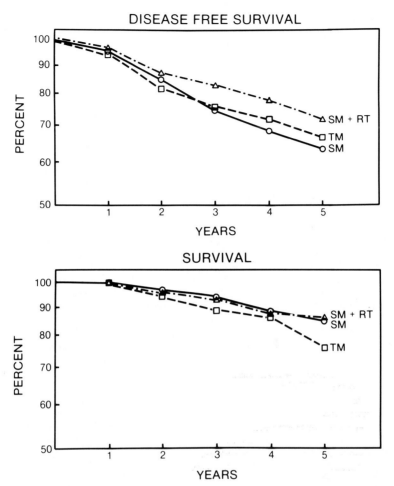

Figure 20.13. NSABP B-06 protocol: Actuarial disease-free survival for patients treated by segmental mastectomy plus radiotherapy (SM+RT), segmental mastectomy alone (SM), or total mastectomy alone (TM). (Adapted from Fisher B, Bauer M, Margolese R, et al: Five year results of a randomized clinical trial comparing total mastectomy and segmental mastectomy with or without radiation in the treatment of breast cancer. N Engl J Med 1985;312:665–673.)

and associates (65) performed a randomized study in patients with operable stage III breast cancers. The patients were treated initially with a modified radical mastectomy and then randomized for completion of treatment with (*a*) postoperative radiation therapy, (*b*) chemotherapy, or (*c*) a combination of postoperative radiation therapy and chemotherapy. The chemotherapy consisted of six cycles of vincristine, doxorubicin, and cyclophosphamide. The radiotherapy consisted of 4500 cGy in 3 weeks to the chest wall and regional lymph nodes. The patients treated with combined radiation therapy and chemotherapy exhibited significantly better local control and survival rates than those in the other two groups (Table 20.10). Only 13% of patients treated with surgery, radiation therapy, and chemotherapy developed

locoregional failures, compared with 20% of those treated with surgery and postoperative radiation therapy and 58% of those treated with surgery and postoperative chemotherapy. On the other hand, the incidence of distant metastasis was lower in the patients that received chemotherapy with or without irradiation.

Inflammatory Carcinoma

Inflammatory carcinoma is a special category of locally advanced breast cancer, and radiation therapy plays an important role in its management. Inflammatory breast cancers are characterized by erythema, heat, peau d'orange, edema, and wheals or ridges indicating extensive dermal lymphatic permeation.

Table 20.10.   Combined Therapy in Technically Operable Stage III Breast Cancer: A Comparison of Adjuvant Treatment Methods in a Randomized Trial[a]

Adjuvant Therapy After Surgery[b]	LF ± DM, %	DM ± LF, %	5-yr DFS, %
Chemotherapy only	58	25	32
	(23/40)	(10/40)	
Radiotherapy only	20	70	25
	(8/40)	(28/40)	
Radiotherapy + chemotherapy	13	28	70
	(5/39)	(11/39)	

LF, locoregional failure; DM, distant metastasis; DFS, disease-free survival.
[a]From Klefström P, Grohn P, Heinonen E, et al: Adjuvant postoperative radiotherapy, chemotherapy, and immunotherapy in stage III breast cancer. II. 5-year results and influence of Levamisole. Cancer 1987;5:936.
[b]Half of the patients in each group also received Levamisole.
[c]Actuarial disease-free survival (alive with no evidence of tumor).

There may be an associated underlying mass, but often there is only a diffuse, ill-defined induration. Histologically, tumor emboli may be seen in the dermal lymphatics.

Patients with inflammatory carcinoma have a rapidly progressive course with a high incidence of local failure and distant metastasis. Barker and associates (66) reported a local recurrence rate of 46% for patients treated with conventional fractionation, compared with 27% for patients treated with twice-daily irradiation. Approximately 80% in each group developed distant metastases. Only 17% of patients treated with conventional fractionation and 27% of those treated with twice-daily irradiation were free of disease at 2 years.

Today, most patients with inflammatory carcinoma are treated initially with chemotherapy and radiotherapy is used later in the course of treatment to improve local control. Median survival times have been increased from 18 to 30 months with the addition of chemotherapy, but long-term survival has not been improved significantly (67). In the past, surgery has not been of value in the treatment of inflammatory carcinoma, but it is being reevaluated as a means of improving local control in patients who respond to chemotherapy with or without radiotherapy (63).

RADIOTHERAPY FOR LOCALLY RECURRENT DISEASE

Locoregional recurrences following a radical or modified radical mastectomy occur in 15 to 25% of patients, and radiation therapy plays a major role in the management of these recurrences. Approximately two-thirds of these patients have a solitary nodule and one-third have multiple sites of recurrence on the chest wall and in the regional lymph nodes.

Locoregional control is important to improve the quality of life for these patients. If chest wall recurrences are not controlled, they enlarge and produce painful ulceration with malodorous discharge. Axillary and supraclavicular recurrences can cause massive arm edema or brachial plexus pain. Locoregional control for these patients also improves survival. In one series, 63% of patients who had control of locally recurrent cancer survived 5 years, compared with only 34% of those with uncontrolled local disease (68).

Bedwinek and associates (20) have emphasized the importance of treating the entire chest wall and lymph-node-bearing areas for patients with isolated locoregional recurrences. Whereas 46% of patients whose initial recurrences were treated with small treatment portals developed a second locoregional recurrence, only 3% of those treated with large field irradiation did (20).

Although elective irradiation of the chest wall and regional lymph nodes can control occult disease in approximately 90% of patients, therapeutic irradiation after local recurrence is less effective in establishing local control. In a series reported from M.D. Anderson Hospital, 194 patients with locally recurrent cancer were treated with radical irradiation with curative intent (68). The best current radiotherapy techniques were used. Nevertheless, local tumor control was achieved in only 64% of these patients. This is understandable because there is a considerably greater tumor burden in patients with locally recurrent cancer.

PALLIATIVE RADIOTHERAPY

Approximately 60% of patients with breast cancer will develop distant metastases sometime during the course of their illness, and these often produce severely debilitating symptoms that can be palliated with radiotherapy. The aim of palliative radiotherapy is to improve the quality of life for these patients. In general, it does not prolong survival significantly.

Radiation therapy is the most useful single agent for the palliation of local symptoms due to metastasis. However, the best results are obtained when radiotherapy and systemic treatment are integrated in a planned program. Hormonal therapy and chemotherapy are useful to suppress generalized metastatic disease, and radiation therapy is indicated for relief of localized symptoms such as pain, hemorrhage, malodorous discharge, impending fracture, neurologic symptoms due to brain metastasis or spinal cord compression, or loss of vision due to retinal metastasis.

The most common metastases from breast cancer are bone metastases, and radiation therapy results in significant pain relief in about 90% of these patients (69, 70). The radiotherapy technique should be based on the site irradiated and the overall prognosis. If a patient has a life expectancy of only a few weeks, a protracted course of treatment is not indicated. However, patients with metastatic breast cancer can survive for extended periods of time, and more permanent palliation can be achieved with higher doses of well-fractionated irradiation.

Spinal cord compression is a devastating late manifestation of breast cancer. It is a medical emergency in which radiation therapy plays a major role. If the patient's general condition is otherwise satisfactory and the cord compression is localized, surgical decompression is warranted, but it should be followed by radiation therapy to secure long-term local control. If decompression is not feasible, radiation therapy should be given within a few hours after the onset of symptoms.

Radiation therapy is also used to treat patients with metastasis to the cerebrum or cerebellum, and those with diffuse meningeal carcinomatosis. Patients with brain metastases have a median survival of approximately 6 months if treated with radiation therapy, compared with only approximately 1 month if left untreated. More important, approximately three-fourths of these patients respond to irradiation with an improvement in mentation and neurologic function. Choroid and retinal metastasis may also occur, and radiation therapy should be initiated early for these patients to avoid further deterioration in vision.

SUMMARY

Radiation therapy is an important part of an oncologist's armamentarium for breast cancer, and it plays a variety of roles in the management of this disease. It is effective as primary therapy following limited resection of early breast cancers and as an adjuvant to radical

surgery in selected patients with a high risk of locoregional failure. It also plays a major role in the management of locally advanced and recurrent breast tumors, and it is the most effective means of palliating local symptoms in patients with distant metastasis.

The usefulness of radiation therapy in breast cancer is based on well-established principles of radiobiology and a knowledge of the natural history of the disease and its patterns of spread. Irradiation is very effective in controlling subclinical disease, and consequently it is useful in improving locoregional control in patients with a high risk of local failure following surgery. Its usefulness in prolonging survival following surgery depends on the relative probabilities of residual locoregional disease and distant metastasis.

REFERENCES

1. Fletcher GH. History of irradiation in the primary management of apparently regionally confined breast cancer. Int J Radiat Oncol Biol Phys 1985;11:2133–2142.
2. Fletcher GH. Combination of irradiation and surgery. In: Murphy GP, ed. International advances in surgical oncology. vol 2. New York: Alan Liss, 1979:55–98.
3. Fletcher GH, ed. Textbook of radiotherapy. 3rd ed. Philadelphia: Lea & Febiger, 1980:194–196.
4. Haagensen CD. The natural history of breast cancer. In: Hagensen CD, ed. Diseases of the breast. 2nd ed. Philadelphia: Saunders, 1971:380–465.
5. Qualheim RE, Gall EA. Breast carcinoma with multiple sites of origin. Cancer 1957;10:460–468.
6. Hermann RE, Esselstyn CB Jr, Cooperman AM, Crile G Jr. Partial mastectomy without radiation therapy. Surg Clin North Am 1984;64:1103–1113.
7. Fisher B, Bauer M, Margolese R, et al. Five year results of a randomized clinical trial comparing total mastectomy and segmental mastectomy with or without radiation in the treatment of breast cancer. N Engl J Med 1985;312:665–673.
8. Fisher B, Wolmark N, Bauer M, Redmond C, Gebhardt M. The accuracy of clinical nodal staging and of limited axillary dissection as a determinant of histologic nodal status in carcinoma of the breast. Surg Gynecol Obstet 1981;152:765–772.
9. Fisher B, Redmond C, Fisher ER, et al. Ten-year results of a randomized clinical trial comparing radical mastectomy and total mastectomy with or without radiation. N Eng J Med 1985;312:674–681.
10. Veronesi U, Rilke F, Luini A, et al. Distribution of axillary node metastases by level of invasion: an analysis of 539 cases. Cancer 1987;59:682–687.
11. Handley RS. Cancer of the breast. Am Surgeon 1975;41(11):667–670.
12. Valagussa P, Bonadonna G, Veronesi U. Patterns of relapse and survival following radical mastec-

tomy: analysis of 716 consecutive patients. Cancer 1978;41:1170–1178.

13. Dahl-Iversen E. Recherches sur les métastases microscopiques des cancers du sein dans les ganglions lymphatiques para-sternaux et sus-clavicularies. Acad Chir 1952;78:651–654.

14. Fisher B, Slack N, Katrych D, Wolmark N. Ten-year follow-up results of patients with carcinoma of the breast in a co-operative clinical trial evaluating surgical adjuvant chemotherapy. Surg Gynecol Obstet 1975;140:528–534.

15. Bross IDJ, Blumenson LE. Predictive design of experiments using deep mathematical models. Cancer 1971;28:1637–1646.

16. Rutqvist LE, Wallgren A. Long-term survival of 458 young breast cancer patients. Cancer 1985;55:658–665.

17. Roth D, Bayat H. The role of residual tumor in the chest wall in the late dissemination of mammary cancer. Ann Surg 1968;168:887–890.

18. Bloom HJG, Richardson WW, Harries EJ. Natural history of untreated breast cancer (1805–1933)—comparison of untreated and treated cases according to histological grade of malignancy. Br Med J 1962;2(suppl):213–220.

19. Tabár L, Fagerberg CJ, Gad A, et al. Reduction in mortality from breast cancer after mass screening with mammography. Lancet 1985;1:829–832.

20. Bedwinek JM, Fineberg AB, Lee J, Ocwieza M. Analysis of failures following local treatment of isolated local-regional recurrence of breast cancer. Int J Radiat Oncol Biol Phys 1981;7:581–585.

21. Haagensen CD. The clinical classification of carcinomas of the breast and the choice of treatment. In: Haagensen CD, ed: Diseases of the breast. 2nd ed. Philadelphia: Saunders, 1971:622–629.

22. Donegan WL, Perez-Mesa CM, Watson FR. A biostatistical study of locally recurrent breast carcinoma. Surg Gynecol Obstet 1966;122:529–540.

23. Tapley ND, Spanos WJ Jr, Fletcher GH, Montague ED, Schell S, Oswald MJ. Results in patients with breast cancer treated by radical mastectomy and postoperative irradiation with no adjuvant chemotherapy. Cancer 1982;49:1316–1319.

24. Fisher B, Montague E, Redmond C, et al. Comparison of radical mastectomy with alternative treatments for primary breast cancer. Cancer 1977;39:2827–2839.

25. Urban JA. Clinical experience and results of excision of the internal mammary lymph node chain in primary operable breast cancer. Cancer 1959;12:14–22.

26. Jackson SM. Carcinoma of the breast—the significance of supraclavicular lymph node metastases. Clin Radiol 1966;17:107–114.

27. Treurniet-Donker AD, Helle PA, Van Putten WLJ. Adjuvant post-operative radiotherapy in operable node positive mammary cancer: a comparison of three treatment protocols. Int J Radiat Oncol Biol Phys 1986;12:2067–2072.

28. Auchincloss H Jr. The nature of local recurrence following radical mastectomy. Cancer 1958;11:611–619.

29. Guttmann R. Radiotherapy in locally advanced cancer of the breast—adjunct to standard therapy. Cancer 1967;20:1046–1050.

30. Paterson R, Russell MH. Clinical trials in malignant disease. Part III—Breast cancer: evaluation of postoperative radiotherapy. (Clin Rad) J Fac Radiol (London) 1959;10:175–180.

31. Robbins GF, Lucas JC, Fracchia AA, Farrow JH, Chu FCH. An evaluation of postoperative prophylactic radiation therapy in breast cancer. Surg Gynecol Obstet 1966;122:979–982.

32. Weichselbaum RR, Marck A, Hellman S. The role of postoperative irradiation in carcinoma of the breast. Cancer 1976;37:2682–2690.

33. Arriagada R, Lê MG, Mouriesse H, Fontaine F, Dewar J, Rochard F, Spielmann M, Lacour J, Tubiana M, Sarrazin D. Long-term effect of internal mammary chain treatment. Results of a multivariate analysis of 1195 patients with operable breast cancer and positive axillary nodes. Radiother Oncol 1988;11:213–222.

34. Leis HP. The other breast. In: Ariel IM, ed. Progress in clinical cancer. vol 1. New York: Grune & Stratton, 1965:507–514.

35. Kurtz JM, Spitalier JM, Amalric R. Late breast recurrence after lumpectomy and irradiation. Int J Radiat Oncol Biol Phys 1983;9:1191–1194.

36. Montague ED. Conservation surgery and radiation therapy in the treatment of operable breast cancer. Cancer 1984;53:700–704.

37. Recht A, Silver B, Schnitt S, Connolly J, Hellman S, Harris JR. Breast relapse following primary radiation therapy for early breast cancer. I. Classification, frequency and salvage. Int J Radiat Oncol Biol Phys 1985;11:1271.

38. Clarke DH, Lê MG, Sarrazin D, et al. Analysis of local-regional relapses in patients with early breast cancers treated by excision and radiotherapy: experience of the Institut Gustave-Roussy. Int J Radiat Oncol Biol Phys 1985;11:137–145.

39. Lacour J, Bucalossi P, Caceres E, et al. Radical mastectomy versus radical mastectomy plus internal mammary dissection. Five-year results of an international cooperative study. Cancer 1976;37:206–214.

40. Lacour J, Lê MG, Hill C, Kramer A, Contesso G, Sarrazin D. Is it useful to remove internal mammary nodes in operable cancer? Eur J Surg Oncol 1987;13:309–314.

41. Rodger A, Montague ED, Fletcher G. Preoperative or postoperative irradiation as adjunctive treatment with radical mastectomy in breast cancer. Cancer 1983;51:1388–1392.

42. Tubiana M, Arriagada R, Sarrazin D. Human cancer natural history, radiation-induced immunodepression and post-operative radiation therapy. Int J Radiat Oncol Biol Phys 1986;12:477–485.

43. Høst H, and Brennnovd IO. The effect of postoperative radiotherapy in breast cancer. Int J Radiat Oncol Biol Phys 1977;2:1061–1067.

44. Høst H, Brennhovd IO, Loeb M. Postoperative radiotherapy in breast cancer—long-term results from the Oslo study. Int J Radiat Oncol Biol Phys 1986;12:727–732.

45. Wallgren A, Arner O, Bergström J, et al. Radiation therapy in operable breast cancer: results from the Stockholm trial on adjuvant radiotherapy. Int J Radiat Oncol Biol Phys 1986;12:533–537.

46. Montague ED, Ames FC, Schell SR, Romsdahl MM. Conservation surgery and irradiation as an alternative to mastectomy in the treatment of clinically favorable breast cancer. Cancer 1984;54:2668–2672.

47. Pierquin B, Marin L. The past and future of conservative treatment of breast cancer. Am J Clin Oncol 1986;9(6):476–480.

48. Calle R, Vilcoq JR, Zafrani B, Vielh P, Fourquet A. Local control and survival of breast cancer treated by limited surgery followed by irradiation. Int J Radiat Oncol Biol Phys 1986;12:873–878.

49. Botnick LE, Harris JR, Hellman S. Experience with breast conserving approaches at the Joint Center for Radiation Therapy, Boston. In: Tobias JS, Pecham MJ, eds. Primary management of breast cancer: alternatives to mastectomy. Baltimore: Edward Arnold, 1985:102–113.

50. Amalric R, Santamaria F, Robert F, et al. Conservation therapy of operable breast cancer—results at five, ten, and fifteen years in 2216 consecutive cases. In: Harris, JR, Hellman S, Silen W, eds. Conservative management of breast cancer: new surgical and radiotherapeutic techniques. Philadelphia: Lippincott, 1983:15–21.

51. Solin LJ, Fowble B, Martz KL, Goodman RL. Definitive irradiation for early stage breast cancer: the University of Pennsylvania experience. Int J Radiat Oncol Biol Phys 1988;14:235–242.

52. Prosnitz LR, Goldenberg IS, Weshler Z, et al. Radiotherapy instead of mastectomy for breast cancer—the Yale experience. In: Harris JR, Hellman S, Silen W, eds. Conservative management of breast cancer; new surgical and radiotherapeutic techniques. Philadelphia: Lippincott, 1983:61–70.

53. Clark RM, Wilkinson RH, Miceli PN, MacDonald WD. Experiences with conservation therapy. Am J Clin Oncol 1987;10:461–468.

54. Veronesi U. Randomized trials comparing conservative techniques with conventional surgery: an overview. In: Tobias JS, Pecham MJ, eds. Primary management of breast cancer, alternatives to mastectomy. Baltimore: Edward Arnold, 1985:131–152.

55. Sarrazin D, Fontaine MJ, Lê MG, Arriagada R. Conservative treatment versus mastectomy in T_1 or small T_2 breast cancer—a randomized clinical trial. In: JR Harris, Hellman S, Silen W, eds. Conservative management of breast cancer: new surgical and radiotherapeutic techniques. Philadelphia: Lippincott, 1983:101–114.

56. Findlay PA, Lippman ME, Danforth JR, et al. Mastectomy versus radiotherapy as treatment for stage I–II breast cancer: a prospective randomized trial at the National Cancer Institute. World J Surg 1985;9:671–675.

57. Pierquin B, Osen R, Maylin C, et al. Radical therapy of breast cancer. Int J Radiat Oncol Biol Phys 1980;6:17–24.

58. Veronesi U, Del Vecchio M, Greco M, et al. Results of quadrantectomy, axillary dissection, and radiotherapy (QUART) in T_1N_0 patients. In: Harris JR, Hellman S, Silen W, eds. Conservative management of breast cancer: new surgical and radiotherapy techniques. Philadelphia: Lippincott, 1983:91–99.

59. Calle R, Pilleron JP, Schlienger P, Vilcoq JR. Conservative management of operable breast cancer: ten years experience at the Foundation Curie. Cancer 1978;42:2045–2053.

60. Harris JR, Connolly JL, Schmitt SJ, et al. The use of pathologic features in selecting the extent of surgical resection necessary for breast cancer patients treated by primary radiation therapy. Ann Surg 1985;201:164–169.

61. Montague ED. Radiation management of advanced breast cancer. Int J Radiat Oncol Biol Phys 1978;4:305–307.

62. Bedwinek J, Rao DV, Perez C, Lee J, Fineberg B. Stage III and localized stage IV breast cancer: irradiation alone vs. irradiation plus surgery. Int J Radiat Oncol Biol Phys 1982;8:31–36.

63. Wilson RE. Surgical management of locally advanced and recurrent breast cancer. Cancer 1984;53(suppl):752–757.

64. Toonkel LM, Fix I, Jacobson LH, Schneider JJ, Wallach CB. Postoperative radiation therapy for carcinoma of the breast: improved results with elective irradiation of the chest wall. Int J Radiat Oncol Biol Phys 1982;8:977–982.

65. Klefström P, Gröhn P, Heinonen E, Holsti L, Holsti P. Adjuvant postoperative radiotherapy, chemotherapy, and immunotherapy in stage III breast cancer. II. 5-year results and influence of Levamisole. Cancer 1987;60:936–942.

66. Barker JL, Montague ED, Peters LJ. Clinical experience with irradiation of inflammatory carcinoma of the breast with and without elective chemotherapy. Cancer 1980;45:625–629.

67. Buzdar AU, Montague ED, Barker JL, Hortobagyi GN, Blumenschein GR. Management of inflammatory carcinoma of the breast with combined modality approach—an update. Cancer 1981;47:2537–2542.

68. Chen KKY, Montague ED, Oswald MJ. Results of irradiation in the treatment of locoregional breast cancer recurrence. Cancer 1985;56:1269–1273.

69. Garmatis CJ, Chu FCH. The effectiveness of radiation therapy in the treatment of bone metastases from breast cancer. Radiology 1978;126:235–237.

70. Allen KL, Johnson TW, Hibbs GG. Effective bone palliation as related to various treatment regimens. Cancer 1976;37:984–987.

21

Systemic Treatment of Breast Cancer

Claude Denham
C. Kent Osborne

The options for systemic therapy in breast cancer have generated substantial optimism as well as controversy over the past 20 years. As a hormonally responsive malignancy, breast cancer has been the focus of intensive laboratory investigations into the mechanisms of hormone-dependent cell proliferation and clinical investigation of the optimal timing of endocrine treatment. The choice, timing, and sequence of cytotoxic agents in the treatment of breast cancer as, one of the more chemotherapy-sensitive solid tumors, have been investigated in many recent and ongoing clinical trials. In addition, other issues have amplified the controversy: (a) the high incidence of breast cancer, (b) the awareness that metastatic breast cancer cannot yet be cured and (c) the extreme heterogeneity of the natural history of breast cancer. This chapter describes and places in perspective the available hormonal and cytotoxic therapies for breast cancer.

CYTOTOXIC CHEMOTHERAPY

Principles of Treatment

Compared with most solid tumors, breast cancer is quite responsive to currently available cytotoxic agents. Unlike colon cancer, malignant melanoma, prostate cancer, and non-small-cell lung cancer, wherein response rates of 10 to 15% are the rule, objective responses will occur in approximately two-thirds of patients with metastatic breast cancer. These responses tend to be short-lived, however, lasting an average of 5 to 12 months. Furthermore, only 5 to 25% of patients have a complete response with total disappearance of all clinically evident tumor. Even complete responses are

temporary, and the disease will eventually recur. The majority of responses are only partial (1).

The following principles should be considered when treating patients with breast cancer with cytotoxic chemotherapy: (a) Combinations of active agents are superior to single agents. (b) Exceedingly high doses of chemotherapy have not yet been proven to be superior to standard therapy. (c) Established metastatic disease cannot be cured with currently available drugs. Thus, a physician's goal in patients with metastatic disease is to choose the treatment regimen that produces the highest likelihood of response of the longest duration with the least short-term and long-term toxicity.

The physician must also keep in mind the extreme variability of the natural history of breast cancer. In some women a rapid fulminant course, not unlike acute leukemia, can be seen. Others, even with established metastatic disease, can have a very indolent course with an extended survival of several years, even if untreated (2). This inherent variability in the clinical course of breast cancer makes evaluation of new treatment strategies difficult, often requiring large groups of patients and many years of follow-up.

Single Agents

Table 21.1 lists the active single agents used to treat breast cancer. Doxorubicin (Adriamycin) is considered generally to be the most active single agent in advanced breast cancer. However, responses are also observed with a variety of other drugs, including alkylating agents, antimetabolites, and vinca alkyloids. On rare occasions, novel schedules, such as continuous infusions of vinblastine or 5-flu-

Table 21.1. Activity of Single Agent Chemotherapy in Metastatic Breast Cancer

Drug	Response Rate[a]
Doxorubicin	35
Cyclophosphamide	32
Thiotepa	30
Methotrexate	25
5-Fluorouracil	25
Mitomycin C	25
Vinblastine	20
L-Phenylalanine mustard	20
Vincristine	10

[a]Approximation based on several studies.

Table 21.2. Combination Regimens Useful Against Breast Cancer

Cyclophosphamide	100 mg/sq m p.o. days 1–14
Methotrexate	40 mg/sq m i.v. day 1, 8 every 4 weeks
5-Fluorouracil	600 mg/sq m i.v. days 1, 8
Cyclophosphamide	500 mg/sq m i.v. day 1
Doxorubicin	50 mg/sq m i.v. day 1 every 3 weeks
5-Fluorouracil	500 mg/sq m i.v. days 1, 8
Cyclophosphamide	100 mg/sq m p.o. days 1–14
Doxorubicin	30 mg/sq m i.v. days 1, 8 every 4 weeks
5-Fluorouracil	500 mg/sq m i.v. days 1, 8
Cyclophosphamide	60 mg/sq m p.o. daily
Methotrexate	15 mg/sq m i.v. weekly
5-Fluorouracil	400 mg/sq m i.v. weekly
Vincristine	0.625 mg/sq m i.v. weekly × 10 weeks
Prednisone	30 mg/sq m p.o. days 1–14, 20 mg/sq m p.o. days 15–28, 10 mg/sq m p.o. days 29–42, then stop

orouracil, have shown improved response rates, compared with those of standard dosing schedules, making them options for salvage chemotherapy. In patients at increased risk of toxicity because of age or organ dysfunction, single agents are sometimes used as initial therapy in patients with metastatic disease. Cyclophosphamide, L-phenylalanine mustard, or even doxorubicin are most often used in this situation. In general, however, both response rates and duration of response are lower with single agents than with combination chemotherapy (1, 3). Combination chemotherapy should always be used when treating patients after mastectomy to inhibit growth of micrometastases (adjuvant therapy).

Combination Chemotherapy

In 1969, Cooper (4) first reported his success with a five-drug combination regimen for metastatic breast cancer, consisting of cyclophosphamide, methotrexate, 5-fluorouracil, vincristine, and prednisone. Since then, variations of this regimen, including elimination of vincristine and prednisone or substitution of doxorubicin for methotrexate, have been devised. Several of the more commonly used regimens are listed in Table 21.2. All of these regimens produce response rates in excess of 50% as initial therapy in advanced breast cancer, but none are clearly superior in terms of overall survival. The combination (cyclophosphamide-methotrexate-5-fluorouracil) regimen (CMF) has a substantial response rate with acceptable toxicity consisting of bone marrow suppression, mild mucositis, mild nausea or vomiting, and alopecia in some patients. Renal dysfunction or the presence of fluid collections such as ascites or pleural effusions can increase the toxicity of methotrexate by prolonging its elimination. Hemorrhagic cystitis can occur with cyclophosphamide therapy unless adequate fluid intake is maintained. This regimen can easily be delivered to outpatients, and it is preferred by many oncologists for first-line treatment of metastatic disease or for adjuvant chemotherapy (1).

Doxorubicin is the single most active drug in advanced breast cancer, and in combination with cyclophosphamide, with or without 5-fluorouracil (CAF), it is associated with the highest reported response rates in this setting. The regimen is more toxic, producing myelosuppression, usually total (although reversible) alopecia, and more severe nausea and vomiting than CMF. In addition, the risk of cardiac toxicity generally limits the total dose of doxorubicin to 450 to 550 mg/sq m or about 6 to 9 months of treatment, depending on dose and schedule. The cardiac toxicity of doxorubicin may be less when the drug is administered by continuous infusion over 48 to 96 hours. In patients who have failed non-doxorubicin-containing regimens, one of the doxorubicin-containing regimens listed in Table 21.2, or doxorubicin alone could be used as a secondary therapy with an expected response rate of between 20 and 50%. In patients refractory to first- or second-line regimens, vinblastine or mitomycin C are sometimes used, although the response rate is low and the remissions are short-lived. The use of high-dose chemotherapy with autologous bone marrow rescue has generated a great deal of enthusiasm recently. Although the response rate with this modality is high, approaching 90%, there are no data at the present time to suggest that survival is prolonged by this aggressive approach, which remains experimental (5).

Adjuvant Chemotherapy

Few areas of medical oncology have generated as much controversy as the issue of adjuvant chemotherapy for breast cancer. The high rate of relapse among patients with primary breast cancer and axillary nodal involvement but without overt distant metastases treated by surgery and/or radiation alone indicates that many breast cancers have already spread systemically by the time of diagnosis (3). The hypothesis was developed that systemic therapy administered shortly after primary surgery might be able to eradicate these micrometastases and cure or at least prolong the survival of patients. Several studies of adjuvant chemotherapy now show more than 10 years of patient follow-up, and definitive conclusions can be made. Most of the initial clinical trials focused on patients with positive axillary nodes who have a high risk for eventual recurrence of disease. More recent studies have examined the potential benefits of adjuvant therapy even in patients with negative axillary nodes. This approach has proven beneficial for some patients but not all.

Enthusiasm for adjuvant chemotherapy increased with the report of a decrease in the relapse rate and improved survival following a single short course of cyclophosphamide therapy in the immediate perioperative period (6). A later National Surgical Adjuvant Breast Project (NSABP) study of melphalan vs. no treatment in patients with positive lymph nodes showed improved disease-free survival that was restricted to premenopausal patients, especially those with one to three positive axillary nodes (7). Another study of node-positive breast cancer by the Milan Cancer Institute comparing the three-drug CMF combination with no adjuvant therapy confirmed this observation and showed improved survival in premenopausal women (8). In this subset, 48% of CMF-treated patients remained disease-free, and 59% remained alive at 10 years of follow-up, as compared with 31% and 45%, respectively, of untreated patients.

The issue of adjuvant chemotherapy for postmenopausal women with positive axillary nodes is less clear. The Milan study showed no disease-free or overall survival advantage for adjuvant CMF in postmenopausal women. A retrospective analysis correlated the lack of benefit with attenuated drug doses in older patients (8). Although uncontrolled studies show improved disease-free and overall survival in postmenopausal women receiving adjuvant chemotherapy, the cumulative data from controlled studies suggest that there is only a modest benefit from adjuvant chemotherapy in postmenopausal women. More recent trials evaluating more aggressive doxorubicin-containing regimens should provide important new information in the near future. Preliminary results suggest that these regimens may be more effective in this subset.

The optimal duration of adjuvant chemotherapy is also an important question that has been addressed in clinical trials. In a follow-up study by the Milan Cancer Institute, women with positive nodes were randomized to 6 months or 12 months of CMF. No reduction of the therapeutic benefit was observed with only 6 months of treatment (8). The optimal duration of other chemotherapy regimens remains to be defined. Furthermore, the value of doxorubicin-containing regimens in the adjuvant setting is currently being investigated.

Most studies of adjuvant chemotherapy have been done in patients with positive axillary nodes who have a high risk for later recurrence. Patients with negative axillary nodes at the time of surgery have a better prognosis, and many are cured by surgery alone. However, about 30 to 35% of these patients will eventually recur and die of their disease. Recently, studies of chemotherapy or endocrine therapy with tamoxifen have been completed in node-negative patients (9–12). Data from three trials that have not yet been published were distributed recently to physicians in the form of a "clinical alert" from the National Cancer Institute (12). The cumulative data from these studies suggest that node-negative patients as a group receive a modest benefit in prolonging disease-free and, perhaps, overall survival with treatment. The challenge now is to develop prognostic factors that can accurately identify those patients whose disease is likely to recur, so that toxic therapies can be avoided in the large proportion of node-negative patients who have already been cured by local therapies.

General guidelines to help make decisions in this controversial area have been provided by an NIH Consensus Conference held in 1985, as listed in Table 21.3 (13). These general recommendations continue to be valid today, although more data are now available in patients with negative axillary nodes. Based on the recent data discussed above, high-risk node-negative patients such as those with large tumors, estrogen receptor-negative tumors, or tumors with aneuploid DNA content or a high proliferative potential determined by flow cytometry should be considered for adjuvant combination chemotherapy. Patients with estrogen recep-

Table 21.3. Recommendations of NIH Consensus Conference for Adjuvant Chemotherapy—1985

Premenopausal, node-positive, ER + or −
  Combination chemotherapy
Postmenopausal, node-positive, ER + tamoxifen
Postmenopausal, node-positive, ER −
  Chemotherapy may be considered
Premenopausal or postmenopausal, node-negative,
  ER + or − Chemotherapy may be considered in
  high-risk patients

tor-positive tumors, especially if the tumor is small, might be candidates for adjuvant endocrine therapy with tamoxifen. Very low-risk, node-negative patients, such as those with very small or mammographically detected tumors or those with diploid DNA content and low proliferative potential by flow cytometry, are problematic. These patients have a very low risk for recurrence, less than 10% at 5 years, and an argument can be made to withhold therapy and to not subject the entire group of patients to the cost and toxicity of treatment for the benefit of so few.

Patients with locally advanced or inflammatory breast cancer present special problems. These patients have large and/or fixed breast masses that can be ulcerated or demonstrate skin erythema, edema, and pathologic evidence of cancer infiltration of the subdermal lymphatics. Mastectomy alone results in a dismal prognosis in these patients, who have a high local recurrence rate and an average survival of 8 to 15 months. Local radiation alone or combined sequentially with surgery becomes an important treatment modality for reducing the risk of local recurrence. Initial treatment with a doxorubicin-based combination chemotherapy may increase disease-free survival over radiation alone (14). Other types of locally advanced disease, including lesions invading the skin (T_4) or with supraclavicular or infraclavicular nodes (N_3), are treated primarily with radiation therapy and chemotherapy as well (15).

Treatment of Metastatic Breast Cancer with Chemotherapy

Chemotherapy is also beneficial and provides important palliation in patients with established metastatic disease. It is used instead of endocrine therapy in (a) patients who have failed prior hormonal therapy; (b) patients who have a low likelihood of responding to hormonal treatments by virtue of being estrogen receptor (ER)-negative, or having extensive visceral disease (especially brain, liver, or

lymphangitic lung metastases); or (c) patients who have rapidly progressive tumor.

In general, combination chemotherapy such as CMF or CAF is used to treat metastatic disease. Single agents are less effective, and the duration of response to combinations is more durable, with response durations ranging from a few months to several years (median ≈1 year).

Most patients with symptoms due to pulmonary, bone, or liver metastases or local skin recurrence are effectively palliated, at least temporarily, with chemotherapy. The effect of chemotherapy on survival remains controversial, however. For patients with life-threatening aggressive disease, there is a clear survival advantage with treatment. The improved quality of life provided by chemotherapy in patients with symptomatic metastases as well as prolonged survival for certain patients justify its use. Cure remains an elusive goal in patients with metastatic disease. The most commonly used regimens are shown in Table 21.2.

ENDOCRINE TREATMENT

Principles of Treatment

Breast cancer, like malignancies of other hormonally responsive organs, often responds to hormonal manipulation. Receptors for estrogen or progesterone are found in two-thirds of breast cancer specimens at diagnosis (16). In the laboratory, the growth of some breast cancer cell lines can be stimulated by estrogens and inhibited by antiestrogens. Presumably, estrogen regulates growth-promoting factors or key metabolic enzymes within the tumor that influence cell growth (17). The exact mechanism of endocrine-mediated changes in tumor size is not well understood, however. Paradoxically, both high doses of estrogen and estrogen antagonists can produce tumor regression. Although our understanding of the biochemical mechanisms of hormone-dependent cell growth has increased dramatically over the past 10 years, the clinical use of endocrine therapy remains largely empiric. Further studies of these mechanisms should provide a more rational basis for the hormonal therapy of breast cancer.

Predicting a Response to Hormones

The likelihood of a response to hormonal therapy in an individual case of breast cancer can be predicted to some degree. The presence of estrogen receptor in the tumor is most reliable predictor of a response to any form of endocrine therapy. Estrogen receptor-positive tu-

Table 21.4.   Factors That Predict a Response to Hormonal Therapy

Estrogen receptor positivity
Long disease-free interval post mastectomy
Skin, bone, or nodular lung metastases
Late postmenopausal status
Indolent disease

mors respond to endocrine therapy in approximately 60% of cases while less than 10% of estrogen receptor-negative tumors respond (16, 18). Table 21.4 lists other factors that predict whether an individual will respond to hormonal therapy. These features are not independent, however. For example, estrogen receptor-positive tumors are more likely to have a long disease-free interval and are more likely to relapse in bone than ER-negative tumors, which are usually more aggressive and have frequent visceral metastases (19). All of these factors may be used to help select appropriate treatment. For instance, an elderly woman with predominant bone disease who is 3 years postmastectomy for breast cancer may warrant a trial of endocrine therapy even though she is estrogen receptor-negative. Conversely, a young woman with rapidly progressive liver metastases should probably receive cytotoxic chemotherapy even though her tumor is estrogen receptor-positive.

Types of Hormonal Therapy

Oophorectomy was the earliest form of systemic cancer therapy. As expected, it is only effective in premenopausal women. Oophorectomy by surgical means or by pelvic irradiation is equally effective, although radiotherapy takes slightly longer for a maximum benefit, and ovarian function may return in some patients.

Surgical oophorectomy is still the preferred first-line endocrine therapy for premenopausal patients by many physicians. Medical castration with the new luteinizing hormone-releasing hormone (LHRH) analogues is currently being studied, and it may eventually obviate the need for surgical castration.

Tamoxifen is the most widely used hormonal therapy in breast cancer, and fortunately, one of the least toxic of all cancer therapies. It is used most often in postmenopausal women, but it is also effective in estrogen receptor-positive premenopausal women with metastatic disease. The standard dose is 10 mg twice per day. Tamoxifen is well-tolerated, with menopausal symptoms being the most common side

effect. Transient leukopenia and thrombocytopenia are reported rarely.

Progestational agents are often used as second-line therapy after a response to tamoxifen in postmenopausal patients. The most commonly used drug, megestrol acetate, is used in a dose of 40 mg four times per day (20). There have been some reports of improved responses with higher doses, but there are more side effects, and this approach remains investigational (21). Medroxyprogesterone acetate, another progestational agent, can be used orally or intramuscularly. Like tamoxifen, progestational agents are well-tolerated. They do cause weight gain due to an anabolic effect, fluid retention, vaginal bleeding, and occasionally a fine tremor and muscle cramps.

Aminoglutethimide was initially developed as an anticonvulsant, but it is useful in treating breast cancer in postmenopausal women. It blocks essential enzymes in adrenocortical steroid synthesis, inhibiting the production of adrenal androgens (22). A more important mechanism is inhibition of aromatization of adrenal androgens such as androstenedione to estrogen in peripheral tissues and in breast cancer cells themselves. The net result is a reduction in the estrogen level. Aminoglutethimide in a dose of 240 mg four times per day is as effective as other hormonal therapies, but because of more prominent side effects, it is often used after progression on tamoxifen or progestational agents. A physiologic replacement dose of hydrocortisone is given with aminoglutethimide to prevent symptoms of adrenal insufficiency and to prevent a rebound rise in ACTH that could override the adrenal block. Lethargy and a pruritic maculopapular rash are common but transient, and they usually respond to a temporary increase of the hydrocortisone dose. Severe cytopenias can rarely occur as well (23).

High-dose estrogens are surprisingly beneficial and were the standard treatment for postmenopausal breast cancer before tamoxifen. Diethylstilbestrol (DES) in a dose of 5 mg three times per day is the most common preparation, but premarin at 2.5 mg three times per day or ethinyl estradiol 1 mg three times per day can be used. A few patients experience a temporary increase in tumor growth or "flare" during the first several weeks of treatment. The flare may herald a subsequent response with continued treatment, and it is not an indication to stop therapy unless it is life-threatening. Approximately one-third of estrogen responders will have a second response on withdrawal of the drug at the time of tumor progression. Some physicians recommend an observation period of 2 to 4 weeks after discontinuing the estrogen before beginning further therapy (23). Fluid retention, thromboembolic sequelae, and nausea are common toxicities, and they preclude use of this drug in certain patients.

Surgical adrenalectomy or hypophysectomy are both effective endocrine therapies for breast cancer. Since other methods are available and since in inexperienced hands the operative morbidity of these procedures can be considerable, they are infrequently used now (24).

Adjuvant Hormonal Therapy

Since the 1940s, several clinical trials have evaluated adjuvant surgical or radiation oophorectomy following mastectomy by either surgery or radiation. In some studies disease-free survival is prolonged in premenopausal women, but no consistent improvement in overall survival has been observed. Oophorectomy is currently being reevaluated in patients selected on the basis of estrogen receptor status.

Both tamoxifen and DES have been evaluated as adjuvant therapy in postmenopausal women. DES is considerably more toxic, so most recent studies have used tamoxifen. Tamoxifen significantly improves the disease-free survival of estrogen receptor-positive, node-positive postmenopausal women. Some studies also show a modest survival benefit in this patient subset. Most studies report that the benefit of adjuvant tamoxifen is greatest in patients with estrogen receptor-positive tumors (24), although estrogen receptor-negative patients have also shown modest benefit in certain studies (10, 11).

The proper duration of adjuvant endocrine therapy with tamoxifen is not yet known, although prolonged therapy for several years may be optimal. Tamoxifen's disease-free and overall survival benefits and its low toxicity have made it standard therapy today in estrogen receptor-positive, node-positive postmenopausal women. Conversely, the consistent improvement in overall survival of premenopausal women has made chemotherapy standard adjuvant treatment for this subset (8, 13). Current studies are evaluating whether more aggressive chemotherapy alone or combined with tamoxifen is superior to tamoxifen alone.

Hormonal Therapy of Metastatic Disease

As outlined previously, a physician can predict the likelihood of a patient responding to hormonal therapy by considering several factors. If these factors suggest that a patient may have a hormonally responsive tumor, then endocrine therapy, which is considerably less toxic than chemotherapy, should be used initially. Chemotherapy is recommended in patients with life-threatening visceral disease, especially if estrogen receptor-negative. Unless there is strong clinical suspicion that a patient might still have a hormonally sensitive tumor, the lack of response to initial endocrine therapy should prompt the physician to change to cytotoxic chemotherapy since there is little likelihood of response to a second endocrine therapy. On the other hand, patients who respond to initial hormonal therapy can frequently be managed at the time of progression with secondary or even tertiary endocrine therapies. The preferred sequence of hormonal therapy varies among physicians, but the following are reasonable guidelines.

In premenopausal women, oophorectomy or tamoxifen can be use as initial therapy or as second-line therapy in responding patients. Third-line endocrine manipulations include medical adrenalectomy with aminoglutethimide, progestational agents, or androgens. If the patient stops responding to endocrine therapy, or if more aggressive disease develops, chemotherapy is indicated.

In postmenopausal women, tamoxifen is the usual initial therapy, although progestins have been used initially by some. Both are less toxic than high-dose estrogens. If the patient responds to this initial therapy, aminoglutethimide is often effective at the time of progression, although the likelihood of toxicity increases. Later responses can sometimes occur with estrogens or androgens.

There are theoretic reasons why combining two or more hormonal agents might be more effective than using a single agent. In clinical practice, however, combinations provide no overall survival advantage, compared with the sequential use of the same agents (25). The combinations often have synergistic toxicity, and they cannot be recommended outside of clinical trials.

The majority of breast cancers are heterogeneous with a mixture of estrogen-receptor-positive and estrogen-receptor-negative cells. Combining chemotherapy and endocrine therapy to eradicate both populations seems logical. In clinical practice, however, combining chemotherapy and hormonal therapy is no more effective than the sequential use of either modality. Furthermore, there are theoretic reasons to suggest that endocrine agents could even antagonize the cytotoxic effects of chemotherapy (26, 27). Thus combined chemoendocrine therapy is not recommended routinely.

In summary, the management of patients with breast cancer with systemic therapy is complicated. The disease differs from patient to patient, and there are many therapeutic modalities that may be appropriate under certain circumstances. Treatment decisions require knowledge of breast cancer biology and natural history, as well as experience and clinical judgment. Today, with proper treatment many breast cancer patients can be cured or the disease can be controlled for extended periods.

REFERENCES

1. Henderson IC. Chemotherapy for advanced disease. In: Harris JR, Hellman S, Henderson IC, et al. eds. Breast diseases. Philadelphia: JB Lippincott, 1987:428–479.
2. Adair F, Berg J, Joubert L, Robbins GF. Long-term followup of breast cancer patients: a thirty year report. Cancer 1974;33:1145–1150.
3. Henderson IC, Canellos GP. Cancer of the breast: the past decade. N Engl J Med 1980;302:17–30, 78–90.
4. Cooper RG. Combination chemotherapy in hormone resistant breast cancer. Proc Am Assoc Cancer Res 1969;10:15.
5. Eder JP, Antman K, Peters WP, et al. High dose combination alkylating agent chemotherapy with autologous bone marrow support for metastatic breast cancer. J Clin Oncol 1986;4:1592–1597.
6. Nissen-Meyer R, Kjellgien K, Malmio K, Mannson B, Norin T. Surgical adjuvant chemotherapy. Cancer 1978;41:2088–2098.
7. Fisher B, Slack N, Katrych D, Wolmark N. Ten-year followup results of patients with carcinoma of the breast in a cooperative clinical trial evaluating adjuvant chemotherapy. Surg Gynecol Obstet 1975;140:528–534.
8. Bonadonna G, Valagussa P, Rossi A, et al. Ten-year experience with CMF based adjuvant chemotherapy in resectable breast cancer. Breast Cancer Res Treat 1985;5:95–115.
9. Bonadonna G, Valagussa P, Tancini G, Current status of Milan adjuvant chemotherapy trials for node-positive and node-negative breast cancer. Natl Cancer Inst Monogr 1986;1:45–49.
10. Nolvadex Adjuvant Trial Organization. Controlled trial of tamoxifen as single adjuvant agent in management of early breast cancer. Lancet 1985;1:836–840.
11. Breast Cancer Trials Committee, Scottish Cancer Trials Office (MRCO), Edinburgh. Adjuvant tamoxifen in the management of operable breast cancer: the Scottish Trial. Lancet 1987;2:171–175.
12. Clinical alert from the National Cancer Institute, 1988.
13. Consensus Conference. Adjuvant chemotherapy for breast cancer. JAMA 1985;254:3461–3463.
14. Sherry MM, Johnson DH, Page DL, Greco FA, Hainsworth JD. Inflammatory carcinoma of the breast: a clinical review and summary of the Vanderbilt experience with multi-modality treatment. Am J Med 1985;79:355–364.
15. Schaake-Koning C, Hamersma van der Linden E, Hart G, Englesman E. Adjuvant chemotherapy and hormonal therapy in locally advanced breast cancer: a randomized clinical study. Int J Radiat Oncol Biol Phys 1985;11:1759–1763.
16. Osborne CK, Yochmowitz MG, Knight WA, McGuire WL. The value of estrogen and progesterone receptors in the treatment of breast cancer. Cancer 1980;46:2884–2888.
17. Lippman ME, Dickson RB, Bates S, et al. Autocrine and paracrine growth regulation of human breast cancer. Breast Cancer Res Treat 1986;7:59–70.
18. Young PCM, Ehrlich CF, Einhorn LH. Relationship between steroid receptors and responses to endocrine therapy and cytotoxic chemotherapy in metastatic breast cancer. Cancer 1980;46:2961–2963.
19. Clark GM, Osborne CK, McGuire WL. Correlations between estrogen receptor, progesterone receptor, and patient characteristics in human breast cancer. J Clin Oncol 1984;2:1102–1109.
20. Hortobagyi GN, Buzdar AU, Frye D, et al. Oral medroxyprogesterone acetate in the treatment of metastatic breast cancer. Breast Cancer Res Treat 1985;5:321–326.
21. Tchekmedyian NS, Tait N, Abrams J, Aisner T. High-dose megestrol acetate in the treatment of advanced breast cancer. Semin Oncol 1988;15(2)S1:44–49.
22. Santen RJ. Suppression of estrogens with aminoglutethimide and hydrocortisone as treatment of advanced breast cancer: a review. Breast Cancer Treat Rep 1981;1:181–188.
23. Henderson IC. Endocrine therapy in metastatic breast cancer. In Harris JR, Hellmann S, Henderson IC, et al., eds. Breast diseases. Philadelphia: JB Lippincott, 1987;398–428.
24. Cummings FJ, Gray RJ, Davis TE, et al. Adjuvant tamoxifen treatment of elderly women with stage II breast cancer. Ann Intern Med 1985;103:324–330.
25. Ingle JN, Twito DI, Schaid DJ, et al. Randomized clinical trial of tamoxifen alone or combined with fluoxymesterone in postmenopausal women with metastatic breast cancer. J Clin Oncol 1988;6(5):825–831.
26. Osborne CK. Combined chemo-hormonal therapy in breast cancer: a hypothesis. Breast Cancer Res Treat 1981;1:121–124.
27. Hug V, Hortobagyi GN, Drewinko B, Finders M. Tamoxifen-citrate counteracts the antitumor effects of cytotoxic drugs in vitro. J Clin Oncol 1985;3(12):1672–1677.

Pregnancy and Breast Cancer

Mara J. Dinsmoor

INCIDENCE AND EPIDEMIOLOGY

The incidence of breast carcinoma occurring in association with pregnancy, usually defined as the time period beginning with conception and ending 1 year postpartum, is as high as 1/1500 to 1/3000 deliveries (1, 2). Fifteen percent of breast carcinomas occur in women younger than 41 years old, and approximately 3% occur during pregnancy (1). Indeed, 11% of those patients under 40 years old and 14% of those under 35 years old will be pregnant at the time of diagnosis (3, 4). Following cervical cancer, cancer of the breast is the second most common malignancy occurring during pregnancy (5). As is the case with most unusual diseases, individual centers' experience with breast cancer in pregnancy is limited, and large controlled studies of treatment, prognosis, and pregnancy outcome are not available. Therapeutic decisions must therefore be based on the limited knowledge that can be gleaned from relatively small series. Unfortunately, since women are now more often delaying childbearing into the fourth and fifth decades, breast carcinoma can be expected to become more common in the obstetric population.

The average age of the pregnant breast carcinoma patient is 32 to 35 years, underscoring the fact that this disease occurs in the "older" pregnant woman (5). However, these patients comprise a relatively young group of breast cancer patients, a group that some feel has a more aggressive disease and a generally poorer prognosis to begin with (6, 7).

Among the accepted risk factors for carcinoma of the breast is advanced age at first term pregnancy. Thus, it appears that a prior pregnancy actually has a protective effect (2, 8). Similar effects are not provided by the "pseudopregnancy" of oral contraceptives, and the protective effects of an early first pregnancy vanish if that pregnancy ends in an early abortion (8–10). An abortion occurring prior to the first full-term pregnancy may increase the risk of breast cancer in young women, although if the abortion follows a full-term pregnancy, risk is not altered (9, 10). There is also some evidence that the risk of recurrence following mastectomy for early breast cancer is increased in patients with a prior abortion (11).

DIAGNOSIS

Delay in Diagnosis

When diagnosed during pregnancy, 65 to 79% of breast carcinomas have advanced beyond stage I, and as many as 19% are at stage IV (3, 12, 13). The relatively advanced stages found at diagnosis in pregnant patients are due in large part to delays in diagnosis. Applewhite and associates (14) estimated that the delay in diagnosis following onset of symptoms averaged 11 months in the pregnant patient, as compared with 4 months in the nonpregnant patient. Although much of this delay was patient related, significant delays were also introduced by the physician (14). Peters (15) noted a median delay of 15 months in the pregnant patient, compared with 9 months in the nonpregnant, premenopausal patient. Some authors have not noted significant delays, including Clark and associates (16), who found that more than one-half of their series of 330 patients had delays in diagnosis less than 6 months. Since most pregnant patients have multiple contacts with medical personnel during this period, these delays are preventable and should not occur.

The presenting symptoms are most commonly those of a nipple discharge or mass (17). The normal breast enlargement that occurs during pregnancy may obscure small tumors, making diagnosis by even the most diligent examiner difficult. As in the nonpregnant patient, most breast abnormalities are first discovered by the patient herself (4, 18, 19). Often the examining physician assumes that breast masses found during pregnancy and lactation are related to normal gestational and/or lactational changes in the breast, and chooses not to perform any diagnostic procedures. A pathologic mass that is palpable initially may seem to disappear with serial examinations, when in fact it simply has become obscured by the enlarging mass of the breast. The physician is then falsely reassured and diagnosis is delayed further.

Diagnostic Evaluation

Mammography should not be relied on as a diagnostic tool during pregnancy. Although the fetal radiation exposure is small, especially with abdominal shielding and in early pregnancy, the increased vascularity and water content of the pregnant breast substantially reduces the quality of the examination. Ultrasound of the breast should not be utilized for the same reason. Pregnancy does not affect the accuracy of histologic diagnosis, and this remains the diagnostic test of choice.

Aspiration under local anesthesia carries minimal risk for both mother and fetus and remains highly accurate in the hands of an experienced cytopathologist (20). If aspiration is nondiagnostic or suspicious, excisional biopsy may be safely performed under local or general anesthesia, preferably local. Vigilance must be maintained, however, as infection and excessive bleeding may be more common following biopsy in the pregnant patient. In addition, during late pregnancy and lactation, biopsy techniques should be modified somewhat to avoid disruption of milk ducts. This includes making the incision parallel to, rather than on, the areolar edge and using blunt rather than sharp dissection (21).

As with the nonpregnant patient in this age group, most breast masses, both cystic and solid, are benign (5, 17, 22). There are several reports of otherwise benign conditions exacerbating during pregnancy and lactation, sometimes mimicking carcinoma. These include unilateral breast hyperplasia, lactational changes in adenomas, and infarction of either hyperplastic breast tissue or adenomas (23–26).

At one time, inflammatory carcinoma was thought to occur more frequently during pregnancy, and the poor prognosis of the pregnant patient was often attributed to this. Further evidence has shown that the histology of breast cancer in pregnancy does not differ significantly from that of the nonpregnant patient (5). Recent large series have reported incidences of inflammatory carcinoma ranging from 2.5 to 8% (12, 16).

MANAGEMENT

Once the diagnosis of carcinoma is made, treatment should not be unduly delayed because of the coexisting pregancy. Tentative or delayed treatment of the pregnant patient may result in what was once local disease becoming advanced and incurable by the time treatment is begun. This factor may be partly responsible for the relatively advanced disease seen in pregnancy (17).

Metastatic Evaluation

Because of risks to the fetus of radiation exposure, most authors recommend modifying the usual metastatic evaluation to minimize fetal exposure to ionizing radiation. Chest radiography in early pregnancy exposes the fetus to minimal radiation, approximately 0.6 mrads (Table 22.1) (27), and should be maintained as part of the initial evaluation. With abdominal shielding, exposure of the term fetus will also be low (28). In the asymptomatic, premenopausal patient the incidence of bone metastases is extremely low (5, 29). Because of the relatively low yield in patients with clinical stage I and II disease, radionuclide bone scans should be reserved for patients with stage III disease and those who exhibit symptoms or laboratory findings suggestive of bone metastases. In 1987, Baker and associates (30) reported a modified bone scanning technique that reduced fetal radiation exposure from 194 mRem to approximately 76 mRem, yet appeared to produce adequate images. Experience with this technique is, however, limited. Although fetal exposure from computed tomography (CT) of the head is low, this procedure should also be reserved for symptomatic patients and those with advanced disease (27). Liver metastases are found in less than 5% of patients with stage I and II disease, so radiographic evaluation of the liver should be performed only when the patient has complaints referrable to those organs or if there are abnormalities in the liver chemistries (29). Although experience with magnetic resonance imaging (MRI) in pregnancy is limited, this diagnostic tool may prove useful in the future.

Surgical Treatment

As in the nonpregnant patient, the treatment of choice for most patients with breast carcinoma is surgical. In general, surgical treatment of the pregnant patient should not vary greatly from that chosen for the nonpregnant patient with similar disease.

Mastectomy appears to be well-tolerated by the developing fetus. Although the spontane-

Table 22.1.   Dose to Embryo or Ovary from Diagnostic Radiologic Procedures in the First Trimester (mrads)[a]

Chest radiograph	0.06
Bone scan	99
Liver scan	14–21
CT of brain	7

[a]Based on data from the Committee on Radiologic Units, Standards, and Protection. Medical Radiation: a good guide to practice. American College of Radiology, 1985; and Wallach MK, Wolf JA, Bedwinek J, et al. Gestational carcinoma in the female breast. Curr Probl Cancer 1983;7:1-58.

ous abortion rate following surgery in the first trimester is slightly increased, most of this increase results from the nature of the operation itself and/or the underlying pathology rather than from the anesthetic (31). Many general anesthetics are potential teratogens when used in the first trimester. Although the risk in humans appears to be low, if possible the use of anesthetics should be avoided during the major period of organogenesis, lasting 8 weeks from conception (5, 31). When performed late in pregnancy, intraabdominal surgery may lead to premature labor or birth; however, the risk of this occurring following mastectomy is minimal (31).

During surgery, care must be taken to avoid vena caval compression by the enlarged uterus and perioperative hypotension, both resulting in decreased uterine blood flow. Vena caval compression and subsequent supine hypotension may be avoided by placing a wedge under the patient's right hip, elevating it 15 to 30°. Prophylactic perioperative tocolytics may reduce the risk of premature delivery and should be used therapeutically if regular uterine contractions occur. Continuous fetal monitoring should be performed intraoperatively and perioperatively to allow intervention should fetal distress occur. In early previable gestations, intervention might consist of increased hydration and oxygenation, position change, or a reduction in uterine manipulation. In the third trimester these maneuvers should also be performed, reserving emergent cesarean delivery for persistent severe distress.

Estrogen and progesterone receptors should be obtained on the neoplastic tissue at the time of surgery, as in the nonpregnant patient, for use as a prognostic indicator and planning adjunctive therapy. There is some evidence that some receptor assays may give false-negative results during pregnancy, due to saturation with endogenous steroid hormones (32).

Adjunctive Therapy

Patients with advanced disease may require treatment with cytotoxic drugs, radiation, or both. Again, the choice of treatment modality should be made following standard protocols, as though the patient were not pregnant. Rather, the patient's pregnancy may affect when treatment is instituted. The antineoplastic drugs commonly used in the treatment of breast cancer (i.e., cyclophosphamide, methotrexate, 5-fluorouracil, doxorubicin, melphalan, chlorambucil, thiotepa, and mitomycin C) cross the placenta and therefore may affect the fetus. Exposure to radiation may also have adverse effects on the fetus. The severity of these effects varies with dose, gestational age at exposure, and type of drug.

First Trimester

If the patient's carcinoma has been diagnosed in the first trimester and chemotherapy is planned, most authors recommend that a therapeutic abortion be performed to avoid potential adverse effects on the fetus (1, 5, 17). There are many reports of normal outcomes following chemotherapy in the first trimester of pregnancy, most following treatment for leukemia or lymphoma (33, 34). Moreover, there are little data as to the teratogenicity of most antineoplastic agents. It appears that aminopterin is highly teratogenic, and methotrexate, a related antimetabolite, has been associated with several congenital malformations following fetal exposure in the first trimester (34, 35). Cyclophosphamide appears to be teratogenic in the first trimester, and multiple congenital malformations have been seen in a fetus following first-trimester exposure to 5-fluorouracil (36, 37). Congenital malformations have been reported following treatment for breast carcinoma with cytotoxic drugs and radiotherapy in the first trimester (38). As summarized by Sweet and Kinzie (37), the overall incidence of malformations following first-trimester exposure to antineoplastic agents in 164 patients was low, about 5%, and almost half of these fetuses had also been exposed to radiotherapy. Unfortunately, there are few studies to which the clinician can refer, and the decision as to abortion remains largely with the patient.

The risks of radiotherapy in the first trimester are also difficult to quantify. With shielding the estimated dose to the developing fetus is approximately 10 to 15 rads after a treatment dose of 5000 rad to the chest area, primarily due to internal scatter (5). Although there does not appear to be a threshold dose below which the fetus is never harmed, doses of this magnitude are usually not associated with adverse effects in humans, although they frequently result in anomalies and embryonal deaths in mice (37). There is conflicting evidence, however, that even small doses of radiation may increase fetal risk for childhood malignancies, especially leukemia (39–42). Substantially higher fetal doses are required to induce abortion, on the order of several hundred rads (43).

Second and Third Trimesters

Although the risk of teratogenicity is much reduced later in pregnancy, the usual chemotherapeutic drugs may still have adverse effects on the rapidly dividing cells of the growing fetus. Multiagent chemotherapy has been used in the past with no immediate discernible adverse fetal or neonatal effects (44, 45). There have been some reports of low birthweight and intrauterine growth retardation following treatment with antineoplastic agents in the second and third trimesters, occurring in up to 40% of neonates (37). There is a recent case report of chromosome gaps and a ring chromosome in a newborn exposed to multiagent chemotherapy during the second and third trimesters (46). There are also several cases of neonatal pancytopenia following maternal chemotherapy in the third trimester (47).

Long-term effects on children exposed in utero to chemotherapy are not known, although possible effects include congenital malformations, chromosomal damage, induction of neoplasia, and slowing of growth and/or mental development. One series with follow-up from 1 to 17 years in 50 infants following exposure to chemotherapeutic agents in utero revealed one infant of a twin pair with congenital malformations. Subsequently the child developed two separate malignancies. All other children, including the other twin, displayed normal growth and development (47).

If possible, delivery should be avoided during the period of maximal bone marrow suppression, as intrapartum complications may lead to life-threatening blood loss or sepsis in the mother. For the same reason, elective abortion should precede initiation of chemotherapy, rather than follow it.

Compared with treatment in the first trimester, radiotherapy in late gestation results in a higher fetal dose, as much as 200 rads in the third trimester (5). Even at this dose, adverse fetal effects in the form of malformations are rare at these later stages of gestation. The major effects are on the still growing central nervous system, sometimes resulting in microcephaly, mental retardation, and growth disturbances (37). After 20 weeks of gestation, the fetal effects of dosages up to 250 rads are limited to the more typical changes of radiation exposure, for example, anemia and dermal erythema (37).

If the pregnancy is approaching fetal viability, therapy may be delayed for a short period (i.e., several weeks) to allow delivery prior to instituting therapy. Neonatal health at delivery should be maximized by administering antenatal steroids when appropriate and planning delivery at an institution with neonatal intensive care facilities. At present, neonatal survival can be expected in most infants born following 28 weeks of gestation. Morbidity, including lung disease, both respiratory distress syndrome and chronic lung disease, blindness, and intraventricular hemorrhage, remains a problem at these gestational ages but is rare beyond 34 weeks of gestation at most institutions. Obviously, decisions as to timing, location, and route of delivery should be made in concert with the perinatologists, neonatologists, and members of the oncology team. Cesarean section should be performed for obstetric indications.

EFFECT OF BREAST CANCER ON PREGNANCY

Other than the previously discussed effects of surgery, chemotherapy and radiotherapy, the diagnosis of breast carcinoma in pregnancy seems to have little impact on the outcome of the pregnancy itself. There are no reports of increased perinatal morbidity or mortality, other than iatrogenic prematurity to allow therapy, or following mastectomy. Although breast carcinoma occasionally metastasizes to the placenta, there are no reported cases of fetal metastases (1, 48, 49).

EFFECT OF PREGNANCY ON BREAST CANCER

Theoretic Concerns

Although the "physiologic immunosuppression" of pregnancy prevents rejection of the fetus as an allograft, physicians have long been concerned about the possible subsequent deleterious effects of a concurrent pregnancy on the course of many illnesses, especially neoplastic and infectious diseases. In normal pregnancy, the cell-mediated immune response is depressed, including a reduced $T_4:T_8$ ratio and a diminished lymphoproliferative response (50). Mechanisms that have been postulated to explain this change include elevated steroid hormone levels and the presence of maternal blocking antibodies (51). These changes in the immune system result in an increased suscepti-

Table 22.2. Breast Cancer in Women <40 Years Old: Stage at Diagnosis and Five-Year Survival[a]

	Nonpregnant n = 155		Pregnant n = 19	
Stage	N%	5-yr survival, %	N(%)	5-yr survival, %
I (negative nodes)	84(54)	70	4(21)	100
II (positive nodes)	57(37)	48	14(74)	50
III (distant disease)	14(9)	7	1(5)	0
Total	100	56	100	57

[a]Adapted from Nugent P, O'Connell TX. Breast cancer and pregnancy. Arch Surg 1985; 120:1221–1224.

bility to certain infectious diseases, although there is little evidence for any adverse effect on the course of malignant disease.

In addition, with a hormonally responsive tumor such as breast carcinoma, the possible trophic effects of the elevated levels of estrogen and progesterone found in pregnancy are important considerations. Elevated levels of prolactin in pregnancy may also have a trophic effect (5, 17). There have also been concerns that the increased vascularity and lymphatic flow of the pregnant breast might favor early metastases (1, 5, 17, 52, 53).

Because of these concerns therapeutic abortion and/or prophylactic oopherectomy were frequently recommended in the past, regardless of planned treatment, in the hope that ending the pregnancy and reducing endogenous steroid hormones would improve survival (53). However, there is no evidence that either procedure improves survival (1, 3, 15–17, 52–54). In this young group of patients, prophylactic oopherectomy may in fact be contraindicated, since the possible benefits of subsequent pregnancies, as discussed later, would then be lost.

Stage of Disease and Survival

It appears that pregnant women in whom the diagnosis of breast cancer is made often have advanced disease at the time of diagnosis. It is difficult to directly compare staging and outcome between different series, as a wide variety of staging classifications have been used in recent years. Stage at diagnosis in pregnant patients was compared with that of nonpregnant patients in women younger than 40 years old in one series. As shown in Table 22.2, advanced stages were significantly more common in the pregnant patient. However, survival did not differ in the two groups once matched in this manner for age and stage at diagnosis (3). In a large series of patients, Peters (15) found that the 5-year survival for patients with a concurrent pregnancy was lower than that for nonpregnant controls matched for stage or age (Table 22.3). However, when

matched for both age and stage at diagnosis, there was little difference in survival (15).

Some series report improved survival when the diagnosis is made or treatment begun at certain stages of pregnancy (15, 55). The data are conflicting and there are many possible biases, so no firm conclusions can be reached as to the possible effect of the stage of gestation at time of diagnosis or treatment.

In addition, axillary nodes are positive in a large number of these patients. In 1956, White and White (54) reported a series of 49 patients with breast cancer associated with pregnancy. Twenty-five of these patients were diagnosed during pregnancy and 12 were diagnosed during lactation. Eighteen (72%) of the patients diagnosed during pregnancy had axillary metastases, including 11/14 (79%) of those who were diagnosed during pregnancy but treated postpartum. Patients diagnosed and treated during lactation also had a high incidence of axillary metastases (7/12, 58%). This compares rather unfavorably with the usual incidence of 20% for tumors smaller than 1 cm in diameter and 60% with large (>5 cm) tumors (56). Of note, however, are the disturbing delays in diagnosis noted in several of the pregnant patients, as long as 48 months from onset of symptoms to treatment in one. Only two patients with nodal metastases were alive 5 years following treatment. Of those who had disease localized to the breast that was treated "promptly," 5-year survival was 50% (6 of 12), quite comparable to

Table 22.3. Survival in Cases Matched for Age and Stage at Diagnosis[a]

Survival, yr	Nonpregnant, %	Pregnant, %	P
1	84	80	NS
3	56	52	NS
5	45	38	NS
8	36	29	NS
10	29	24	NS

[a]From Peters MV. The effect of pregnancy in breast cancer. In: Forrest APM, Kunkler PB, eds. Prognostic factors in breast cancer. Baltimore: Williams & Wilkins, 1968:65–80.

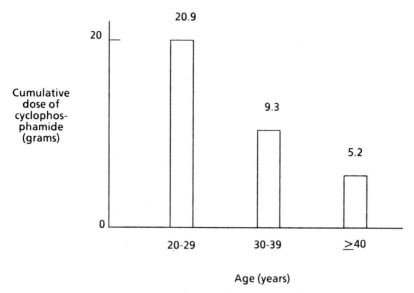

Figure 22.1. Cumulative dose of cyclophosphamide at onset of amenorrhea.

nonpregnant patients in the prechemotherapy era (54). Byrd and associates (22) also noted a relationship between the length of delay in diagnosis and the frequency of positive axillary nodes. In another series, 62% (18/29) of the patients had axillary metastases, only five of whom (28%) survived for 5 years. The 11 patients without nodal metastases were all alive 5 years later (22). Even after excluding those patients with inflammatory carcinoma, all of whom had nodal metastases, King and associates (12) found axillary metastases in 56% (31/55) of their pregnant patients with carcinoma. This was much higher than the 38% incidence in nonpregnant patients at the same center (12).

In a series of women under age 35, the incidence of axillary metastases was much higher in the pregnant patient than in the group as a whole (77 vs. 59.1%). In those patients with positive nodes, the clinical cure rates did not differ (20 vs. 21%) (4). In other series, 72 to 80% of pregnant breast carcinoma patients have had positive axillary lymph nodes (13, 16).

Estrogen Receptors

As noted previously, measurement of estrogen receptors (ER) in the pregnant patient may be misleading. Nevertheless, in small series of pregnant patients in whom ER were measured, 0 to 29% were positive (3, 32). Estrogen receptors in carcinoma patients 35 years old or younger are positive in 30% (57). In contrast, approximately 80% of breast cancers overall are ER positive (58). In the nonpregnant patient at any age, lack of ER is associated with

a hormonally unresponsive tumor and a poorer prognosis (57, 59). At present, this has not been specifically studied in the pregnant patient.

PREGNANCY AFTER BREAST CANCER

Fertility

Due partly to the relatively advanced age of the usual breast carcinoma patient, there is little information in the literature specifically addressing the fertility of these patients after treatment. Following treatment with alkylating agents, including cyclophosphamide, melphalan, and nitrogen mustard, many women develop amenorrhea. Ovarian biopsies have revealed an arrest of follicular maturation and a reduction in primordial follicles in many of these women (60). The alkylating agent most commonly used in the treatment of breast cancer is cyclophosphamide, which leads to premature ovarian failure in more than one-half of patients treated with doses of 40 to 120 mg/day (60). Effects are more pronounced in older patients and those treated with higher doses. (Fig. 22.1). Once amenorrhea develops, less than 10% of patients will have resumption of menses within 12 months (60). Oligomenorrhea or amenorrhea with hormonal evidence of ovarian hypofunction following treatment appears to be predictive of future infertility (60). Following treatment of Hodgkin's disease, 59% of those women desiring pregnancy who had regular menses without menopausal symptoms became pregnant. Although the an-

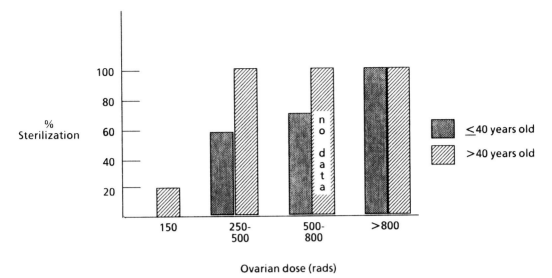

Figure 22.2.   Incidence of sterilization following ovarian irradiation.

timetabolites may affect reproductive function during treatment, they do not appear to have long-term effects on fertility (60).

The human ovary is less sensitive to ionizing radiation than is the human testis. Menopause occurring as a result of radiation therapy occurs at relatively low doses in older women, while higher doses are required in women in their 20s and 30s (Fig. 22.2). Ovarian doses of 450 to 800 rads are required to bring about menopause in most young women, far above the exposures following irradiation of the chest wall or axilla (60).

There is evidence that the risk of spontaneous abortion or congential malformations is increased in a pregnancy conceived following either radiotherapy or multiagent chemotherapy (60).

Recurrence

In most series, there has been no evidence that a pregnancy subsequent to treatment for breast carcinoma adversely affects outcome in any manner (3, 4, 14, 16, 54, 61). Most authors recommend delaying pregnancy for at least 2 years following initial treatment, as the majority of recurrences will occur in this time period (3, 12, 16, 17). In addition, Clark and Reid (16) showed that patients who became pregnant within 6 months of diagnosis had a poorer prognosis with fewer 5-year survivors, compared with those who delayed pregnancy for 2 to 5 years (53.8 vs. 100% survival). There has been some concern that a simple comparison of outcome for patients with and without a subsequent pregnancy may introduce a bias, in that

only patients who are free from disease for an extended period of time and therefore at a lower risk for recurrence will become pregnant. Comparing this group with the remainder of the carcinoma patients might then suggest that a subsequent pregnancy had no effect on or even improved survival.

Cooper and Butterfield (63) studied 32 patients with a pregnancy following treatment and compared them with a group of controls matched for age, stage, and initial survival after mastectomy. Stage 1 patients with negative axillary nodes who subsequently became pregnant had a 5-year survival of 94%, while those who did not had a 5-year survival of 71%. When compared year by year following pregnancy, there again was no evidence of an adverse effect of pregnancy on prognosis (63). In a similarly matched group, Peters (15) found that 5-year survival rates were higher in the subsequent pregnancy group (72%) than in the matched control group (49.5%). This difference persisted at 10 years survival and appeared to be more pronounced in those patients under 35 years of age, the age group in which prophylactic castration is also least beneficial (15, 62). Reporting a series of 53 patients, Rissanen (64) concluded "the results seem clearly to suggest that pregnancy after the treatment of mammary carcinoma affects the prognosis favourably . . . provided there are no metastases when the pregnancy begins." In another study of 57 women who became pregnant following treatment of breast carcinoma, the most important factor influencing survival was node status at diagnosis (13). Other variables, including interval between treatment and pregnancy, clinical stage at diagnosis and pregnancy termination, did not aid in predicting survival (13).

These data suggest that not only is survival not compromised by a pregnancy subsequent to breast carcinoma, it may even be enhanced. Because most data are limited to patients with no evident disease at the onset of pregnancy, these conclusions do not necessarily apply to the patient with residual or recurrent disease.

Other Issues

As with any woman with a life-threatening disease who is considering pregnancy, the patient contemplating pregnancy following breast cancer should be counseled extensively as to her long-term prognosis. The absence of nodal disease at diagnosis and the receptor status of the tumor appear to be strong predictors of survival (5). Pregnancy should be strongly discouraged in patients with involved axillary nodes or evidence of recurrent disease, as the chance of the pregnancy reaching viability is substantially decreased and long-term maternal survival is unlikely.

REFERENCES

1. Donegan WL. Cancer and pregnancy. CA 1983;33:194–214.
2. McMahon B, Cole P, Brown J. Etiology of human breast cancer: a review. J Natl Cancer Inst 1973;50:21–42.
3. Nugent P, O'Connell TX. Breast cancer and pregnancy. Arch Surg 1985;120:1221–1224.
4. Treves N, Holleb AI. A report of 549 cases of breast cancer in women 35 years of age or younger. Surg Gynecol Obstet 1958;107:271–283.
5. Wallack MK, Wolf JA, Bedwinek J, et al. Gestational carcinoma of the female breast. Curr Probl Cancer 1983;7:1–58.
6. Ribeiro G, Swindell R. The prognosis of breast carcinoma in women aged less than 40 years. Clin Radiol 1981;32:231–236.
7. Kleinfeld G, Haagensen CD, Cooley E. Age and menstrual status as prognostic factors in carcinoma of the breast. Ann Surg 1963;157:600–605.
8. Kelsey JL, Hildreth NG. Causative factors in breast cancer. In: Margolese RG, ed. Contemporary issues in oncology. Vol. I. Breast cancer, New York: Churchill Livingstone, 1983:26.
9. Hadjimichael OC, Boyle CA, Meigs JW. Abortion before first live birth and risk of breast cancer. Br J Cancer 1986;53:281–284.
10. Pike MC, Henderson BE, Casagrande JT, Rosario I, Gray GE. Oral contraceptive use and early abortion as risk factors for breast cancer in young women. Br J Cancer 1981;43:72–76.
11. Ownby HE, Martino S, Roi LD, et al. Interrupted pregnancy as an indicator of poor prognosis in $T_{1,2}, N_0, M_0$ primary breast cancer. Breast Cancer Res Treat 1983;3:339–344.
12. King RM, Welch JS, Martin JK, Coulam CB. Carcinoma of the breast associated with pregnancy. Surg Gynecol Obstet 1985;160:228–232.
13. Ribeiro G, Jones DA, Jones M. Carcinoma of the breast associated with pregnancy. Br J Surg 1986;73:607–609.
14. Applewhite RR, Smith LR, Di Vincenti F. Carcinoma of the breast associated with pregnancy and lactation. Am Surg 1973;39:101–104.
15. Peters MV. The effect of pregnancy in breast cancer. In: Forrest APM, Kunkler PB, eds. Prognostic factors in breast cancer. Baltimore: Williams & Wilkins, 1968:65–80.
16. Clark RM, Reid J. Carcinoma of the breast in pregnancy and lactation. Int J Radiat Oncol Biol Phys 1978;4:693–698.
17. Donegan WL. Breast cancer and pregnancy. Obstet Gynecol 1977;50:244–252.
18. Parente JT, Amsel M, Lerner R, Chinea F. Breast cancer associated with pregnancy. Obstet Gynecol 1988;71:861–865
19. Zinns JS. The association of pregnancy and breast cancer. J Repro Med 1979;22:297–301.
20. Bottles K, Taylor RN. Diagnosis of breast masses in pregnant and lactating women by aspiration cytology. Obstet Gynecol 1985;66:76S–78S.
21. Newton ER. Complications of diagnostic and therapeutic procedures. In: Newton M, Newton ER, eds. Complications of gynecologic and obstetric management. Philadelphia: Saunders, 1988:293.
22. Byrd BF, Bayer DS, Robertson JC, Stephenson SE. Treatment of breast tumors associated with pregnancy and lactation. Ann Surg 1962;155:940–947.
23. Jimenez JF, Ryals RO, Cohen C. Spontaneous breast infarction associated with pregnancy presenting as a palpable mass. J Surg Oncol 1986;32:174–178.
24. O'Hara MF, Page DL. Adenomas of the breast and ectopic breast under lactational influences. Hum Pathol 1985;16:707–712.
25. Skaane P, Skjennald A, Solberg LA. Unilateral breast hyperplasia in pregnancy simulating neoplasm. Br J Radiol 1987;60:407–409.
26. Rickert Rr, Rajan S. Localized breast infarcts associated with pregnancy. Arch Pathol 1974;97:159–161.
27. Committee on Radiologic Units, Standards, and Protection. Medical radiation: a guide to good practice. Reston, Va: American College of Radiology, 1985.
28. Laws PW, Rosenstein M. A somatic dose index for diagnostic radiology. Health Physics 1978;35:629–642.
29. Danforth DN, Lichter AS, Lippman ME. The diagnosis of breast cancer. In: Lippman ME, Lichter AS, Danforth DN, eds. Diagnosis and management of breast cancer. Philadelphia: Saunders,1988:85, 87.
30. Baker J, Ali A, Groch MW, Fordham E, Economou ST. Bone scanning in pregnant patients with breast carcinoma. Clin Nucl Med 1987;12:519–524.
31. Brodsky JB. Anesthesia and surgery during early pregnancy and fetal outcome. Clin Obstet Gynecol 1983;26:449–457.

32. Holdaway IM, Mason BH, Kay RG. Steroid hormone receptors in breast tumours presenting during pregnancy or lactation. J Surg Oncol 1984;25:38–41.

33. Mulvihill JJ, McKeen EA, Rosner F, Zarrabi MH. Pregnancy outcome in cancer patients. Cancer 1987;60:1143–1150.

34. Nicholson HO. Cytotoxic drugs in pregnancy. J Obstet Gynaec B Cwlth 1968;75:307–312.

35. Milunsky A, Graef JW, Gaynor MF. Methotrexate-induced congenital malformations. J Pediatr 1968;72:790–795.

36. Stephens J, Golbus M, Miller T, et al. Multiple congenital anomalies in a fetus exposed to 5-fluorouracil during the first trimester. Am J Obstet Gynecol 1980;137:747–749.

37. Sweet DL, Kinzie J. Consequences of radiotherapy and antineoplastic therapy for the fetus. J Reprod Med 1976;17:241–246.

38. Stewart A, Webb J, Hewitt D. A survey of childhood malignancies. Br Med J 1958;1:1495–1508.

39. Murray CL, Reichert JA, Anderson J, Twiggs LB. Multimodal cancer therapy for breast cancer in the first trimester of pregnancy. JAMA 1984;252:2607–2608.

40. MacMahon B. Prenatal x-ray exposure and childhood cancer. J Natl Cancer Inst 1962;28:1173–1191.

41. Green ML, Meiser P, Dobben GD. Analysis of morbidity and mortality of children irradiated in fetal life. Radiology 1967;88:347–349.

42. Diamond EL, Schmerler H, Lilienfeld AM. The relationship of intra-uterine radiation to subsequent mortality and development of leukemia in children: a prospective study. Am J Epidemiol 1973;97:283–313.

43. Brent, RL. The effects of ionizing radiation, microwaves, and ultrasound on the developing embryo: clinical interpretations and applications of the data. Curr Probl Pediatr 1984;14:61-87.

44. Jones RT, Weinerman BH. MOPP given during pregnancy. Obstet Gynecol 1979;54:477.

45. Volkenandt M, Buchner T, Hiddemann W, Van de Loo J. Acute leukemia during pregnancy [Letter]. Lancet 1987;2:1521-1522.

46. Schleuning M, Clemm C. Chromosomal aberrations in a newborn whose mother received cytotoxic treatment during pregnancy. N Engl J Med 1987;317:1666-1667.

47. Reynoso EE, Shepard FA, Messner HA, Farquharson HA, Garvey MB, Baker MA. Acute leukemia during pregnancy: the Toronto leukemia study group experience with long term follow-up of children exposed in utero to chemotherapeutic agents. J Clin Oncol 1987;5:1098-1106.

48. Potter JF, Schoeneman M. Metastasis of maternal cancer to the placenta and fetus. Cancer 1970;25:380-388.

49. Sedgely MG, Ostor AG, Fortune DW. Angiosarcoma of breast metastatic to the ovary and placenta. Aust NZ J Obstet Gynaecol 1985;25:299-302.

50. Sridama V, Pacini F, Yang SL, Moawad A, Reilly M, DeGroot LJ. Decreased levels of helper T cells: a possible cause of immunodeficiency in pregnancy. N Engl J Med 1982;307:352-356.

51. Weinberg ED. Pregnancy-associated depression of cell-mediated immunity. Rev Infect Dis 1984;6:814-831.

52. Sahni K, Sanyal B, Agrawal MS, Pant GC, Khanna NN, Khanna S. Carcinoma of the breast associated with pregnancy and lactation. J Surg Oncol 1981;16:167-173.

53. Holleb AI, Farrow JH. The relation of carcinoma of the breast and pregnancy in 283 patients. Surg Gynecol Obstet 1962;115:65-71.

54. White TT, White WC. Breast cancer and pregnancy: report of 49 cases followed 5 years. Ann Surg 1956;144:384-383.

55. Ribeiro GG, Palmer MK. Breast carcinoma association with pregnancy: a clinician's dilemma. Br Med J 1977;2:1524-1527.

56. Danforth DN, Lipman ME. Surgical treatment of breast cancer. In: Lippman ME, Lichter AS, Danforth DN, eds. Diagnosis and management of breast cancer. Philadelphia: Saunders, 1988:141.

57. Rosen PP, Lesser ML, Kinne DW, Beattie EJ. Breast carcinoma in women 35 years of age or younger. Ann Surg 1984;199:133-142.

58. LeClercq G, Heuson JC. Estrogen receptors in the spectrum of breast cancer. Curr Prob Cancer 1976;1:1-34.

59. Hubay CA, Pearson OH, Marshall JS, et al. Adjuvant therapy of stage II breast cancer: 48-month follow-up of a prospective randomized clinical trial. Breast Cancer Res Treat 1981;1:77-82.

60. Damewood MD, Grochow LB. Prospects for fertility after chemotherapy or radiation for neoplastic disease. Fertil Steril 1986;45:443-459.

61. Harvey JC, Rosen PP, Ashikari R, Robbins GF, Kinne DW. The effect of pregnancy on the prognosis of carcinoma of the breast following radical mastectomy. Surg Gynecol Obstet 1981;153:723-725.

62. Taylor SG. Endocrine ablation in disseminated mammary carcinoma. Surg Gynecol Obstet 1962;115:443-448.

63. Cooper DR, Butterfield J. Pregnancy subsequent to mastectomy for cancer of the breast. Ann Surg 1970;171:429-433.

64. Rissanen PM. Pregnancy following treatment of mammary carcinoma. Acta Radiol Ther 1962;8:415-422.

Index

Page numbers in *italics* denote figures; those followed by "t" denote tables.

A

Abscess of breast, 67, *67*, 83
  mammographic features of, 135, *135*
  sonographic features of, *157*, 158
Acromegaly, 36–37
Actin, 114
Addison's disease, 35t, 36
Adenocarcinoma, 90t. *See also* Ductal adenocarcinoma; Lobular adenocarcinoma
  aspirates from, 116–117
  ductal, 100–110, *102–110*
  lobular, 110–111, 111t–112t, *111–113*
Adenoid cystic carcinoma, 112
Adenoma
  florid nipple, 96, *96*
  lactating, 96, *96*
  of medium ducts, 96
  pituitary. *See* Prolactinoma
  pleomorphic, 97
  tubular, 96
Adenosis, 87
  blunt duct, 87
  microglandular, 87
  sclerosing, *89*, 89–90, 90t
    mammographic appearance of, 134–135
Adhesins, 51
Adjuvant therapies
  chemotherapy, 268–269, 269t
  hormone therapy, 271
  radiotherapy, 251–255, 253t–254t, *253–255*
Adrenal insufficiency, 36
Adriamycin. *See* Doxorubicin
Agalactia, 34
Aging
  cancer risk and, 219, *221*
  stromal fibrosis of, 86–87, *87*
Ahumada-del Castillo syndrome, 14
Allergy, breast milk prophylaxis against, 53–54
Amastia, 9, *10*, 82
Ambulatory surgery, 185–194. *See also* specific procedures
  aspiration of cyst, *185*, 185–186
  axillary lymph node dissection, *191–193*, 192
  cutting needle biopsy, 187, *187*
  fine-needle aspiration of solid lesion, *186*, 186–187

needle localization and biopsy of nonpalpable lesions, 192–193, *194*
  open biopsy, 187–192
  resection of intraductal lesions, 192, *193*
Amino acids, in milk sources, 48
Aminoglutethimide, 270
  for metastatic disease, 271
Aminopterin, in pregnancy, 275
Anatomy of breast, 4–6
  arteries, 5, *6*
  lymphatics, 6–7, *7*, *244*
  milk duct system, 4, *5–6*
  nerves, 7
  patient education about, 79
  veins, 6
Androgens, role in breast cancer development, 221–222
Angiosarcoma, 113
Anisomastia, 10, *10*
Antibiotics, during breast-feeding, 72
Antihypertensive drugs, during breast-feeding, 72
Anxiety-nursing failure syndrome, 77
Apocrine duct carcinoma, 109, *110*
Apocrine metaplasia, 85–86, *86*
Appearance of breast, 8, *8–9*
Architectural distortion, 145, *145*
Areola
  at birth, 1
  reconstruction of, *216*, 216–217
Arteries, 5, *6*
Aspiration biopsy, 97–98, *97–98*, *116–117*, 116–118, 117t
Asymmetry of breasts
  after augmentation mammoplasty, 200
  after reduction mammoplasty, 205
Athelia, 9, 82
Augmentation mammoplasty, 196–201
  aspiration of lump/cyst after, 201
  cancer risk and, 201
  complications of, 199–201
    asymmetry, 200
    capsular contracture, 198–201
    hematoma, 199
    implant breakage, 200
    infection, 199
    loss of sensation, 199
    malpositioned implant, 200